The Deeper Dimension of Yoga

The
Deeper
Dimension
of Yoga

THEORY AND PRACTICE

Georg Feuerstein

SHAMBHALA
BOSTON & LONDON
2003

Shambhala Publications, Inc.
Horticultural Hall
300 Massachusetts Avenue
Boston, Massachusetts 02115
www.shambhala.com

9 8 7 6 5 4 3 2 1

First Edition
Printed in the United States of America

♾ This edition is printed on acid-free paper that meets the
American National Standards Institute z39.48 Standard.
Distributed in the United States by Random House, Inc.,
and in Canada by Random House of Canada Ltd

Library of Congress Catologing-in-Publication Data

Feuerstein, Georg.
The deeper dimension of Yoga: theory and practice /
Georg Feuerstein.
p. cm
Includes bibliographical references and index.
ISBN 1-57062-935-8
1. Yoga. I. Title.
B132.Y6 F48752003
181'.45—dc21
2002014201

Dedication

I dedicate this volume to all the friends and students who have been instrumental in helping me realize my vision for our Yoga Research and Education Center, and especially to my traveling partner Trisha, who, for the past twenty years, has steadfastly, effectively, and uncomplainingly labored mostly behind the scene. May everyone be blessed with a joyous heart and peaceful mind!

Contents ✣

Acknowledgments

PREPARING A BOOK for the press always gives me the welcome opportunity to thank some of those friends who have contributed to it directly or indirectly. In the case of the present work, I would like to express my gratitude especially to the following people:

Swami Veda Bharati whom I feel privileged to be able to call a friend on the spiritual path and whose amazing knowledge, wisdom, tranquility, helpfulness, and not least ever-ready humor have become a growing force in my life;

Richard Rosen whose friendship has been unstinting and steadfast for many years

friends and fellow teachers Patricia Walden, John Friend, Liisa O'Maley, and Janice Gates for supporting my efforts on behalf of traditional Yoga;

all my students and friends at Yoga Research and Education Center whose numerous questions prompted me to write many of the more recent essays in this volume;

my wife and spiritual companion, Trisha, who reads and critiques almost everything that flows from my pen, even when it happens to be late at night, and always manages to bring another perspective to my thoughts and their expression;

Peter Turner for his vision and support of my writings, and the friendly editorial spirits at Shambhala Publications, notably Eden Steinberg, Ben Gleason, and Joel Segel, for serving as midwives at the birthing of my fifth Shambhala book.

May all be blessed with peace and happiness!

Preface ✿

POSSIBLY 30 MILLION to 40 million people around the world practice Yoga today. By and large, they approach Yoga as physical fitness training. As one Yoga teacher observed: Yoga has been reduced to fitness, more specifically stretching, and yet more specifically stretching of the hamstrings. This comment would be funny if it were not sadly true. While any approach to Yoga practice is a potential gateway to the real thing, there is clearly a continued need to emphasize that Yoga is a *spiritual* tradition, which seeks to bestow happiness and inner freedom rather than merely physical fitness and health.

For the past thirty or more years, I have championed *traditional* Yoga. This book is yet another effort in the same direction. It consists of 78 essays—long and short—27 of which stem from my long-out-of-print *Sacred Paths*, with the rest either taken from the website of the Yoga Research and Education Center (YREC) or newly written especially for this volume. All of them are concerned with various aspects of Yoga's magnificent heritage extending over a span of 5,000 years. This translates into about 200 generations, as compared to the ten generations that make up the history of the United States. We can readily see how Yoga is a condensate of massive experience and knowledge. It is undoubtedly the greatest product of the genius of the Indic people, who have created the oldest continuous spiritually based civilization on Earth. Nowadays India is groaning under the growing burden of its 1 billion citizens and the onslaught of Western capitalism and consumerism, which clash with the Indic spiritual heritage. But there are still many noble individuals who, like the world-famous "Mahatma" Gandhi, look to the inherited ideals of wisdom for guidance and inspiration. They are never disappointed. For the ancient wisdom passed down from the Vedic seers and sages to modern seekers is as valid today as it was then.

Even today, despite widespread industrialization, India is still a land of religion and spirituality. It is rich in temples, shrines, saints, sages, yogins, and pious folk. The sacred festival of the *kumbha-melā*, celebrated in Allahabad in February 2001, attracted no fewer than 100 million. Skepticism and cynicism are rampant mostly in the sprawling urban environments. But increasingly those Indians who have received a Western-type education are ignorant and even dismissive of their spiritual heritage. Little is being done to preserve either the temples or the sacred literatures written in Sanskrit, Tamil, Marathi, and other Indic languages. Thus every year, many treasures are destroyed and lost forever. In 2000, in conjunction with Babaji's Kriya Yoga Ashram in Montreal, YREC launched a project that will help preserve, edit, translate, and publish in book form as many Tamil Siddha Yoga manuscripts as can be found in South India. Swami Veda Bharati, the spiritual head of the Rama Ashrama in Rishikesh, is endeavoring to do the same relative to Sanskrit Yoga manuscripts. There are a sporadic few other efforts, but these all fall short of what ought to be done to preserve India's spiritual heritage.

On the other hand, it is encouraging to see so many Westerners turning to Yoga and experiencing its benefits. Current estimates suggest that there are up to 20 million Yoga practitioners in the United States alone. In at least 99 percent of cases, their Yoga practice consists of "doing" Hatha-Yoga postures one or more times per week. Clearly, even this limited approach is producing some good results. According to a report by Intersurvey Inc. dated May 12, 2000, 9 percent of Americans (that is, some 25 million people) have tried "Yoga," as opposed to 14 percent who have experimented with meditation of an unspecified nature and 3 percent who have tried Tai Chi. Yoga's effectiveness has been rated 87 percent, as opposed to meditation, which came in at 85 percent, and Tai Chi at 73 percent, though it is not clear what criteria were used to determine this. Presumably "Yoga" stands here for the yogic postures (*āsana*).

Yoga, of course, is so much more than postures, and its real power lies in the domain of mind training and self-transformation. It has been said that contemporary Yoga is highly reductionistic. This is true enough, yet I also see "fitness Yoga" as an opportunity for discovering Yoga's deeper side. That deeper side is concerned with our spiritual destiny. The postures, if done correctly, will calm our nervous system and perhaps create sufficient space in our psyche to explore breath control. Then, when yogic breathing has put us in touch with the body's life force (*prāna*), we also may become open to the spiritual aspects of our being.

I am less indulgent in my view of teachers who impart Yoga as a mere fitness system. Anyone who calls himself or herself a Yoga teacher should know the tradition for which they speak. Yoga has had a glorious history and offers a sophisticated understanding of the human mind, profound moral and philosophical teachings, and a great many practices apart from the postures. Yoga teachers have an obligation to be grounded in all of that and at least to endeavor to faithfully communicate the whole of Yoga. Only to the degree that Yoga teachers are committed to preserving the total heritage of Yoga can the Western Yoga movement make a lasting contribution to modern humanity. I am critical of the trend to reinvent Yoga without first having achieved mastery in the traditional teachings. For the past thirty-five years, I have advocated traditional Yoga in my books, articles, seminars, and interviews. In 1996, I founded Yoga Research and Education Center to help bring to the contemporary Yoga movement more of an understanding and appreciation of the traditional forms of Yoga, so that practitioners can benefit more from Yoga's incredible potency.

Yoga definitely has come west. Now the challenge before us is to unlock its full potential, which is possible only when we are willing to practice it in depth. I like to contemplate the possibility of a future civilization that lives by such lofty yogic principles as nonharming, kindness, tolerance, cooperation, forgiveness, contentment, peace, and genuine happiness.

Like most of my other books, this volume is also addressed to the growing number of seekers who are turning to the various yogic traditions for answers to the Big Questions. Those who enjoyed the essays in *Sacred Paths* will no doubt relish the many new essays in the present volume. In particular, I have included essays that examine aspects of Buddhist and (less so) Jaina Yoga. All yogic traditions are full of wisdom and practical advice, and therefore we should not neglect any. Study (*svādhyāya*) is very important, especially for Westerners unfamiliar with the Indic civilization. Besides, it has always been an integral part of Yoga. Contrary to the opinion of some seekers, the intellect is not intrinsically destructive of spirituality. The opposite is the case: Without a clear, sharp, and focused mind, we are unlikely to reach our spiritual destination. Some of the greatest masters of India— Gautama, Nāgārjuna, Shankara, Abhinava Gupta, Haribhadra—have also been intellectually very gifted.

In any case, regardless of our present physical, emotional, mental, moral, or spiritual condition, we can always improve our situation by resorting to the yogic disciplines. Yoga is a potent antidote to suffering (*duhkha*) and, if consistently practiced, can fulfill our deep-seated impulse toward inner freedom, peace of mind, and lasting happiness.

GEORG FEUERSTEIN
Yoga Research and Education Center

AUM TAT SAT—OM AH HUM

PART ONE

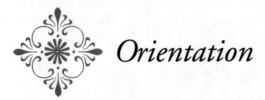 *Orientation*

What Is Yoga?

IN THE WEST, YOGA is widely practiced as a form of calisthenics or fitness training. The headstand, which many newcomers eagerly aspire to master, has become a symbol of this approach. For the outsider, this posture (*āsana*) looks intriguing and difficult to do. In fact, it is reasonably easy to learn, and there are far more difficult postures that require many months, or even years, of daily practice before they are fully mastered.

More importantly, the postures are only the "skin" of Yoga. Hidden behind them are the "flesh and blood" of breath control and mental techniques that are still more difficult to learn, as well as moral practices that require a lifetime of consistent application and that correspond to the skeletal structure of the body. The higher practices of concentration, meditation, and unitive ecstasy (*samādhi*) are analogous to the circulatory and nervous system.

At the core of Yoga is the realization of the transcendental Reality itself, however it may be conceived. This aspect of the yogic work is not at all obvious when we watch someone perform complicated postures with great flexibility and elegance. To be sure, many Western (and Eastern) practitioners are themselves not particularly aware of the spiritual dimension of Yoga. Without it, however, Yoga remains on the level of a pastime. The traditional purpose of Yoga, however, has always been to bring about a profound transformation in the person through the transcendence of the ego. It is therefore good to remind ourselves of the purpose of authentic Yoga.

Yoga is not easy to define. In most general terms, the Sanskrit word *yoga* stands for "spiritual discipline" in Hinduism, Jainism, and certain schools of Buddhism. Even when the term is not explicitly used, these three great traditions are essentially Yoga. Thus Yoga is the equivalent of Christian *mysticism*, Moslem *Sufism*, or the Jewish *Kabbalah*. A spiritual practitioner is known as a *yogin* (if male) or a *yoginī* (if female).[1] Viewed more narrowly, Yoga is a *particular* branch on the huge tree of Hindu spirituality, with

Vedānta and Sāmkhya forming the two most prominent other branches. The word *yoga* is derived from the verbal root *yuj* ("to yoke" or "to harness"). What must be yoked or harnessed is attention, which ordinarily flits from object to object.

As I have shown in my book *The Yoga Tradition*, the roots of Yoga reach back into the distant past.[2] Probably arising from archaic Shamanism, Yoga developed into an immensely complex tradition with rather fuzzy edges, which makes it difficult at times to demarcate it from the other branches of Hindu spirituality.

In its earliest identifiable form, Yoga was connected with the sacrificial ritualism of the Vedic peoples, who created the world's oldest extant literature—the *Vedas*—and apparently also were the authors of the so-called Indus-Sarasvati (or Harappan) civilization.[3] Vedic Yoga consisted primarily in techniques of mental concentration, breath control, chanting, and ritual worship. It served the purpose of invoking, envisioning, and even merging with various deities. The Vedic male and female deities (*deva*) were considered great allies in the invisible realm without whose benediction life could not run smoothly. Only by focusing attention, by turning it into a laser beam, could the barrier between the visible and the invisible be melted and the deities contacted.

It is widely held that the early Vedic worldview was plainly polytheistic, gradually giving way to religious monotheism and metaphysical nondualism. But this opinion has been called into question by some researchers, who see monotheistic and even nondualist notions already in the archaic hymns of the *Rig-Veda*.[4] Some think that the early hymns reflect polytheism while the later hymns (especially those in books 1 and 10) express nondualist ideas. The idea that the invisible realm is populated with beings (deities = angels) who are somehow relevant to human beings in the visible realm does not necessarily exclude a felt sense that behind all manifestation is just One Being. In monotheism, that Singularity is given a personal face (usually that of the "Creator"). In philosophical nondualism, the same Singularity is understood in abstract terms as an impersonal "It." Both orientations have coexisted in India since time immemorial.

Yoga operates with both a personalist conception of a Supreme Person (be it God or Goddess) and an impersonalist notion of an Absolute (often called *brahman*). Sometimes, as in the *Bhagavad-Gītā* (Lord's Song), an attempt is made to integrate both ideas. Thus some forms of Yoga are more religiously oriented, while others tend to be more philosophical. For example, there are numerous religious elements connected with Bhakti-Yoga, the path of devotional self-surrender to the Higher Reality, whereas Jnāna-Yoga, the path of self-transcending wisdom, tends to be more philosophical or metaphysical.

However, Yoga's growing technology of physical and mental practices came to be associated with a nondualist (*advaita*) metaphysics. According to the earliest teachings of Hindu nondualism, as contained in the *Upanishads*, the multifaceted world is an emanation from the singular transcendental Reality called *brahman* ("that which thrives").[5] Yoga was introduced as a way back to that Singularity (*eka*).

The sages experienced that unitary Reality, which is supraconscious and utterly blissful, as being the core not only of the whole universe but also of the human personality. As the core of the personality it was called "Self," or *ātman*. The Sanskrit term *yoga* was accordingly redefined as the "union" between the lower or embodied self and the transcendental Self (*ātman*), and this is still the prevalent understanding of the word inside and outside India. However, even Yoga as union includes an element of yoking, for the lower self cannot merge into the higher Self without proper focusing of attention.

With the exception of a single but influential school—that of Classical Yoga—all Hindu schools of Yoga are based on the metaphysical idea of nonduality.[6] The same is essentially true of Mahāyāna and Vajrayāna Buddhism. Classical Yoga, also called "Royal Yoga" (*rāja-yoga*), was formulated by Patanjali some time in the second century C.E.,[7] apparently in dialogue with Mahāyāna Buddhism. As is obvious from the *Yoga-Sūtra*, a work consisting of 195 short aphorisms (*sūtra*), Patanjali taught a dualistic metaphysics. He pitched the Spirit or Self (*purusha*) against Nature/Cosmos (*prakriti*), regarding both as irreconcilable ultimate principles.

According to Patanjali, there are many (perhaps even innumerable) transcendental Selves, just as Nature comprises countless individual forms. However, only the Selves are conscious. Nature is insentient, and this includes the mind! The seemingly independent consciousness of the mind (*citta*) is thought to be entirely due to the "proximity" of the Self's supraconscious awareness (*cit*). Nature and its products can never evolve to become the Self, and the Self does not emanate the different categories of Nature. Creation is a process whereby the transcendental foundation (*pradhāna*) of Nature gives rise to lower levels and forms of existence.

The Self, or Spirit, is merely a witness of this cosmic process, which runs its course automatically, just as the ultimate destruction of the visible and invisible universe is preprogrammed. The Self is neither born nor dies. It is indestructible because it does not consist of any parts. Only from the viewpoint of the unenlightened mind does the Self, or transcendental Consciousness, appear to be implicated in the various realms of Nature.

For Patanjali, the purpose of Yoga was to extricate the Spirit from its involvement in the processes of Nature. That involvement is a case of mistaken identity: the Self falsely identifies with the body-mind, thus causing the phenomenon of individuated consciousness, which suffers its presumed limitations.

Patanjali's dualist philosophy is unconvincing but it does have a certain practical merit, because from our finite viewpoint, the conscious subject, or Self, does indeed appear to be an "other" that must be carefully distinguished from the objective world and matter. Through progressive discrimination (*viveka*), we cease to identify with what we are not in truth. Finally, the Self awakens to its true status as an eternally free and independent Consciousness. This condition is not merely an altered state of consciousness, because even high ecstatic states still occur within the orbit of Nature. Rather, Self-realization is an utterly transcendental "nonevent." It is a nonevent because the Self is never actually in bondage to Nature but is essentially and perpetually free. It only *deems* itself attached to a body-mind and therefore seemingly suffers all the limitations of embodiment. The whole drama of bondage followed by liberation is enacted on the stage of the mind alone.

In Classical Yoga, Self-realization is called *kaivalya*, which means literally "aloneness." That which is "alone" (*kevala*), or separate from Nature, is the transcendental Self. But the Self is not a windowless monad, which would be a dreary prospect and hardly worthy of the kind of sustained spiritual aspiration that marks all authentic Yoga. Although Patanjali says nothing about this, we must assume that the many eternal Selves are all copresent and thus intersecting in infinity. In Patanjali's understanding, Self-realization presupposes the demise of the body-mind. This is the ideal of *videha-mukti* or "disembodied liberation." Not surprisingly, one of the traditional commentators on his *Yoga-Sūtra* defined Yoga as *viyoga* or "disunion" or "disjunction," that is, the separation from Nature/Cosmos.

By contrast, most nondualist schools of Yoga teach the ideal of *jīvan-mukti* or "living liberation." According to this teaching, we do not need to die before we can realize our true identity, the Self. Rather, liberation is a matter of recovering the Self in the midst of the hustle and bustle of life and then transforming life in the light of that realization. This is the ideal celebrated in the nondualist tradition of Vedānta, which has long been closely associated with Yoga.

Yoga, whether dualist or nondualist, is concerned with the elimination of suffering (*duhkha*). Here suffering does not mean the pain resulting from a cut or the emotional torment experienced through political oppression. These are simply manifestations of a deeper existential suffering. That suffering is the direct outcome of our habitual sense of being locked into a body-mind that is separate from all others. Yoga seeks to prevent future suffering of this kind by pointing the way to the unitary consciousness that is disclosed in ego-transcending ecstatic states.

From the viewpoint of traditional Yoga, even the pleasure or well-being (*sukha*) experienced as a result of the regular performance of yogic postures, breath control, or meditation is suffused with suffering. First of all, the pleasure is bound to be only temporary, whereas the innate bliss (*ānanda*) of the Self is permanent. Second, pleasure is relative: We can compare our present sense of enjoyment with similar experiences at different times or by different people. Thus, our experience contains an element of envy. Third, there is always the hidden fear that a pleasurable state will come to an end, which is a reasonable assumption.

Yoga is a systematic attempt to step out of this whole cycle of gain and loss. When the *yogin* or *yoginī* is in touch with the Reality beyond the body-mind, and when he or she has a taste of the unalloyed delight of the Self, all possible pleasures that derive from objects (rather than the Self) come to lose their fascination. The mind begins to be more equanimous. As the *Bhagavad-Gītā* (2.48), the most popular Hindu Yoga scripture, puts it: "Yoga is balance (*samatva*)." This notion of balance is intrinsic to Yoga and occurs on many levels of the yogic work. Its culmination is in the "vision of sameness" (*sama-darshana*), which is the graceful state in which we see everything in the same light. Everything stands revealed as the great Reality, and nothing excites us as being more valuable than anything else. We regard a piece of gold and a clump of clay or a beautiful person and an unattractive individual with the same even-temperedness. Nor are we puffed up by praise or deflated by blame.

This condition, which is one of utter lucidity and serenity, must not be confused with one of the many types of ecstasy (*samādhi*) known to *yogins*. Ecstasies, visions, and psychic (paranormal) phenomena are not at all the point of spiritual life. They can and do occur when we earnestly devote ourselves to higher values, but they are by-products rather than the goal of authentic spirituality. They should certainly not be made the focus of our aspiration.

Thus, Yoga is a comprehensive way of life in which the ultimate Reality, or Spirit, is given precedence over other concerns. It is a sacred path that conducts us, in the words of an ancient *Upanishad*, from the unreal to the Real, from falsehood to Truth, from the temporal to the Eternal.

The yogic way of life exists in two fundamental forms. One can be said to be marked by the mystical ascent from the ordinary consciousness to the supraconsciousness, as it is revealed at the peak of ecstasy, the state of *nirvikalpa-samādhi*. The Sanskrit word *nirvikalpa* can mean either "formless" or "beyond conception." When the movements of the mind are completely pacified in the ecstatic state, the ultimate Reality flashes forth. The bliss of this temporary realization is so powerful and attractive that the *yogin* becomes quite indifferent to ordinary life and desires to spend more and more time in the state of transconceptual ecstasy (*nirvikalpa-samādhi*). This approach, which I have dubbed "verticalist," coincides with the way of external renunciation (*samnyāsa*), consisting in the abandonment of the world. Spiritual verticalism—as opposed to integralism—adopts an "in, up, and out" attitude: Through yogic practices, the individuated consciousness (in the form of attention) is withdrawn from the external world and focused on itself (or its contents), then raised to ever higher levels of functioning (i.e., "higher" states of awareness), and then made to exit the body and Nature/Cosmos altogether. In the drug culture of the 1960s, this theme resurfaced at a lower level under the motto "turn on, tune in, drop out."

The second fundamental form of the yogic path does not lead away from the world in some mystical flight. On the contrary, it affirms life and creativity but brings a new perspective to them. This supramystical orientation is not primarily interested in the fleeting eclipse of the ego that mystical experience provides. It recognizes all experiences, including the elevated state of *nirvikalpa-samādhi*, as being merely that: an experience. Rather, it is based on the continuous transcendence of the ego to the point where the deliberate act of self-transcendence becomes a spontaneous gesture, which is known as *sahaja-samādhi*.

Because this second, supramystical or integral form of the yogic path does not deny life, it also does not reject the faculty of reason, as is typically the case with mystical Yoga. This has been clearly understood and elaborated by the Western sage Paul Brunton, who drank deep from the fountain of Hindu Yoga and Vedānta. In his *Notebooks*, he wrote:

> It is not enough to negate thinking; this may yield a mental blank without content. We have also to transcend it. The first is the way of ordinary yoga; the second is the way of philosophic yoga. In the second way, therefore, we seek strenuously to carry thought to its most abstract and rarefied

point, to a critical culminating whereby its whole character changes and it merges of its own accord in the higher source whence it arises. If successful, this produces a pleasant, sometimes ecstatic state—but the ecstasy is not our aim as with ordinary mysticism. With us the reflection must keep loyally to a loftier aim, that of dissolving the ego in its divine source.[8]

We certainly cannot *think* our way to spiritual liberation. The reflection Brunton speaks of is a matter of wisdom or higher understanding, called *jnāna* in Sanskrit. This faculty corresponds to the Greek concept of *gnosis*, which is central to the esoteric tradition of Gnosticism. Such higher understanding alone can guide us to a realization that is full and that, in turn, can transfigure our ordinary life. Then, whether we are visited by ecstasies or, as is inevitable, by experiences of sorrow and pain, we remain steadfast in our adherence to the all-encompassing Reality. Thus we succeed in bringing some of its glory and brilliance down to Earth.

𝕾 2 𝕾
Mapping Yoga

YOGA IS THE CURRENT of spirituality that has developed on the Indian peninsula over a period of some five thousand years. Its three major *forms* are Hindu Yoga, Buddhist Yoga, and Jaina Yoga. Within each of these great spiritual cultures, Yoga has assumed various forms. Hindu Yoga is the most diversified branch of the yogic tree, and its most important branches are:

Rāja-Yoga (Royal Yoga), also known as Pātanjala-Yoga or Classical Yoga
Hatha-Yoga (Forceful Yoga)
Karma-Yoga (Yoga of Action)
Jnāna-Yoga (Yoga of Wisdom)
Bhakti-Yoga (Yoga of Devotion)
Mantra-Yoga (Yoga of Potent Sound)
Tantra-Yoga (Continuity Yoga), which includes Kundalinī-Yoga (Yoga of the Serpent Power), Laya-Yoga (Yoga of Absorption)

For explanations of these and other forms of Yoga, please refer to chapters 12 ("Forty Types of Yoga") and 13 ("The Tree of Hindu Yoga") in this volume. Other groupings are possible. For instance, in Buddhism Mantra-Yoga and Tantra-Yoga are often equated.

Underlying all forms and branches of Yoga is the understanding that the human being is more than the physical body and that, through a course of discipline, it is possible to discover what this "more" is. Hindu Yoga speaks of a transcendental Self (*ātman, purusha*), which is eternal and inherently blissful, as our true identity. Buddhism and Jainism have their own distinct ways of describing the goal of the transformative path of Yoga.

Yoga entered the Western hemisphere mainly through the missionary work of Swami Vivekananda, who represented Hinduism at the Parliament of Religions in 1893. Since then Yoga has undergone a unique metamorphosis. In the hands of numerous Western Yoga teachers, most of whom have learned (Hatha-)Yoga from other Western teachers rather than native Indian gurus, Yoga has been tailored to suit the specific needs of their countrymen and -women. Thus, by and large and under the protest of but few purists, Yoga has been secularized and turned from a rigorous spiritual discipline into an "instant" fitness system. However, there also has been a continuous influx of Indian teachers, who, with varying degrees of success, have tried to communicate the traditional teachings of Yoga.

Among the best known Indian gurus spreading Hindu Yoga in the Americas and Europe are the following:

Swami Rama Tirtha (no organization)
Paramahansa Yogananda (Self-Realization Fellowship)
Swami Satchidananda (Satchidananda Ashram, Yogaville)
Swami Venkatesananda (Divine Life Society)
Swami Muktananda (Siddha Yoga Dham)
Maharishi Mahesh Yogi (Transcendental Meditation)
Swami Satyananda Saraswati (Bihar School of Yoga)
Swami Rama (Himalayan International Institute)
Shrila Prabhupada (International Society for Krishna
    Consciousness)
Bhagwan Rajneesh (later "Osho," Osho International Foundation)
Swami Vishnudevananda (Sivananda Yoga Centers)
Swami Jyotirmayananda (Yoga Research Foundation)
Sri Chinmoy (Chinmoy Mission)
B. K. S. Iyengar (Iyengar Yoga Association)
Jiddu Krishnamurti (Brockwood Park)

A century after Swami Vivekananda's successful mission in the United States and Europe, the Western Yoga movement can claim perhaps 30 million members. Most of them are practitioners of one or the other system of Westernized Hatha-Yoga, with those who are spiritually motivated in their Yoga practice forming a small minority. Whatever the inherent problems of the Western Yoga movement may be, it has grown steadily over the past hundred years, and more rapidly since the late 1960s. This is undoubtedly due to a combination of factors, not least the Baby Boomers' interest in alternative healthcare and their spiritual and moral confusion.

Whether or not the Western Yoga movement will continue to hold appeal for Westerners depends on the degree of integrity and authenticity with which practitioners pursue it. Not only must Western Yoga be informed by the knowledge of modern science and medicine, but, above all, it must properly secure its roots in the traditional psychospiritual teachings of India. I venture to suggest that Yoga, having survived the vicissitudes of at least five millennia, will hold its own in our modern world.

❖ 3 ❖
Yoga: What For?

WE CAN PRACTICE YOGA for all sorts of reasons: to remain fit; to stay healthy or recover our health; to balance our nervous system; to calm our busy mind; and to live in a more meaningful way. All these goals are worthy of our attention and pursuit.

Yet, traditionally, Yoga has for several millennia been employed as a pathway out of suffering (*duhkha*) and to liberation (*moksha, nirvāna*), or enlightenment (*bodhi*). Long ago, the masters of Yoga recognized that we can never be completely satisfied with life until we have found the source of happiness beyond pleasure and pain. Even when we are completely fit and healthy, enjoy a relatively balanced nervous system, and live in an apparently meaningful way, deep down we still feel ill at ease. We just have to dig deep enough to go past all the layers of limited satisfaction—the kind of satisfaction that depends on having just the right sort of external circumstance. We can easily discover whether we are truly content and happy when we lose our job, have our marriage break up, or have a good friend suddenly turn against us. In the case of a great Yoga master, these events will not cause as much as a ripple in his or her mind.

Upon enlightenment, when the mind is free from obscurations, neither pleasure nor pain will diminish our inner freedom. We are pure Consciousness and at one with the Source of all things. This is what the Hindu Yoga tradition also calls "Self-realization." The Self, or Spirit, is supraconscious, immortal, eternally free, and unspeakably blissful. From a yogic point of view, there is no higher attainment than this; nor is there a pursuit more worthy than this. For when we have realized our true nature, as pure Consciousness or Awareness, whatever we do will be infused with the freedom and bliss of that realization. We are all right in any circumstance and can enrich all circumstances with wisdom and compassion so as to benefit other beings.

Whatever our personal reasons for practicing Yoga may be, it is good to bear Yoga's traditional goal in mind. This will prevent us from getting stuck with a particular limited achievement. Yoga seeks to tap into our *full* potential.

❈ 4 ❈
Yoga: For Whom?

Even though Yoga originated and for thousands of years developed on Indian soil, it understands itself as a liberation tradition for *all* humanity. Its moral foundations are held to be universally true; its physical and mental practices are designed for our common human body and mind; its goal—the transcendental Reality—is the ground of all existence. Whatever yogic teachings are specific to India's culture, these represent only a fraction of Yoga's total heritage. Therefore Yoga is in principle as relevant to contemporary humanity as it was to our remote ancestors.

There is no evidence that the human mind or psyche has changed significantly over the last 5,000 years.[1] "Progress" has shown itself to be a flimsy concept. We have not become more moral or intelligent; we definitely have not become wiser. Certainly our knowledge of the universe has reached unparalleled proportions through the efforts of science, but this has not changed the quality of our thinking. The best thinkers of the ancient world compare favorably with the best thinkers of modernity. The most that we could claim is that today a larger number of people participate in scientific knowledge and the wonders of technology. But all this knowledge has not contributed to us living freer and happier lives. Most members of our species, sadly enough, are quite dysfunctional despite science and technology. This can easily be seen from the statistics on mental health, crime, and war.

We know a great deal more about many more things than our forebears, but exceedingly few of us have a clear picture of life. If anything, knowledge has made us more confused. We have lost track of the essentials by which we can live more meaningfully and with contentment. Our lives have become incredibly complicated, with stress relentlessly undermining our health and sanity.

In other words, the yogic work of self-transformation encounters similar challenges to bygone ages, which had their own pathologies. Yoga is a well-trodden path to inner freedom, peace, and happiness. It puts us in touch with what Abraham Maslow called "being values," without which our lives are superficial and ultimately unfulfilling.[2] Yoga offers answers to the fundamental questions of human existence: Who am I? Why am I here? Where do I go? What must I do? Whenever we pause long enough in the midst of our hectic lives, these questions surface from oblivion. When they do, few people have plausible answers for them. But without such answers, we are merely adrift.

Yoga can provide direction today as efficiently as it did five or more millennia ago. It is for everyone. Its various approaches are not only not antithetical but positively complementary. They make up a spectrum of possible engagement of the yogic path to liberation. Whatever our particular temperament or orientation, we can find a resonating yogic approach that will lead us out of confusion and unhappiness.

Shri Yogendra, founder-president of the Yoga Institute in Santa Cruz (a suburb of Bombay, India) addressed the notion that ancient Yoga is unsuitable for modern life as part of a larger pattern of prejudice:

> . . . a busy man regards it as a waste of time which he could utilize to better purpose; the normally healthy man believes he has no need for it; the non-conformist and the unconventional dislike the very idea of following anything which demands their loyalty or devotion; the youth believes it is for the old, and the luxury-loving persons could not think of being simple, while many opine that Yoga and modern life are self-contradictory and need not be attempted.[3]

These excuses say nothing about Yoga but everything about the ordinary individual, who is always looking to preserve the status quo.

Yoga, of course, actively undermines conventional patterns of existence, at least insofar as they prevent inner freedom, peace, and happiness. In that sense it is a *radical* teaching, which goes to the root (*radix*) of the problem: lethargy, fear of change, prejudice, self-delusion—all of which can be summarized as ignorance (*avidyā*). The whole purpose of Yoga is to remove ignorance, which is in the way of enlightenment. Therefore Yoga speaks to every single unillumined person in the world.

Guidelines for Selecting a Yoga Teacher, Yoga Therapist, or Class

CAN I TEACH MYSELF YOGA OR SHOULD I FIND A SUITABLE TEACHER?

First of all, we should determine our goal or goals in pursuing Yoga, whether we wish to practice it as one or more of the following approaches: a spiritual discipline, a healthy lifestyle, rigorous fitness training, occasional flexibility training, a way to decompress, or a system of therapeutic exercises for self-healing.

Obviously the greater our expectations, the more of a commitment to actual practice we will have to make and the more instruction or guidance we will need. If we intend to practice Yoga for fitness, it will suffice in most cases to practice several sessions of postures at least thirty minutes a week. If we hope to use Yoga for therapeutic purposes, we should allow for at least one daily session (but ideally two sessions) of postures and breath control, each lasting thirty to sixty minutes, as well as dietary and other lifestyle changes recommended to us by a Yoga therapist. If we want to practice Yoga as a lifestyle, we must pay attention to all its teachings on physical and mental health. If we are interested in Yoga as a spiritual discipline, we must prepare to engage it round the clock for the rest of our life.

Preferably, beginners should learn Yoga (of whatever kind) from a qualified teacher rather than from books, videotapes, or audiocassettes. In the case of yogic postures, even two or three sessions can be helpful in acquiring the correct approach from the outset. We may have individual needs that a good teacher will recognize or take into account when helping us develop a personal program. Once we have experienced a couple of classes and have had the benefit of a qualified teacher's advice, we can continue practicing and exploring Yoga postures, etc., under our own steam. In that case, we would benefit from checking in with a teacher every so often, just to make sure we have not acquired any bad habits in executing the various postures and other practices.

In the case of meditation, it is advisable to practice with a qualified teacher until we can reproduce the meditative state, using that teacher's particular method, without outside help. In the beginning, it is helpful to practice in a group, which produces a kind of field effect that makes meditation somewhat easier for everyone.

Before deciding on a teacher or class, we must be clear about what we wish to gain, be it to get a basic sense of how Yoga works, so that we can do its various exercises on our own; receive expert instruction on an ongoing basis; boost our motivation by practicing in the company of other people; receive instruction about the spiritual aspects of Yoga; or obtain spiritual initiation from a qualified teacher.

If we have any health concerns or have not had a physical in a while, we should get a physician's okay before taking up Yoga postures or breath control (or any physical exercise system). This is not necessary for the practice of meditation.

How Do I Find a Qualified Teacher or Yoga Therapist?

It is difficult to recommend individual teachers, because personalities and approaches differ widely, and the same personality or approach does not work for everyone. Most importantly, practitioners ought to understand that there is a big difference between a Yoga teacher and a guru. The latter will have a lot more expectations of a student. As far as Hatha-Yoga is concerned, which is what most people seem to be interested in, there are as yet no state or national requirements for what should be taught in a class and how. Consequently we can find all sorts of orientations, formats, and standards. Some "Yoga teachers"—especially those found in health clubs—are fitness instructors with only a few days of training in the Hatha-Yoga postures. *Caveat emptor!*

The Yoga Alliance, located in West Reading, Pennsylvania, is attempting to establish common standards for Yoga teachers in this country. Currently it registers Yoga professionals with a minimum training of 200 hours, which includes techniques, teaching methodology, anatomy, physiology, and some philosophy and history. In January 2002, Yoga Research and Education Center (YREC) pushed the envelope by launching a 700-hour training program extending over two years. YREC also recognizes the need for ongoing training and is in the process of designing teaching intensives for its graduates and other qualified Yoga teachers.

To find a teacher or class, we can ask friends or local librarians, look up bulletin boards in health food stores or listings in Yoga magazines, and there are plenty of online resources. Next we should feel free to ask tough questions (e.g., What are the teacher's credentials?) and air any concerns we might have. If our interest is primarily in Hatha-Yoga postures, we must especially ask about the *style* of Hatha-Yoga offered. Some styles—notably the so-called Power Yoga, Ashtanga-Yoga, or "Hot Yoga"—call for athletic fitness and are very demanding. The Iyengar style is quite exacting, while the Viniyoga style of postures is a tailor-made flow of *āsanas* for each individual.

As with Yoga teachers, there are as yet no commonly agreed-upon standards for Yoga therapy training. Many so-called Yoga therapists are simply Yoga teachers using postures and controlled breathing for therapeutic purposes. Fully qualified Yoga therapists are a rarity. The International Association of Yoga Therapists (IAYT) is making an effort to improve the situation. It was founded by Richard Miller, Ph.D., and Larry Payne, Ph.D., in 1989 and became a division of YREC ten years later. Among other things, IAYT offers an annual journal, a triannual newsletter, and a website containing articles and research bibliographies (*www.iayt.org*). It also operates a referral service for the public.

WHAT CAN I DO IF I DON'T HAVE ACCESS TO A TEACHER OR CLASS?

Traditionally, Yoga has always been an initiatory discipline in which a guru closely supervised the spiritual progress of a disciple. Nowadays, however, few people are either interested in or capable of true discipleship. But even Hatha-Yoga, when practiced more seriously, requires a qualified teacher at least in the beginning.

If a person lives in an isolated area, books, magazines, videos, audiocassettes, and television can provide valuable information about the yogic postures. But we must be clear that information is not the same as guidance. Since people tend to be impatient and want to practice advanced postures or even breath control right away, injuries can and do happen. Therefore I strongly recommend proceeding slowly and step by step. Because the yogic postures involve motor skills, most people without access to a teacher will select a video. There are a large number of audio- and videotapes on the market. Please consult Richard Rosen's review article on Yoga Research and Education Center's website at *www.yrec.org/audiovideo.html*. Good practical Hatha-Yoga books for beginners are:

Yoga for Dummies by Georg Feuerstein and Larry Payne (IDG Books)
Yoga for Body, Breath, and Mind by A. G. Mohan (Shambhala Publications)
Relax and Renew by Judith Lasater (Rodmell Press)
Yoga Journal's Yoga Basics by Mara Carrico (Henry Holt)
The New Yoga for People Over 50 by Suza Francina (Health Communications)
How Yoga Works: An Introduction to Somatic Yoga by Eleanor Criswell (Freeperson Press)

As for magazines that cover the practicalities of day-to-day Yoga, the following periodicals (in alphabetical order) can be recommended:

Spectrum: The Journal of the British Wheel of Yoga. A quarterly magazine published by the British Wheel of Yoga and edited by Rosemary Turner. Address: BWY, 1 Hamilton Place, Coston Road, Sleaford, Lincs. NG 34 7ES, England. Tel.: (01529) 306851.
Yoga & Health. A monthly magazine published by Yoga Today Ltd. and edited by Jane Sill. Address: *Yoga & Health*, 21 Caburn Crescent, Lewes, East Sussex BN7 1NR.
Yoga and Total Health. A monthly magazine published by the Yoga Institute and edited by Jayadeva Yogendra. Address: The Yoga Institute, Santa Cruz East, Bombay 400 055, India. Tel.: 6122185-6110506.
Yoga Bulletin. A quarterly newsletter published by the Kripalu Yoga Teachers Association and edited by Laurie Moon. Address: Kripalu Center, P.O. Box 793, Lenox, MA 01240. Tel.: (413) 448-3400.
Yoga International. A bimonthly magazine published by the Himalayan International Institute and edited by Deborah Willoughby. Address: *Yoga International*, Rural Route 1, Box 407, Honesdale, PA 18431. Tel.: (717) 253-6241.
Yoga Journal. A bimonthly magazine published by the California Yoga Teachers Association and edited by Kathryn Arnold. Editorial offices: 2054 University Avenue, Berkeley, CA 94704. Subscription address: *Yoga Journal*, P.O. Box 469018, Escondido, CA 92046-9018. Tel.: (510) 841-9200.

Yoga Life. A monthly magazine full of helpful practical advice and local color produced by the Yoga Jivana Satsangha (established by the late Dr. Swami Gitananda Giri) and edited by Meenakshi Devi Bhavanani. Address: *Yoga Life*, c/o ICYER, 16-A Mattu Street, Chinnamudaliarchavady, Kottakuppam (via Pondicherry), Tamil Nadu 605 104, India.

Yoga Rahasya. A quarterly magazine dedicated to the teachings of B. K. S. Iyengar and traditional Yoga, published by Light on Yoga Research Trust and edited by Rajvi Mehta. Address in the United States: IY-NAUS c/o Laura Allard, 1420 Hawthorne Avenue, Boulder, CO 80304. Address for subscriptions from other parts of the world: Yoga Rahasya, c/o Sam N. Motiwala, Palia Mansion, 622 Lady Jehangir Road, Dadar, Mumbai 400 014, India.

Yoga: Revue Bimestrielle. A French bimonthly magazine published and edited by André van Lysebeth. Address: *Yoga*, rue des Goujons 66-72, B-170 Bruxelles, Belgium.

Yoga Studies. The official online newsletter of YREC/International Association of Yoga Therapists, intended for Yoga teachers and students and published three times a year by Yoga Research and Education Center. The newsletter is available to YREC/IAYT members only.

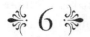

Ten Fundamental Principles of Yoga

YOGA IS A COMPLEX tradition with a history of five thousand or more years. Beginners are easily overwhelmed by the vastness and richness of Yoga's practice, philosophy, and literature. But there are a few underlying principles that, once grasped, provide easier access to all the numerous aspects of Yoga. Here are ten such fundamental principles.

1. Yoga is what is traditionally called a liberation teaching (*moksha-shāstra*). It seeks to liberate us from our limited notion of who we are. We habitually identify with our particular body, mind, possessions, and relationships (which we often treat like possessions). But this mental-emotional habit, according to Yoga, is really a profound and fateful *misidentification*. It keeps us stuck in our behavioral grooves, causing us to experience suffering (*duhkha*) over and over again. Who we are in truth is *something* or *someone* beyond our particular body, mind, possessions, and relationships. From a yogic perspective, we are immortal, supraconscious Being. As that singular Being, we are unlimited and free. All of Yoga's teachings aim at helping us to realize this fundamental truth.

2. Because human beings have different strengths and weaknesses, the masters of Yoga have designed various approaches, so that Yoga can be helpful to everyone. Thus there are different branches, which correspond to specific emotional and mental capacities or preferences. Generally, within Hindu Yoga, seven such branches are distinguished:

> *Rāja-Yoga* is the "Royal Yoga"—the eightfold path of Patanjali's *ashta-anga-yoga*, also called "Classical Yoga"—aiming at liberation through meditation, which is for practitioners who are capable of intense concentration accompanied by renunciation of the world.
> *Hatha-Yoga* is the "Forceful Yoga" aiming at liberation through physical transformation.
> *Jnāna-Yoga* is the "Yoga of Wisdom" aiming at liberation through the

steady application of higher wisdom that clearly discerns between the real and the unreal and, like Rāja-Yoga, emphasizes renunciation.

Karma-Yoga is the "Yoga of Action" aiming at liberation through self-transcending service, often considered especially suitable for those who lack the necessary qualities for concentration and meditation, but really a necessary orientation for all Yoga practitioners.

Bhakti-Yoga is the "Yoga of Devotion" aiming at liberation through self-surrender in the face of the Divine, which holds appeal for those who feel deeply and look upon the transcendental Reality in personal rather than impersonal terms.

Mantra-Yoga is the "Yoga of Potent Sound" aiming at liberation through the recitation (aloud or mental) of empowered sounds (such as *om, hum, ram, hare krishna,* etc.), which is often considered an aspect of Tantra-Yoga.

Tantra-Yoga is the "Continuity Yoga" aiming at liberation through ritual, visualization, subtle energy work, and the perception of the identity (or continuity) of the ordinary world and the transcendental Reality.

These seven branches are alternative portals into the mysteries of Yoga and thus our own consciousness.

3. All branches and forms of Yoga have as their foundation a sound moral life. Such a life is guided by the principle of *dharma*, which means "morality," "law," "order," and "virtue." It stands for moral virtues like nonharming (*ahimsā*), truthfulness (*satya*), abstention from theft (*asteya*), chastity (*brahmacarya*), compassion (*karunā*), and kindness (*maitrī*). Without a firm grounding in these moral principles, Yoga cannot lead us to its ultimate goal of liberation. For so long as we pursue a lifestyle that falls short of these moral virtues, our energies are scattered and we continue to harvest the negative repercussions of our actions. A morally sound life, however, allows us to stop the creation of negative effects and to focus our energies like a laser beam, so that we can fully discover or realize our true nature.

4. Yoga is a continuum of theory and practice. That is to say, Yoga is not mere armchair philosophy, nor is it merely a battery of practices. In order to engage Yoga properly and successfully, one must pay due attention to the ideas behind its practical disciplines and, vice versa, to the exercises and techniques embodying its theories. This calls for *thoughtful* and *mindful* practice. For instance, regular and correct practice of the yogic postures will undoubtedly help us maintain good physical health. Yet, to tap into their deeper potential, we must understand them as being merely one small

aspect of Yoga's integrated approach toward spiritual liberation. Similarly, meditation definitely balances the nervous system and calms the mind. However, only when we understand the nature of the mind—thanks to the yogic theories—can we hope to overcome the inherent limitations of our mental make-up and discover transcendental Consciousness. For this reason, study (*svādhyāya*) has been held in high esteem by most schools of Yoga; it complements steady application to the practical disciplines.

5. However simple a particular yogic approach may be, all approaches require a profound commitment to self-transformation. If we fear change and tend to cling to our established ways, we cannot succeed in Yoga. The practice of Yoga calls for considerable personal effort (*vyāyāma*), which involves self-discipline (*ātma-nigraha*). As we endeavor to replace undesirable habit patterns with positive ones, we inevitably experience a measure of frustration. However, this frustration is creative rather than self-destructive. The Sanskrit word for this process is *tapas*, meaning "glow" or "heat." The term also stands for "asceticism," which is based on self-restraint.

6. Yoga comprises numerous practices—both physical and mental. These can be reduced to two major categories: *abhyāsa* and *vairāgya*. Abhyāsa is the repeated performance of exercises or techniques that are intended to produce a positive state of mind in us. *Vairāgya* is the complementary practice of letting go of old behavior patterns or attachment. *Abhyāsa* gradually reveals to us the deeper, hidden aspects of the mind, while *vairāgya* moves us step by step beyond appearances and toward Reality.

7. The closer we are to Self-realization, or enlightenment, the more ordinary we become. Only seekers striving for liberation as if it were a trophy glamorize the yogic process and themselves. They want to be extraordinary, whereas liberated beings are perfectly ordinary. They are as happy washing dishes as they are sitting quietly in meditation or teaching their disciples. For this reason, Yoga has from the beginning celebrated not only the path of the world-renouncing ascetic (*samnyāsin*) but also that of the world-engaging householder (*grihastha*) who uses the opportunities of daily life to practice the virtues of a yogic lifestyle.

8. In all Yoga practice, there is an element of pleasant "surprise" or favorableness. In the theistic schools of Yoga, this is explained as the grace (*prasāda*) of the Divine Being; in nontheistic schools, such as Jaina Yoga or certain schools of Buddhist Yoga, help is said to flow from liberated beings (called *arhats, buddhas, bodhisattvas, tīrthankaras,* or *mahā-siddhas*). Also, gurus are channels of benevolent energies, or blessings, intended to ripen their disciples. The process by which a guru blesses a disciple is called

"transmission" (*samcāra*). In some schools, it is known as *shakti-pāta*, meaning "descent of the power." The power in question is the Energy of Consciousness itself.

9. All Yoga is initiatory. That is, initiation (*dīkshā*) by a qualified teacher (guru) is essential for ultimate success in Yoga. It is possible to benefit from a good many yogic practices even without initiation. Thus, most exercises of Hatha-Yoga—from postures to breath control to meditation—can be successfully practiced on one's own, providing the correct format has been learned. But for the higher stages of Yoga, empowerment through initiation is definitely necessary. The habit patterns of the mind are too ingrained for us to make deep-level changes without the benign intervention of a Yoga master. All yogic practices can usefully be viewed as preparation for this moment.

10. Yoga is a gradual process of replacing our unconscious patterns of thought and behavior with new, more benign patterns that are expressive of the higher powers and virtues of enlightenment. It takes time to accomplish this far-reaching work of self-transformation, and therefore practitioners of Yoga must first and foremost practice patience. Enlightenment, or liberation, is not realized in a matter of days, weeks, or months. We must be willing to commit to an entire lifetime of yogic practice. There must be a basic impulse to grow, regardless of whether or not we will achieve liberation in this lifetime. It is one of Yoga's fundamental tenets that no effort is ever wasted; even the slightest attempt at transforming ourselves makes a difference. It is our patient cumulative effort that flowers into enlightenment sooner or later.

7

Is Yoga a Religion?

SOME WESTERNERS WHO ARE practicing Christians or Jews are concerned about Yoga being an Eastern religion. They fear that by taking up the practice of Yoga, they might undermine their own religious faith. Are their fears warranted? Is Yoga a religion? The quick answer to both questions is: Instead of undermining their personal faith, Yoga can actually deepen it. In the following I will offer a more detailed explanation.

Let me begin with the extremist position of Christian fundamentalism, which regards Yoga as a dangerous import from the East that should under all circumstances be shunned. Often Yoga is lumped together with New Age teachings, which are seen as a threat to the Christian establishment.[1]

Yoga, it is quite true, has historically been associated with India's three great religious-cultural traditions—Hinduism, Buddhism, and Jainism. Thus the teachings of Yoga are infused with many concepts that have a Hindu, Buddhist, or Jaina flavor. The most striking examples, which often are a stumbling block for Westerners, are the ideas of karma and rebirth and the notion that there are numerous deities in addition to the one ultimate Reality. First of all, there have been Yoga masters who dismissed the twin ideas of karma and reincarnation,[2] and the deities (*deva*) of Hinduism, Buddhism, and Jainism can be compared to the angels of Christianity and Judaism. Clearly, such beliefs are not essential to Yoga practice. In fact, we need not believe in anything other than the possibility that we can transform ourselves: that we can go beyond our present understanding and experience of the world and, more significantly, beyond our current egocentric state of being.

At the heart of all forms of Yoga is the assumption that we have not yet tapped into our full potential as a human being. In particular, Yoga seeks to put us in touch with our spiritual core—our innermost nature—that which or who we truly are. That nature is described differently by the various schools of Yoga. Rather than being expected to believe in any of the traditional explanations, we are free to allow our personal experience and realization to shape our understanding.

Over the millennia, Yoga has become associated with various philosophical and theological systems—none of which can be said to define Yoga
itself. For Yoga is first and foremost a practical spiritual discipline that emphasizes personal experimentation and verification. In other words, direct
personal experience or spiritual realization is considered senior to any theory or conceptual system.

For this reason, Yoga can and in fact has been practiced by people with
widely differing philosophies and beliefs. Some Yoga practitioners believe
in a personal God who created the universe, others favor a metaphysics that
regards the world as illusory and the ultimate Reality as singular and formless. Yet others (notably the practitioners of Theravāda Buddhism) refuse to
speculate about metaphysical matters. Accordingly, some Yoga practitioners
are more religious than others. But Yoga itself is primarily a tool for exploring the depth of our human nature, of plumbing the mysteries of the body
and the mind. Of course, as we delve into the practice of Yoga, we will find
that certain ideas about the world and human nature are more useful than
others. So, possibly, the notions of karma and rebirth might resurface, because they have a certain explanatory force. Or we might have experiences
that lend credence to the age-old teaching that "all is one" (*sarvam ekam*).

How can Yoga enrich the religious or spiritual life of a practicing Christian or Jew? The answer is the same as for a practicing Hindu, Buddhist, or
Jaina. Yoga aids all who practice religion, regardless of their persuasion, by
balancing the nervous system and stilling the mind through its various exercises (from posture to breath control to meditation). Yoga's heritage is
comprehensive enough so that anyone can find just the right techniques
that will not conflict with his or her personal beliefs. More than that, reli-
gious-minded folk will find in Yoga many ideas and sentiments, especially
about moral life, with which they will easily resonate. Who could find fault,
for instance, with the yogic recommendation to pursue a virtuous life dedicated to nonharming, truthfulness, compassion, charity, tolerance, and freedom from greed, anger, jealousy, and so forth?

Millions of Christians and Jews around the world are already practicing
Yoga, and there is even a "Christian Yoga." Yoga—mostly a simplified version of Hatha-Yoga—is being taught at many branches of the YMCA, and
various Jewish centers also offer Yoga classes.

So, practicing Christians or Jews (or practitioners of any other religious
tradition), should take from Yoga what makes sense to them and deepen
their own faith and spiritual commitment. But they also should keep an
open mind about their spiritual experiences and insights arising from the

practice of Yoga. After all, all theories, explanations, and beliefs are merely conceptual frameworks superimposed on reality. We ought not to cling to them too tenaciously lest they should prevent us from seeing what is really the case.

All the great religious traditions of the world have their spiritual explorers. Yoga is India's gift to those wishing to become psychonauts—travelers in the inner space of consciousness. If we genuinely desire to know ourselves more profoundly and make sense of the world in which we live, Yoga is a reliable, well-tested vehicle.

Yoga as Art and Science

B. K. S. IYENGAR, the most influential Hatha-Yoga master of our time, wrote: "Yoga is an art, a science and a philosophy."[1] In what way can Yoga be characterized both as an art and a science?

The definition of art is problematic, but, simplistically, it is the application of skills to the creation of aesthetic values. Science can be defined as the methodical pursuit of knowledge about the phenomena of the physical world on the basis of unbiased observation and systematic experimentation. Roughly speaking, the objects of art and science are beauty and truth, respectively.

Yoga is an art because it evidently does not have the mathematical exactitude of the natural sciences. The British-American mathematician-philosopher Alfred North Whitehead once remarked: "Art flourishes when there is a sense of adventure, a sense of nothing having been done before, of complete freedom to experiment; but when caution comes in you get repetition, and repetition is the death of art."[2] These comments apply to Yoga quite well. It is an incredible adventure of the spirit, which seeks to create an altogether new destiny. Each time the practitioner applies the wisdom of Yoga to life's many situations, he or she must engage the process as if it were the first time. Thus Yoga is continuous self-application but not merely repetition. The Sanskrit term *abhyāsa*, which literally means "repetition," has the primary meaning of "practice" in the context of Yoga, and practice calls for what the Zen masters call "beginner's mind."

Any efforts to squeeze Yoga into the much-celebrated scientific method is doomed to failure, which is not to say that Yoga cannot or should not be studied rigorously from a scientific perspective. In fact, since the 1920s various research organizations and individual researchers have conducted such research, especially medical investigations, with varying degrees of success, and their findings have definitely been helpful in appraising Yoga's effectiveness.[3]

Yet, Yoga is not completely subjective and inexact either. It proceeds according to careful rules established over a long period of (repeatable) personal experimentation. The outcome of steady practice of Yoga's various techniques is reasonably predictable. The yogic authorities are fond of emphasizing that if a student does A, B, and C in the prescribed manner, he or she will realize enlightenment in a specified period of time. Depending on which authority one listens to, on the "fast" path of Tantra-Yoga, the dedicated practitioner (*sādhaka*) can expect enlightenment in the span of only three years, seven years, or three lifetimes. There are many traditional biographies of Buddhist adepts whose development led to enlightenment in a comparatively short period of time.

But we must not forget that spiritual growth depends very much on personal factors that are not readily quantifiable, and therefore the time frame of a person's success also is not easily determinable. The traditional schedules are suggestive rather than indicative.

In his book *The Art of Yoga*, B. K. S. Iyengar calls Yoga a "disciplinary art which develops the faculties of the body, mind and intellect" and whose "purpose is to refine man."[4] Initially he practiced Yoga for health reasons, but gradually he developed the yogic postures into an art form bringing "charm and delicacy, poise and peace, harmony and delight in presentations."[5] Undoubtedly he relates in this artistic way to the rest of Yoga as well. At the same time, Iyengar—whose method of *āsana* practice is the most exacting of all—makes it clear that the yogic techniques, if practiced correctly, have predictable results.

Iyengar sees the relationship between art and science as follows: "Art in its initial stages is science; science in its highest form is art."[6] That is to say, at first the artist must master technique (the scientific part of art), just as the scientist who wants to master science must see beauty in truth. The delight and awe of mathematicians when looking at a particularly concise formula is a well-known manifestation of artistic sensibility. Long ago, Pythagoras knew of the meeting place of science (in the form of mathematics) and art (in the form of music). Even before him, the Indians had discovered the same connection, as expressed in their *Shulba-Sūtras*.

Yoga practitioners look upon their own body-mind as an artistic instrument that can be explored fairly precisely by carefully observing the time-honored rules of the yogic heritage. This effort yields what the Western esoteric traditions call the "music of the spheres"—the mystical sound *om* reverberating throughout the cosmos followed by the wondrous realization of absolute oneness (*ekatva*) beyond all qualities.

The Yoga of Science

THE GOAL OF SCIENCE, observed Carl Friedrich von Weizsäcker, is not to transform the world; rather the primary motivation is the quest for truth.[1] And yet, in my view, this quest remains incomplete without its translation into the realm of practical life. If not the world, science—the knowledge gained from science—surely must transform the scientist. Knowledge in the abstract is merely a titillation of the intellect, an inconsequential stimulation of a segment of our total humanness.

To fulfill itself, knowledge must find expression in the body. More than that, it must transmute the body by the power of its truth. And it is truth, not knowledge, which is replete with power. The power associated with knowledge is manipulative power, such as political leverage or overpowering influence. The power inherent in truth, however, is transformative in the deepest sense. It is capable of remaking the person in the light of truth.

What truth? Or should we be speaking of truths? To hold true, truth must be singular. Always. A multiplicity of truths is a contradiction in terms. The custom of speaking of many truths arose out of the loss of truth and its substitution by countless facts. But facts are not truth. Only wisdom (*prajñā*) is truth-bearing (*ritambharā*) and therefore liberating. Truth is Reality without conceptual blinders.

To the degree that the path of science is illumined by the ideal of truth, it has the capacity of guiding the scientist, step by step, to the discovery of truth—not merely factual truth but the kind of truth that sees everything in context and also preserves that context. A consideration of the larger context of human life must include reference to humanity's evolutionary potential, including its possible spiritual destiny. Thus science can serve as a stepping-stone to the "evolutionary science" of Yoga, that is, to spiritual discipline through which our full potential is revealed.

Yoga's techniques of concentration and meditation, if mastered, disclose the transcendental possibilities of the mind, which allows us to experience truth at the highest level, as "ultimate Truth" (*paramārtha-satya*).

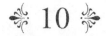

Traditional Definitions of Yoga

"Yoga is the control of the whirls of the mind (*citta*)." — *Yoga-Sūtra* (1.2)

"Yoga is skill in [the performance of] actions." — *Bhagavad-Gītā* (2.50)

"Yoga is ecstasy (*samādhi*)." — *Yoga-Bhāshya* (1.1)

"Yoga is said to be the oneness of breath, mind, and senses, and the abandonment of all states of existence." — *Maitrī-Upanishad* (6.25)

"Yoga is the union of the individual psyche (*jīva-ātman*) with the transcendental Self (*parama-ātman*)." — *Yoga-Yājnavalkya* (1.44)

"Yoga is said to be the unification of the web of dualities (*dvandva-jāla*)." — *Yoga-Bīja* (84)

"Yoga is known as the disconnection (*viyoga*) of the connection (*samyoga*) with suffering." — *Bhagavad-Gītā* (6.23)

"Yoga is said to be control." — *Brahmānda-Purāna* (2.3.10.115)

"Yoga is the separation (*viyoga*) of the Self from the World-Ground (*prakriti*)." — *Rāja-Mārtanda* (1.1)

"Yoga is said to be the unity of exhalation and inhalation and of blood and semen, as well as the union of sun and moon and of the individual psyche with the transcendental Self." — *Yoga-Shikhā-Upanishad* (1.68-69)

"This they consider Yoga: the steady holding of the senses." — *Katha-Upanishad* (6.11)

"Yoga is called balance (*samatva*)." — *Bhagavad-Gītā* (2.48)

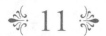

Yoga in Hinduism, Buddhism, and Jainism

BOTH THE WORD AND the concept *yoga* are known to and used by India's three major cultural complexes—Hinduism, Buddhism, and Jainism. Yoga lies at their very heart. Thus it is not only completely possible to speak of a Hindu Yoga, Buddhist Yoga, and Jaina Yoga, but these cultural complexes do so themselves.

HINDU YOGA

The Hindu cultural complex, which comprises many religious and spiritual-philosophical traditions, is the earliest to arise on the Indian peninsula. The Indic civilization has recently been dated back to the seventh millennium B.C.E., which makes it the oldest *continuous* civilization on Earth.[1] Judging from the archeological artifacts unearthed in what is now Pakistan, the people of Vedic times (fifth to third millennium B.C.E.) and earlier have laid the foundations for all future developments on the peninsula. The continuity between the artifactual evidence of Mehrgarh (seventh to fifth millennium B.C.E.), Mohenjo Daro and Harappa (fourth to second millennium B.C.E.), and contemporary Hinduism is absolutely remarkable.

"Hinduism" is the name given to the cultural complex that is based on the Vedic culture (embodied in the *Rig-Veda*) or related traditions of that early age. Some scholars identify this complex with the so-called Indus or Harappan civilization, recently renamed as the Indus-Sarasvati civilization by a growing group of archaeologists, historians, and indologists. Hindu Indians themselves call their cultural complex *sanatāna-dharma*, or "eternal law." The term is also often applied specifically to the post-Vedic cultural complex as developed since the time of the Bharata war (c. 1500 B.C.E.), which is chronicled in the vast *Mahābhārata* epic. Some limit the term to the developments since the Gupta era (c. 300–650 C.E.) Here I understand "Hinduism" in a more comprehensive way as applying to the cultural complex of the *Vedas* themselves and all the later developments based on these archaic scriptures. "Hindu Yoga" refers to the spiritual or liberation teachings within the cultural complex of Hinduism, which comprise many branches, schools, and lineages.

Yogic teachings made their first appearance in the four Vedic hymnodies, but at that time were still called *tapas* (austerity). The term *yoga* in the technical sense known today did not emerge until the middle *Upanishads*, notably the *Katha-Upanishad* (c. 800–600 B.C.E.). The further evolution can be seen in the Sāmkhya-Yoga teachings of the extensive *Mahābhārata* epic (especially the *Bhagavad-Gītā*). Around 100–200 C.E., under the influence of Buddhism, Patanjali codified the yogic path in his *Yoga-Sūtra*. The subsequent development of Yoga was greatly influenced by Tantra (emerging c. 300 or 400 C.E.), finally leading to the creation of Hatha-Yoga (c. 1000 C.E.), which today is the most popular branch. Largely through the Tantric masters, the term and concept of *yoga* was carried over also into Buddhism and Jainism, though both these cultural complexes have from the outset been suffused with yogic ideals, ideas, and practices.

JAINA YOGA

The cultural complex of Jainism entered upon the stage of history with Vardhamāna Mahāvīra (Great Hero), who lived from 599 to 527 B.C.E. and was an older contemporary of Gautama the Buddha. He apparently carried on a tradition whose beginnings extend far back in time, and the Jaina canon itself speaks of Mahāvīra's twenty-three enlightened predecessors. With the possible exception of Pārshva, the twenty-third illumined teacher of Jainism, Western scholars tend to dismiss the earlier *tīrthankaras* (fordmakers, i.e., spiritual pioneers) as fictional characters. There are, however, no particular grounds for doing so, the impossible lifespans of those teachers notwithstanding.

Mahāvīra, of royal descent, practiced the most severe kind of asceticism (*tapas*), including nudity, and attained enlightenment after only twelve years of uninterrupted practice. Unfortunately, the earliest recorded version of his teaching (the fourteen *Pūrvas*) has been lost, and the still-extant canonical scriptures (forty-five or, according to another tradition, eighty-four in all) were assembled as late as 300 B.C.E. and perhaps not written down for another 150 years or so.

While the early scriptures apply the label *kevalin* (transcender) to Mahāvīra, there can be no doubt that he in essence practiced a form of Yoga. In the famous *Tattva-Artha-Adhigama-Sūtra*, authored by Umāsvāti in

c. 100 C.E., the term *yoga* is used in the generic sense of "activity." Here we find, however, also a long list of moral qualities attributed to a Jaina adept, which perfectly match those expected of a Hindu *yogin*.

Then, in the eighth century, Haribhadra Sūri freely referred to the Jaina teaching as Yoga, as can be seen in his *Yoga-Bindu* and *Yoga-Drishti-Samuc-caya*. In the former text (37), he calls Yoga "the best wish-fulfilling tree (*kalpa-taru*)" and "the foundation for realizing Reality (*tattva*)." This great philosopher and logician, who reputedly wrote no fewer than 1,440 works, describes the Jaina path in a way not unlike Patanjali.

Several centuries later, Hemacandra (1089-1172 C.E.), another great scholar-practitioner, wrote the *Yoga-Shāstra*, which also treats the Jaina path as a form of Yoga. This text even offers descriptions of several postures (*āsana*) that are strikingly similar to those given by Hindu Yoga masters.

BUDDHIST YOGA

Of the numerous ascetics who lived in India around the middle of the second millennium B.C.E., only two left behind teachings that achieved a lasting influence also outside of India. One was Vardhamāna Mahāvīra, the other Gautama the Buddha. The latter is generally believed to have lived from 563 to 483 B.C.E. Like Mahāvīra, he was born into a ruling family but abandoned the privileges of his social status in favor of a life devoted entirely to self-discipline and self-knowledge. Like Mahāvīra, he is remembered as having become liberated, or enlightened. In common with Mahāvīra, the Buddha never wrote anything down, and his sermons (*sūtra*; Pali: *sutta*) were condensed into the written word long after he had passed. Unlike Mahāvīra, however, his teaching (*dharma*) has won a significant following, now in the Western hemisphere largely as an unintended by-product of the Chinese invasion of Tibet.

At the core of the cultural-spiritual complex of Buddhism is spiritual discipline, or Yoga. Buddhist Yoga is taught in three major forms:

1. Hīnayāna (Small Vehicle), the path of the *arhat* (worthy one) and *pratyeka-buddhi* or solitary realizer, emphasizing the moral disciplines and meditation;

2. Mahāyāna (Great Vehicle), the path of the *bodhisattva*, who aspires to enlightenment in order to benefit all beings;

3. Vajrayāna (Diamond Vehicle), or Tantric Buddhism, which incorporates elements from the other two vehicles, especially the *bodhisattva* ideal,

but adds many new elements, especially the notion to achieve enlightenment as rapidly as possible to alleviate the suffering of all beings.

The followers of Hīnayāna rely exclusively on the Pali canon said to represent the authentic words of the Buddha. They tend not to use the word
yoga for their practice. Today the Theravāda school is the only remaining
school of the Hīnayāna branch of Buddhism. It flourishes particularly in Sri
Lanka (former Ceylon) and Burma and, in the form of the *vipassana* meditation practice, is also being practiced by thousands of Westerners.

The followers of Mahāyāna, relying on sacred scriptures written in Sanskrit (specifically the *Prajñā-Pāramitā-Sūtras*), are more familiar with the
idea of Yoga, especially since one of Mahāyāna's best known schools is
called Yogācāra (Yoga Conduct).

The word and concept of *yoga* are thoroughly familiar to practitioners of
Tibetan Vajrayāna, as the Tantric scriptures understand the Buddhist
dharma as a yogic path. The supreme class of Tantra, in fact, is known as
anuttara-yoga-tantra, or "Highest Yoga Tantra." The texts belonging to this
class widely employ the term *yoga* and often call the Tantric practitioner a
yogin. Perhaps the most famous discipline of Vajrayāna is the sixfold Yoga of
Nāropa, which includes the spectacular practice of inner heat (Tibetan:
tumo) demonstrated in TV documentaries: Through visualization, *mantra*
recitation, and breath control, *tumo* practitioners can dry a wet blanket in
the middle of an icy Himalayan night, and melt the snow around their bodies at the same time. It is this branch of Buddhism, which, under the leadership of the Dalai Lama, is attracting a growing number of seekers in
Western countries.

COMMON GROUND

It is useful to think of the spiritual ideas and practices at the core of Hinduism, Buddhism, and Jainism as representing *forms* of Yoga, because this
will allow us to notice the common ground between these great traditions.
Once we have come to appreciate that Hindu, Buddhist, and Jaina Yoga
share many important features, we might also be more willing to learn from
their differences. Thus we can foster the spirit of tolerance, dialogue, and
ecumenism.

✦ 12 ✦
Forty Types of Hindu Yoga

THE SANSKRIT WORD *yoga* stems from the verbal root *yuj* meaning either "to yoke" or "to unite." Thus, in a spiritual context, *yoga* stands for "training" or "unitive/integrative discipline." The Sanskrit literature contains numerous compound terms ending in *-yoga*. These stand for various yogic approaches or features of the path. The following is a descriptive list of forty such terms. Not all of these form full-fledged branches or types of Yoga, but they represent at least emphases in diverse contexts. All of them are instructive insofar as they demonstrate the vast scope of Hindu Yoga.

1. *Abhāva-Yoga:* The unitive discipline of nonbeing, meaning the higher yogic practice of immersion into the Self without objective support such as *mantras*; a concept found in the *Purānas*.

2. *Adhyātma-Yoga:* The unitive discipline of the inner self; sometimes said to be the Yoga characteristic of the *Upanishads*.

3. *Agni-Yoga:* The unitive discipline of fire, causing the awakening of the serpent power (*kundalinī-shakti*) through the joint action of mind (*manas*) and life force (*prāna*).

4. *Ashtānga-Yoga:* The unitive discipline of the eight limbs (*anga*), also called Rāja-Yoga, Pātanjala-Yoga, or Classical Yoga.

5. *Asparsha-Yoga:* The unitive discipline of "noncontact," which is the nondualist Yoga propounded by Gaudapāda in his *Māndūkya-Kārikā*; cf. Sparsha-Yoga.

6. *Bhakti-Yoga:* The unitive discipline of love/devotion, as expounded, for instance, in the *Bhagavad-Gītā*, the *Bhāgavata-Purāna*, the *Shvetāshvatara-Upanishad*, and numerous other scriptures of Vaishnavism and Shaivism.

7. *Buddhi-Yoga:* The unitive discipline of the higher mind, first mentioned in the *Bhagavad-Gītā*.

8. *Dhyāna-Yoga:* The unitive discipline of meditation.

9. *Ghatastha-Yoga:* The unitive discipline of the "pot" (*ghata*), meaning the body; a synonym for Hatha-Yoga mentioned in the *Gheranda-Samhitā*.

10. *Guru-Yoga:* The unitive discipline relative to one's teacher, which is fundamental to almost all forms of Yoga.

11. *Hatha-Yoga:* The unitive discipline of the force (meaning the serpent power or *kundalinī-shakti*); or forceful unitive discipline.

12. *Hiranyagarbha-Yoga:* The unitive discipline of Hiranyagarbha (Golden Germ), who is considered the original founder of the Yoga tradition.

13. *Japa-Yoga:* The unitive discipline of *mantra* recitation.

14. *Jnāna-Yoga:* The unitive discipline of discriminating wisdom, which is the approach of the *Upanishads.*

15. *Karma-Yoga:* The unitive discipline of self-transcending action, as first explicitly taught in the *Bhagavad-Gītā.*

16. *Kaula-Yoga:* The unitive discipline of the Kaula school, a Tantric Yoga.

17. *Kriyā-Yoga:* The unitive discipline of ritual; also the combined practice of asceticism (*tapas*), study (*svādhyāya*), and worship of the Lord (*īsh-vara-pranidhāna*) mentioned in the *Yoga-Sūtra* of Patanjali.

18. *Kundalinī-Yoga:* The unitive discipline of the serpent power (*kundalinī-shakti*), which is fundamental to the Tantric tradition, including Hatha-Yoga.

19. *Lambikā-Yoga:* The unitive discipline of the "hanger," meaning the uvula, which is deliberately stimulated in this yogic approach to increase the flow of "nectar" (*amrita*) whose external aspect is saliva.

20. *Laya-Yoga:* The unitive discipline of absorption or dissolution (*laya*) of the subtle elements (*bhūta*) prior to their natural dissolution at death.

21. *Mahā-Yoga:* The great unitive discipline, a concept found in the *Yoga-Shikhā-Upanishad,* where it refers to the combined practice of Mantra-Yoga, Laya-Yoga, Hatha-Yoga, and Rāja-Yoga.

22. *Mantra-Yoga:* The unitive discipline of numinous sounds that help protect the mind, which has been a part of the Yoga tradition ever since Vedic times.

23. *Nāda-Yoga:* The unitive discipline of the inner sound, a practice closely associated with original Hatha-Yoga.

24. *Pancadashānga-Yoga:* The unitive discipline of the fifteen limbs (*pancadasha-anga*): (1) moral discipline (*yama*), (2) restraint (*niyama*), (3) renunciation (*tyāga*), (4) silence (*mauna*), (5) right place (*desha*), (6) right time (*kāla*), (7) posture (*āsana*), (8) root lock (*mūla-bandha*), (9) bodily equilibrium (*deha-samya*), (10) stability of vision (*dhrik-sthiti*), (11) control of the life force (*prāna-samrodha*), (12) sensory inhibition (*pratyāhāra*), (13) concentration (*dhāranā*), (14) meditation upon the Self (*ātma-dhyāna*), and (15) ecstasy (*samādhi*).

25. *Pāshupata-Yoga:* The unitive discipline of the Pāshupata sect, as expounded in some of the *Purānas.*

26. *Pātanjala-Yoga:* The unitive discipline of Patanjali, better known as Rāja-Yoga or Yoga-Darshana.

27. *Pūrna-Yoga:* The unitive discipline of wholeness or integration, which is the name of Sri Aurobindo's Integral Yoga.

28. *Rāja-Yoga:* The royal unitive discipline, also called Pātanjala-Yoga or Ashtānga-Yoga.

29. *Samādhi-Yoga:* The unitive discipline of ecstasy.

30. *Sāmkhya-Yoga:* The unitive discipline of insight, which is the name of certain liberation teachings and schools referred to in the *Mahābhārata.*

31. *Samnyāsa-Yoga:* The unitive discipline of world renunciation, which is contrasted against Karma-Yoga in the *Bhagavad-Gītā.*

32. *Samputa-Yoga:* The unitive discipline of sexual congress (*maithunā*) in Tantra-Yoga.

33. *Samrambha-Yoga:* The unitive discipline of hatred, as mentioned in the *Vishnu-Purāna,* which illustrates the profound yogic principle that one becomes what one constantly contemplates (even if charged with negative emotions).

34. *Saptānga-Yoga:* The unitive discipline of the seven limbs (*sapta-anga*), also known as Sapta-Sādhana in the *Gheranda-Samhitā:* (1) six purificatory practices (*shat-karma*), (2) posture (*āsana*), (3) seal (*mudrā*), (4) sensory inhibition (*pratyāhāra*), (5) breath control (*prānāyāma*), (6) meditation (*dhyāna*), and (7) ecstasy (*samādhi*).

35. *Shadanga-Yoga:* The unitive discipline of the six limbs (*shad-anga*), as expounded in the *Maitrāyanīya-Upanishad:* (1) breath control (*prānāyāma*), (2) sensory inhibition (*pratyāhāra*), (3) meditation (*dhyāna*), (4) concentration (*dhāranā*), (5) examination (*tarka*), and (6) ecstasy (*samādhi*).

36. *Siddha-Yoga:* The unitive discipline of the adepts, a concept found in some of the *Tantras.*

37. *Sparsha-Yoga:* The unitive discipline of contact; a Vedantic Yoga mentioned in the *Shiva-Purāna,* which combines *mantra* recitation with breath control; cf. Asparsha-Yoga.

38. *Tantra-Yoga:* The unitive discipline of the *Tantras,* a *kundalinī*-based Yoga.

39. *Tāraka-Yoga:* The unitive discipline of the "deliverer" (*tāraka*); a medieval Yoga based on light phenomena.

40. *Yantra-Yoga:* The unitive discipline of focusing the mind upon geometric representations (*yantra*) of the cosmos.

❧ 13 ❧

The Tree of Hindu Yoga

PREAMBLE

Yoga can be pictured as a major branch of a gigantic tree whose roots are anchored deep in the neolithic age, with the highest branches of its canopy still growing in our own era. The base of its stem is formed by the Vedic culture, as we know it from the surviving four hymnodies—the *Rig-Veda, Yajur-Veda, Sāma-Veda,* and *Atharva-Veda.* Careful study of these works reveals that the seers (*rishi*) who composed them were steeped in Yoga, which they still called *tapas,* often rendered as "asceticism" (from the verbal root *tap,* "to glow"). Their Yoga was entirely a solar Yoga, with the Sun being the focus of their spiritual aspirations. Much later, in the *Bhagavad-Gītā* (4.1), the Sun is remembered as the original teacher of Yoga.

The profound teachings of the Vedic seers, whose words of wisdom came to be regarded as "revelation" (*shruti*) by subsequent generations, were developed in the *Brāhmanas* (ritual texts), *Āranyakas* (ritual texts for forest-dwelling ascetics), and the *Upanishads* (gnostic texts). The last-mentioned scriptures—which, like the other works, were transmitted orally for a long time before they were put in writing—embody the diversified teachings of Vedānta (meaning "*Veda's* end"), which in essence are nondualist (*advaita*).

Shortly after the time of the *Upanishads* of the middle period (notably the *Katha-Upanishad* and *Shvetāshvatara-Upanishad*), the trunk of our figurative tree split in three. The thick middle trunk continued the Vedic tradition leading to what came to be called Hinduism; the second trunk evolved the small but ramifying tradition of Jainism; and the third trunk unfolded the complex tradition of Buddhism.

The middle stem—that of Hinduism—gave rise to numerous branches, each with its own sub-branches and twigs. Apart from the metaphysical tradition of Vedānta, which is at the heart of Hinduism and which in due course came to be regarded as one of the six philosophical systems

39

(*shad-darshana*), the most important branch is that of Sāmkhya-Yoga, which subsequently split into the philosophical systems of Sāmkhya and Yoga. (Yoga is spiritual discipline in general, but the name is also used to designate a particular philosophical system, namely that of Patanjali, the compiler of the *Yoga-Sūtra*.) The other major branches of the Hindu stem are made up of the philosophical traditions of Mīmāmsā (ritualism), Vaisheshika (natural philosophy), and Nyāya (logic).

Other major branches are the religious traditions of Shaivism (focusing on Shiva), Vaishnavism (focusing on Vishnu and his various incarnations, notably Rāma and Krishna), and Shaktism (focusing on the feminine Divine in its numerous forms, especially Kālī and Sundarī).

When we look more closely at the Hindu Yoga branch of our figurative tree, we find that there are many sub-branches and twigs. Seven major sub-branches can be distinguished as follows: Rāja-Yoga, Hatha-Yoga, Jnāna-Yoga, Bhakti-Yoga, Karma-Yoga, Mantra-Yoga, and Tantra- or Laya-Yoga.

RĀJA-YOGA

The designation *rāja-yoga*, meaning "Royal Yoga," is a comparatively late coinage that came in vogue in the sixteenth century C.E. It refers specifically to the Yoga system of Patanjali, created in the second century C.E., and is most commonly used to distinguish Patanjali's eightfold path of meditative introversion from Hatha-Yoga. Rāja-Yoga is also known as the Yoga-Darshana (view/system of Yoga) and Classical Yoga. Patanjali's own name for his yogic path is Kriyā-Yoga, the Yoga of transformative action. It is the high road of meditation, contemplation, and renunciation, consisting of the following eight limbs (*ashta-anga*), or categories of practice:

1. *yama*—moral discipline comprising nonharming (*ahimsā*), nonstealing (*asteya*), truthfulness (*satya*), chastity (*brahmacarya*), and nongrasping or greedlessness (*aparigraha*)
2. *niyama*—self-restraint comprising purity (*shauca*), contentment (*samtosha*), asceticism (*tapas*), self-study (*svādhyāya*), and devotion to the Lord (*īshvara-pranidhāna*)
3. *āsana*—posture (specifically for meditation)
4. *prānāyāma*—breath control
5. *pratyāhāra*—sensory inhibition
6. *dhāranā*—concentration
7. *dhyāna*—meditation, or sustained and deepening concentration

8. *samādhi*—ecstasy, or merging in consciousness with the object of meditation

Together the eight limbs lead practitioners out of the maze of their own preconceptions and confusions to a sublime state of freedom. This is accomplished through the progressive control of the mind (*citta*). Beyond the highest ecstatic state lies the freedom of the transcendental Self, which is the pure Witness (*sākshin*) of all mental processes. For Patanjali, Self-realization is *kaivalya*, or the "isolation" or "aloneness" of that transcendental Witness. The many free Selves (*purusha*) all intersect in infinity and eternity. Enlightenment, or liberation, consists in simply waking up to our true nature, which is the transcendental Spirit, or Self.

HATHA-YOGA

The word *hatha* means "force" or "forceful." Thus Hatha-Yoga is the "forceful Yoga" or "Yoga of Force," meaning the Yoga of the inner *kundalinī* power. This branch of Yoga, which is particularly associated with Matsyendra Nātha and Goraksha Nātha, two perfected masters or *siddhas*, is a medieval development arising out of Tantra. It approaches Self-realization through the vehicle of the physical body and its energetic (pranic/etheric) template. In the first instance, Hatha-Yoga seeks to strengthen or "bake" the body so that practitioners have a chance to cultivate higher realizations. Secondly, it means to transubstantiate the body into a "divine body" (*divya-deha*) or "adamantine body" (*vajra-deha*), which is endowed with all kinds of paranormal capacities. Thus, the disciplines of Hatha-Yoga are designed to help manifest the ultimate Reality in the finite human body-mind. Sri Aurobindo put it this way:

> The chief processes of Hathayoga are *āsana* and *prānāyāma*. By its numerous Asanas or fixed postures it first cures the body of that restlessness which is a sign of its inability to contain without working them off in action and movement the vital forces poured into it from the universal Life-Ocean, gives to it an extraordinary health, force and suppleness and seeks to liberate it from the habits by which it is subjected to ordinary physical Nature and kept within the narrow bounds of her normal operations. . . . By various subsidiary but elaborate processes the Hathayogin next contrives to keep the body free from all impurities and the nervous system unclogged for those exercises of respiration which are his most important instruments.[1]

In addition to posture, breath control, sensory inhibition, concentration, meditation, and ecstasy, the *Gheranda-Samhitā*, a seventeenth-century manual, also recognizes the following preparatory practices:

- *dhauti* (cleansing), consisting of cleansing the teeth, tongue, ears, frontal sinuses, throat, stomach, intestinal tract, and rectum
- *vasti* (or *basti*, "bladder"), consisting in contracting and dilating the sphincter muscle to cure constipation, etc.
- *neti* (untranslatable word), consisting in inserting a thin thread or rubber tube into the nostrils to remove rheum
- *lauli* or *nauli* ("rolling"), a technique of rotating the abdominal muscles to massage the inner organs
- *trātaka* ("rolling"), or steady, relaxed gazing at a small object, such as the flame of a candle, which is thought to stabilize the mind and cure certain eye diseases
- *kapāla-bhāti* (lit., "skull-luster"), consisting in a breathing technique and the practice of drawing up water through the nostrils and expelling it through the mouth or sipping it and then expelling it through the nasal passages, which is thought to rid the body of rheum

These practices are held to purify the subtle channels (*nādī*) through which the life force (*prāna*) circulates. When the life force is mastered via the breath, the mind also is mastered, since breath and mind are most intimately associated. When the mind is subdued, the higher practices can be cultivated leading to ecstatic merger with the object of one's contemplation.

It is evident from the above sequence of practices that Hatha-Yoga is a self-contained path to liberation, not merely an adjunct to Rāja-Yoga, as some traditional authorities maintain.

Aurobindo, himself a master of Jnāna-Yoga, readily admitted that dedicated practitioners of Hatha-Yoga can accomplish extraordinary feats. Yet he also asked, What have we gained "at the end of all this stupendous labour"?[2] As he saw it, Hatha-Yoga makes a huge demand on the practitioner's time and energy and hardly seems worth all the effort and difficulties. In his words, "Hathayoga attains large results, but at an exorbitant price and to very little purposes."[3] Aurobindo's critique fails to take into account that Hatha-Yoga not merely aims at health, vitality, and longevity but also at liberation, specifically liberation in an immortal body. It does not really apply to the highest traditional expressions of Hatha-Yoga, though it is valid for much of its contemporary manifestations.

JNĀNA-YOGA

The word *jnāna* means "knowledge," "insight," or "wisdom," and in spiritual contexts has the specific sense of what the ancient Greeks called *gnosis*, a special kind of liberating knowledge or intuition. Jnāna-Yoga is the path of Self-realization through the exercise of gnostic understanding, that is, the discernment of the Real (*sat*) from the unreal (*asat*) or illusory (*māyā*). Practitioners of this Yoga rely on the higher mind (*buddhi*) to guide them out of the thicket of ignorance (*avidyā*), which fragments the One into the multiple beings and things of ordinary perception. In contrast to Rāja-Yoga, which operates on the basis of a dualist (*dvaita*) metaphysics that distinguishes between the many transcendental Selves (*purusha*) and Nature (*prakriti*), the metaphysics of Jnāna-Yoga is strictly nondualist (*advaita*). It is the path of the Vedānta tradition par excellence, as first taught in the *Vedas* and articulated more specifically in the *Upanishads*.

The path of Jnāna-Yoga, which has been described as "a straight but steep course,"[4] is outlined with elegant conciseness by Sadānanda in his *Vedānta-Sāra*, a fifteenth-century text. Sadānanda lists four principal means (*sādhana*) for attaining emancipation:

1. Discernment (*viveka*) between the permanent and the transient; that is, the constant practice of seeing the world for what it is—a finite and changeable realm that, even at its most enjoyable, must never be confused with the transcendental Bliss.

2. Renunciation (*virāga*) of the enjoyment of the fruit (*phala*) of one's actions; this is the high ideal of Karma-Yoga, which asks students to engage in appropriate actions without expecting any personal reward.

3. The "six accomplishments" (*shat-sampatti*), which are detailed below.

4. The urge toward liberation (*mumukshutva*); that is, the cultivation of the spiritual impulse, or self-transcendence.

The six accomplishments are:

1. Tranquillity (*shama*), or the art of remaining serene even in the face of adversity.

2. Sense-restraint (*dama*), or the curbing of one's senses, which are habitually hankering after stimulation.

3. Cessation (*uparati*), or abstention from actions that are not relevant either to the maintenance of the body or to the pursuit of enlightenment.

4. Endurance (*titikshā*), which is specifically understood as the stoic ability to be unruffled by the play of opposites (*dvandva*) in Nature, such as heat and cold, pleasure and pain, or praise and censure.

5. Mental collectedness (*samādhāna*), or concentration, the discipline of single-mindedness in all situations but specifically during periods of formal education.

6. Faith (*shraddhā*), a deeply inspired, heartfelt acceptance of the sacred and transcendental Reality. Faith, which is fundamental to all forms of spirituality, must not be confused with mere belief, which operates only on the level of the mind.

In some works a threefold path is expounded:

1. Listening (*shravana*), or reception of the sacred teachings
2. Considering (*manana*) the import of the teachings
3. Contemplation (*nididhyāsana*) of the truth, which is the Self (*ātman*)

Step by step, the practitioner peels away all the veils concealing the ultimate Truth, which is the singular Spirit. This realization brings peace, bliss, and inner freedom.

BHAKTI-YOGA

Rāja-Yoga and Jnāna-Yoga approach Self-realization chiefly through the transcendence and transformation of the mind, whereas Hatha-Yoga aspires to the same goal through the transmutation of the body. In Bhakti-Yoga, the emotional force of the human being is purified and channeled toward the Divine. To the *bhāktas*, or devotees, the transcendental Reality is usually conceived as a supreme Person rather than as an impersonal Absolute. Many practitioners of this path even prefer to look upon the Divine as the Other. They speak of communion and partial merging with God rather than total identification, as in Jnāna-Yoga.

The term *bhakti*, derived from the root *bhaj* ("to share" or "to participate in"), is generally rendered as "devotion" or "love." Bhakti-Yoga is thus the Yoga of loving self-dedication to, and love-participation in, the divine Person. It is the way of the heart. Shāndilya, the author of one of two extant *Bhakti-Sūtras* (1.2), defines *bhakti* as "supreme attachment to the Lord." It is the only kind of attachment that does not reinforce the egoic personality and its karmic destiny. Attachment is a combination of placing one's attention on something and investing it with great emotional energy. It is such energized love-attachment (*āsakti*) that *bhakti-yogins* consciously harness in their quest for communion or union with the Divine.

In Bhakti-Yoga, the practitioner is always a devotee (*bhakta*), a lover, and the Divine is the Beloved. There are different degrees of devotion, and the *Bhāgavata-Purāna*, composed in the ninth or tenth century C.E., delineates nine stages. These have been formalized by Jīva Gosvāmin, the great sixteenth-century preceptor of Gaudīya Vaishnavism, in his *Shat-Sandarbha* (Six Compositions) as follows:

1. Listening (*shravana*) to the names of the divine Person (*purusha-uttama*). Each of the hundreds of names highlights a distinct quality of God, and hearing them creates a devotional attitude in the receptive listener.

2. Chanting (*kīrtana*) praise songs in honor of the Lord. Such songs generally have a simple melody and are accompanied by musical instruments. Again, the singing is a form of meditative remembrance of the Divine and can lead to ecstatic breakthroughs.

3. Remembrance (*smarana*) of God, the loving meditative recalling of the attributes of the divine Person, often in his human incarnation—for instance, as the beautiful cowherd Krishna.

4. "Service at the feet" (*pāda-sevana*) of the Lord, which is a part of ceremonial worship. The feet are traditionally considered a terminal of magical and spiritual power (*shakti*) and grace. In the case of one's living teacher, self-surrender is frequently expressed by bowing at the *guru's* feet. Here service at the Lord's feet is understood metaphorically, as one's inner embrace of the Divine in all one's activities.

5. Ritual (*arcanā*), the performance of the prescribed religious rites, especially those involving the daily ceremony at the home altar on which the image of one's chosen deity (*ishta-devatā*) is installed.

6. Prostration (*vandana*) before the image of the Divine.

7. "Slavish devotion" (*dāsya*) to God, which is expressed in the devotee's intense yearning to be in the company or proximity of the Lord.

8. Feeling of friendship (*sākhya*) for the Divine, which is a more intimate, mystical form of associating with God.

9. "Self-offering" (*ātma-nivedana*), or ecstatic self-transcendence, through which the worshiper enters into the immortal body of the divine Person.

These nine stages form part of a ladder of continuous ascent to ever more fervent devotion and thus, ultimately, to merging with the Divine.

Remarkably, the *Bhāgavata-Purāna* (7.1.30) acknowledges the liberating power of emotions other than love — such as fear, sexual desire, and even hatred — so long as their object is the Divine. The secret behind this is simple enough: In order to fear God (as did Kamsa), feel hatred for the Divine (as did Shishupāla), or approach the Lord with burning sexual love (as did the cowgirls of Vrindavāna in the case of the God-man Krishna), a person must place his or her attention on the Divine. This focus creates a bridge across which the eternally given grace can enter and transform that person's life, even to the point of enlightenment, provided the emotion is intense enough.

The final moment of realization, when the devotee merges with the Divine, is described in the *Bhagavad-Gītā* as supreme love-participation (*para-bhakti*). Prior to that event, devotion requires that God be faced as separate from oneself, so that He/She can be worshiped in song, ritual action, or meditation. After that moment, however, the Divine and the devotee are inseparably merged in love, though most schools of Bhakti-Yoga insist that this mystical merging is not one of total identification with God. The Divine is experienced as infinitely more comprehensive than the devotee, who is rather like a conscious cell within the incommensurable body of God.

KARMA-YOGA

To exist is to act. Even an inanimate object such as a rock has movement, as it expands and contracts with changes in temperature. And the building blocks of matter, the atomic particles, are in fact no building blocks at all but incredibly complex patterns of energy in constant motion. Thus, the universe is a vast vibratory expanse. In the words of philosopher Alfred North Whitehead, the world is *process*. It is on this insight, commonplace as it may seem, that Karma-Yoga is founded.

The word *karma* (or *karman*), derived from the root *kri* ("to make" or "to do"), has many meanings. It can signify "action," "work," "product," "effect," and so on. Thus Karma-Yoga is literally the Yoga of Action. But here the term *karma* stands for a particular kind of action. Specifically, it denotes an inner attitude toward action, which is itself a form of action. What this attitude consists in is spelled out in the *Bhagavad-Gītā*, which is the earliest scripture to teach Karma-Yoga.

> Not by abstention from actions does a person enjoy action-transcendence, nor by renunciation alone does one approach perfection. (3.4)

For, not even for a moment can anyone ever remain without perform-ing action. Everyone is unwittingly made to act by the qualities (*guna*) is-suing from Nature. (3.5)

He who restrains his organs of action but sits remembering in his mind the objects of the senses is called a self-bewildered hypocrite. (3.6)

So, O Arjuna, more excellent is he who, controlling the senses with his mind, embarks unattached on Karma-Yoga with his organs of action. (3.7)

You must do the allotted action, for action is superior to inaction; not even your body's processes (*yātrā*) can be accomplished by inaction. (3.8)

This world is action-bound, save when this action is [intended] as sacrifice. With that purpose, O son of Kuntī, engage in action devoid of attachment. (3.9)

. . . .

Therefore always perform unattached the proper (*kārya*) deed, for the man who performs action without attachment attains the Supreme. (3.19)

The God-man Krishna continues:

Always performing all [allotted] actions and taking refuge in Me, he attains through My grace the eternal, immutable State. (18.56)

Renouncing in thought all actions to Me, intent on Me, resorting to Buddhi-Yoga, be constantly "Me-minded." (18.57)

The objective of Karma-Yoga is stated to be "action freedom." The actual Sanskrit term is *naishkarmya*, which literally means "nonaction." But this literal meaning is misleading, because it is not inactivity that is intended here. Rather, *naishkarmya-karman* corresponds to the Taoist notion of *wu-wei*, or inaction in action. That is to say, Karma-Yoga is about freedom *in* ac-tion, or the transcendence of egoic motivations. When the illusion of the ego as acting subject is transcended, then actions are recognized to occur spontaneously. Without the interference of the ego, their spontaneity ap-pears as a smooth flow. Hence truly enlightened beings have an economy and elegance of movement about them that is generally absent in unen-lightened individuals. Behind the action of the enlightened being there is no author; or we could say that Nature itself is the author.

Action performed in the spirit of self-surrender has benign invisible effects. It improves the quality of our being and makes us a source of spiritual uplift for others. Lord Krishna, in the *Bhagavad-Gītā*, speaks of the *karma-yogin's* working for the welfare of the world. The Sanskrit phrase he uses is *loka-samgraha*, which literally means "world gathering" or "pulling people together." What it refers to is this: Our own personal wholeness, founded in self-surrender, actively transforms our social environment, contributing to its wholeness.

"Mahatma" Gandhi was modern India's most superb example of a *karma-yogin* in action. He worked tirelessly on himself and for the welfare of the Indian nation. In pursuing the lofty ideal of Karma-Yoga, Gandhi had to give up his life. He did so without rancor, with the name of God—"Rām"— on his lips. He embraced his destiny, trusting that none of his spiritual efforts could ever be lost, as is indeed the solemn promise of Lord Krishna in the *Bhagavad-Gītā*, which Gandhi read daily. Gandhi believed in the inevitability of karma, but he also believed in free will.

MANTRA-YOGA

Sound is a form of vibration, and it was known as such to the yogis of ancient and medieval India. According to the dominant theory of the science of sacred sound—known as *mantra-vidyā* or *mantra-shāstra*—the universe is in a state of vibration (*spanda* or *spandana*). A mantra is sacred utterance, numinous sound, or sound that is charged with psychospiritual power. A mantra is sound that empowers the mind, or that is empowered by the mind. It is a vehicle of meditative transformation of the human body-mind and is thought to have magical potency.

The most widely employed and recognized mantric sound is the sacred syllable *om*, which symbolizes the ultimate Reality. It is found in Hinduism, Buddhism, and Jainism. But, traditionally, a mantra is a mantra only when it is imparted by a teacher to a disciple during an initiatory ritual. Thus, the sacred syllable *om* is not a mantra when used by an uninitiated person. It acquires its mantric power only through initiation.

Mantras, which may consist of single sounds or a whole string of sounds, can be employed for many different purposes. Originally, mantras were presumably used to ward off undesirable powers or events and to attract those that were deemed desirable, and this is still their predominant application. In other words, mantras are used as magical tools. But they are also employed in spiritual contexts as instruments of empowerment, where they aid the aspirant's search for identification with the transcendental Reality.

The beginnings of Mantra-Yoga lie far back in the era of the *Vedas*. But Mantra-Yoga proper is a product of the same philosophical and cultural forces that also gave rise to Tantra in medieval India. In fact, Mantra-Yoga is a principal aspect of the Tantric approach and is treated in numerous works belonging to that spiritual heritage.

According to the *Mantra-Yoga-Samhitā*, Mantra-Yoga has sixteen limbs:

1. Devotion (*bhakti*), which is threefold: (1) prescribed devotion (*vaidhi-bhakti*), (2) devotion involving attachment (*rāga-ātmika-bhakti*)—that is, which is tainted by egoic motives, and (3) supreme devotion (*para-bhakti*), which yields superlative bliss.

2. Purification (*shuddhi*), which is distinguishable by the following four factors: body, mind, direction, and location. This practice entails (a) cleansing the body, (b) purifying the mind (through faith, study, and the cultivation of various virtues), (c) facing in the right direction during recitation, and (d) using an especially consecrated location for one's practice.

3. Posture (*āsana*), which is meant to stabilize the body during meditative recitation; it is said to comprise two principal forms, namely *svastika-āsana* and the lotus posture (*padma-āsana*), which are both described in chapter 18.

4. "Five-limbed service" (*panca-anga-sevana*), the daily ritual of reading the *Bhagavad-Gītā* (Lord's Song) and the *Sahasra-Nāma* (Thousand Names) and reciting songs of praise (*stava*), protection (*kavaca*), and heart-opening (*hridaya*). These five practices are understood as powerful means of granting attention and energy to the Divine and thereby becoming assimilated into it.

5. Conduct (*ācāra*), which is of three kinds: divine (*divya*), or that which is beyond worldly activity and renunciation; "left-hand" (*vāma*), which involves worldly activity; and "right-hand" (*dakshina*), which involves renunciation.

6. Concentration (*dhāranā*), which may have an external or an internal object.

7. "Serving the divine space" (*divya-desha-sevana*), which has sixteen constituent practices that convert a given place into consecrated space.

8. "Breath ritual" (*prāna-kriyā*), which is said to be singular but accompanied by a variety of practices, such as the various types of placing (*nyāsa*) the life force into different parts of the body.

9. Gesture or "seal" (*mudrā*), which has numerous forms. These hand gestures are used to focus the mind. One such gesture is the *anjali-mudrā*, which is executed by placing the palms together in front of the chest.

10. "Satisfaction" (*tarpana*), which is the practice of offering libations of water to the deities (*deva*), thereby delighting them and making them favorably disposed toward the *yogin*.

11. Invocation (*havana*), or calling upon the deity by means of *mantras*.

12. Offering (*bali*), which consists in making gifts of fruit, etc., to the deity. The best offering is deemed to be the gift of oneself.

13. Sacrifice (*yāga*), which can be either external or internal. The inner sacrifice is praised as superior.

14. Recitation (*japa*), which is of three kinds: mental (*mānasa*), quiet (*upāmshu*), and voiced (*vācika*).

15. Meditation (*dhyāna*), which is manifold, because of the great variety of possible objects of contemplation.

16. Ecstasy (*samādhi*), which is also known as the "great state" (*mahā-bhāva*) in which the mind dissolves into the Divine itself or into the chosen deity as a manifestation of the Divine.

As is evident from this outline of the sixteenfold path of Mantra-Yoga, this school has a pronounced ritualistic orientation. This reflects well the overall orientation of Tantra. Today, when mantras are widely sold and published, it is perhaps good to remember that they originated in a sacred setting. Mantra-Yoga has through the ages been presented as the easiest of all approaches to Self-realization. What could possibly be easier than to recite a mantra? Yet, it is obvious that this Yoga, in the final analysis, is as demanding as any other. The mindless repetition of mantras, especially by the uninitiated, can hardly lead to enlightenment or bliss. Paradoxically, we must be intensely attentive in order to go beyond the mechanism of attention and realize the ultimate Being-Consciousness-Bliss. Mantra-Yoga demands the same self-transcendence as all other forms of Yoga.

LAYA-YOGA (TANTRA-YOGA)

Laya-Yoga, which is at the heart of Tantra-Yoga, focuses on meditative "absorption" or "dissolution" (*laya*) of the subtle elements and other factors of the psyche or mind to the point of ecstatic realization (*samādhi*) and, finally, liberation. The word *laya* is derived from the root *lī*, meaning "to become dissolved" or "vanish" but also "to cling" and "to remain sticking." This dual connotation of the verbal root *lī* is preserved in the word *laya*. The *laya-yogins* seek to meditatively *dissolve* themselves by *clinging* solely to the transcendental Self. They endeavor to transcend all memory traces and sensory experiences by dissolving the microcosm, the mind, into the transcendental Being-Consciousness-Bliss. Their goal is to progressively dismantle their inner universe by way of intense contemplation, until only the singular transcendental Reality, the Self, remains.

Laya-Yoga is a frontal attack on the illusion of individuality. As Shyam Sundar Goswami, who has written the most authoritative book on the subject, explained:

> Layayoga is that form of yoga in which yoga, that is *samādhi*, is attained through *laya*. *Laya* is deep concentration causing the absorption of the cosmic principles, stage by stage, into the spiritual aspect of the Supreme Power-Consciousness. It is the process of absorption of the cosmic principles in deep concentration, thus freeing consciousness from all that is not spiritual, and in which is held the divine luminous coiled power, termed *kundalinī*.[5]

The *laya-yogins* are concerned with transcending these karmic patterns within their own mind to the point at which their inner cosmos becomes dissolved. In this endeavor they utilize many practices and concepts from Tantra-Yoga, which also can be found in Hatha-Yoga, especially the model of the subtle body (*sūkshma-sharīra*) with its psychoenergetic centers (*cakra*) and currents (*nādī*).

Central to Laya-Yoga, moreover, is the important notion of the *kundalinī-shakti*, the serpent power, which represents the universal life force as manifested in the human body. The arousal and manipulation of this tremendous force also is the principal objective of the *hatha-yogin*. In fact, Laya-Yoga can be understood as the higher, meditative phase of Hatha-Yoga.

As the awakened *kundalinī* force ascends from the psychoenergetic center at the base of the spine to the crown of the head, it absorbs a portion of the life energy in the limbs and trunk. This is esoterically explained as the reabsorption of the five material elements (*bhūta*) into their subtle counterparts. The body temperature drops measurably in those parts, whereas the crown feels as if on fire and is very warm to the touch. The physiology of this process is not yet understood. Subjectively, however, *yogins* experience a progressive dissolution of their ordinary state of being, until they recover the ever-present Self-Identity (*ātman*) that knows no bodily or mental limits.

INTEGRAL YOGA

All the branches of Yoga described so far were creations of premodern India. With Sri Aurobindo's Integral Yoga we enter the modern era. This Yoga is a vivid demonstration that the Yoga tradition, which has always been highly adaptive, is continuing to develop in response to the changing cultural conditions. Integral Yoga is the single most impressive attempt to reformulate Yoga for our modern needs and abilities.

While intent on preserving the continuity of the Yoga tradition, Sri Aurobindo was eager to adapt Yoga to the unique context of the Westernized world of our age. He did this on the basis not only of his own European education but also his profound personal experimentation and experience with spiritual life. He combined in himself the rare qualities of an original philosopher and those of a mystic and sage. Aurobindo saw in all past forms of Yoga an attempt to transcend the ordinary person's enmeshment in the external world by means of renunciation, asceticism, meditation, breath control, and a whole battery of other yogic means. By contrast, Integral Yoga—which is called *pūrna-yoga* in Sanskrit—has the explicit purpose of bringing the "divine consciousness" down into the human body-mind and into ordinary life.

While Aurobindo certainly did not deny the value of asceticism, he sought to assign to it its proper place within the context of an integral spirituality. He argued that the ancient Hindu thinkers and sages took very seriously the Vedāntic axiom that there is only a single Reality but failed to do proper justice to the correlated axiom that "all this is Brahman." In other words, they typically ignored the presence of the nondual Divine in and as the world in which we live. Aurobindo's "supramental Yoga" revolves around the transformation of terrestrial life. He wanted to see paradise on Earth— a thoroughly transmuted existence in the world.

Integral Yoga has no prescribed techniques, since the inward transformation is accomplished by the divine Power itself. There are no obligatory rituals, mantras, postures, or breathing exercises to be performed. The aspirant must simply open himself or herself to that higher Power, which Sri Aurobindo identified with The Mother. This self-opening and calling upon the presence of The Mother is understood as a form of meditation or prayer. Aurobindo advised that practitioners should focus their attention at the heart, which has anciently been the secret gateway to the Divine. Faith, or inner certitude, is deemed a key to spiritual growth. Other important aspects of Integral Yoga practice are chastity (*brahmacarya*), truthfulness (*satya*), and a pervasive disposition of calm (*prashānti*).

❧ 14 ❧
Styles of Hatha-Yoga

HATHA-YOGA IS A relatively late arrival in the evolution of Yoga, dating back little more than one thousand years. Hatha-Yoga entered the Western hemisphere in the 1920s and today it is the most widely practiced branch of Hindu Yoga, with tens of millions of practitioners who are primarily interested in health and fitness and know little about its traditional goals of self-transcendence, self-transformation, and Self-realization. In its voyage from medieval India to the modern West, Hatha-Yoga has undergone a number of transmutations. The most significant adaptations were made during the past several decades in order to serve the needs of Western students.

Hatha-Yoga, as practiced so widely today, goes back to just a handful of contemporary teachers—Swami Kuvalayananda (1883–1966) of the Kaivalyadhama Institute in Lonavla (South India), Swami Sivananda (1887–1963) of Rishikesh (North India), T. S. Krishnamacharya (1887–1998) of Mysore, Swami Shyam Sundar Goswami (1891–1978) of Bengal and then Sweden, Shri Yogendra (1897–1989) of Bombay, the American Yoga pioneer Theos Bernard (1908–1947), Selvarajan Yesudian (1916–1998), Swami Dev Murti (dates not known), Swami Gitananda Giri (1907–1993) of South India, and controversial Dhirendra Brahmachari (1924–1994), who taught Indian Prime Minister Indira Gandhi.

Easily the most influential of these adepts was Krishnamacharya, a Yoga master and pundit, who taught his son T. K. V. Desikachar (Viniyoga style), brother-in-law B. K. S. Iyengar (Iyengar Yoga style), brother-in-law Pattabhi Jois (Ashtanga Yoga style), and also Indra Devi (1899–2002), the "First Lady of Yoga" in America—all of whom came to represent different styles of Hatha-Yoga. Krishnamacharya can be said to have launched a veritable Hatha-Yoga renaissance in modern times that is still sweeping the world.

The second most influential source of contemporary Hatha-Yoga was Swami Sivananda, a physician turned renouncer, who trained numerous disciples. Foremost among those whose teaching includes Hatha-Yoga are Swami Satyananda (1923–   ), founder of the Bihar School of Yoga; Swami

Sivananda Radha (1911–1995), who created Hidden Language Hatha-Yoga; Swami Vishnudevananda (1927–1993), and Swami Satchidananda (1914–2002), one of the spiritual heroes of the Woodstock era and creator of the Integral Yoga style.

Of the many styles of Hatha-Yoga available today, the following are the best known (roughly in order of their popularity):

Iyengar Yoga, which is the most widely recognized approach to Hatha-Yoga, was created by B. K. S. Iyengar (1918–   ), the younger brother-in-law and disciple of Shri Krishnamacharya. This style is characterized by precision performance and the aid of various props, such as cushions, stuffed bags, benches, wood blocks, and straps, and hence is sometimes called "furniture Yoga." Iyengar has trained thousands of teachers, many of whom are in the United States. His Ramamani Iyengar Memorial Yoga Institute, founded in 1974 and dedicated to his late wife Ramamani, is located in Pune, India, and serves many of his Western students as the destination of an annual pilgrimage.

Ashtanga (or Power) Yoga originated with K. Pattabhi Jois (1915–   ), who studied with Shri Krishnamacharya for twenty-five years and whose Ashtanga Yoga Institute is located in Mysore, India. Ashtānga Yoga, though based on the *Yoga-Sūtra*, differs from Patanjali's eight-limbed path.

Bikram Yoga is the style taught by Bikram Choudhury (1944–   ). Bikram Choudhury, who studied with Bishnu Gosh (the brother of famous Paramahansa Yogananda, author of *Autobiography of a Yogi*), won a gold medal in weightlifting at the 1964 Olympics. His system features 26 postures performed in a standard sequence in a room heated to 100–110 degrees Fahrenheit (hence also "Hot Yoga."). This approach is fairly vigorous and requires a certain level of fitness on the part of students.

Integral Yoga was developed by Swami Satchidananda, a disciple of the famous Swami Sivananda of Rishikesh, India. Swami Satchidananda made his debut at the Woodstock festival in 1969, where he taught the Baby Boomers to chant *om*, and over the years has attracted thousands of students. As the name suggests, this style aims to integrate the various aspects of the body-mind through a combination of postures, breathing techniques, deep relaxation, and meditation. Function is given preeminence over form. Integral Yoga is taught at Integral Yoga International, headquartered at Satchidananda (or Yogaville) Ashram in Buckingham, Virginia, and its over forty branches worldwide.

Kripalu Yoga, inspired by Swami Kripalvananda (1913–1981) and developed by his disciple Yogi Amrit Desai (1932–   ), is a three-stage Yoga tailored for the needs of Western students. In the first stage, postural alignment and coordination of breath and movement are emphasized, and the postures are held for a short duration only. In the second stage, meditation is included into the practice and postures are held for prolonged periods. In the final stage, the practice of postures becomes a spontaneous "meditation in motion." Kripalu Yoga is taught by numerous teachers around the world, and the Kripalu Center in Lenox, Massachusetts, offers a battery of classes, workshops, and retreats for beginners and advanced students. Every year, some 12,000 individuals go through the "Kripalu experience" at the Center's 300-acre property.

Viniyoga is one of the approaches developed by Shri Krishnamacharya and continued by his son T. K. V. Desikachar (1938–), whose school is located in Madras, India. Viniyoga works with what is called "sequential process," or *vinyāsa-krama*. The emphasis is not on achieving an external ideal form but on practicing a posture according to one's individual needs and capacity. Regulated breathing is an important aspect of Viniyoga, and the breath is carefully coordinated with the postural movements.

Sivananda Yoga is the creation of the late Swami Vishnudevananda, also a disciple of Swami Sivananda, who established his Sivananda Yoga Vedanta Center in Montreal in 1959. He trained over 6,000 teachers, and there are numerous Sivananda centers around the world. This style includes a series of twelve postures, the Sun Salutation sequence, breathing exercises, relaxation, and mantra chanting.

Ananda Yoga is anchored in the teachings of Paramahansa Yogananda (1893–1952; author of *Autobiography of a Yogi*) and was developed by Swami Kriyananda (1926–), one of Yogananda's direct disciples. This is a gentle style designed to prepare the student for meditation, and its distinguishing features are the affirmations associated with postures. It includes Yogananda's unique energization exercises (*kriyā*), first developed in 1917, which involve consciously directing the body's energy (life force or *prāna*) to different organs and limbs. The center for Ananda Yoga is the Ananda World Brotherhood Village situated in Nevada City, California, and has around 300 residents.

Kundalinī-Yoga is not only an independent approach of Yoga but is also the name of a style of Hatha-Yoga, originated by the Sikh master Yogi Bhajan (1929–), a disciple of Sant Hazara Singh, Swami Dev Murti, and Dhirendra Brahmachari. Its purpose is to awaken the serpent power (*kundalinī*) by means of postures, breath control, chanting, and meditation. Yogi Bhajan, who came to the United States in 1969, is the founder and spiritual head of the Healthy, Happy, Holy Organization (3HO), which is headquartered in Los Angeles but has numerous branches around the world.

Hidden Language Yoga was developed by Swami Sivananda Radha (1911–1995), a German-born woman student of Swami Sivananda. This style seeks to promote not only physical well-being but also self-understanding by exploring the symbolism inherent in the postures. Hidden Language Yoga is taught by the teachers of Yasodhara Ashram in Kootenay Bay, British Columbia, and its various branches.

Somatic Yoga is the creation of Eleanor Criswell-Hanna, a professor of psychology at Sonoma State University in California who has taught Yoga since the early 1960s. She is managing editor of *Somatics* journal, which was launched by her late husband, Thomas Hanna, inventor of Somatics. Somatic Yoga is an integrated approach to the harmonious development of body and mind, based both on traditional yogic principles and modern psychophysiological research. This gentle approach—which is explained in Criswell-Hanna's book *How Yoga Works*—emphasizes visualization, very slow movement into and out of postures, conscious breathing, mindfulness, and frequent relaxation between postures.

Other prominent styles of Hatha-Yoga are Anusara Yoga (developed by John Friend), Tri Yoga (developed by Kali Ray), White Lotus Yoga (developed by Ganga White and Tracey Rich), Jivamukti (developed by Sharon Gannon and David Life), and Ishta Yoga (developed by Mani Finger and made popular in the United states by his son Alan).

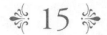

Crossing the Boundary between Hinduism and Buddhism via Tantra-Yoga

FOR MOST OF MY LIFE I studied and practiced a Hindu *sādhana*—primarily versions of Rāja-Yoga and Karma-Yoga, with a dab of Bhakti-Yoga and (in my youth) Hatha-Yoga. A major change occurred when, in 1993, I took up the practice of Tibetan Vajrayāna Buddhism (Buddhist Tantra). When my friends and students learned of my "conversion," they became understandably curious, and I explained to them that I have long had a tremendous respect for Gautama the Buddha and his liberation teaching but that my karma had always steered me toward Hindu Yoga. Had I discovered Buddhism before I became deeply interested in Ramana Maharshi and Hindu Yoga at the age of fourteen, I would in all likelihood have embarked on the study and practice of Buddhism instead.

Later, in the early 1970s, when I became acquainted with Buddhist literature,[1] I was already firmly entrenched in my research and practice of Hindu Yoga. At that time, I also felt that so much work had been done on Buddhist Yoga that I could hardly hope to contribute anything original or useful.

This feeling continued until very recently when I began to think that, perhaps in the near future, I ought to turn my attention as a writer also to Buddhist Yoga in the form of Tibetan Buddhism. Since then I have made small forays into the teachings of Vajrayāna and Mahāyāna. These explorations have led, among other things, to my translating the *Heart Sūtra* and portions of Shāntideva's *Bodhicaryāvatāra*, and writing a short commentary on the *Eight Verses of Mind Training*.

People often ask me whether I experience cognitive dissonance as a result of my continuing work on Hindu Yoga and my personal practice of Vajrayāna. My answer is always the same: No, I experience no conflict at all. My approach to spiritual life is integrative rather than sectarian. I hold all liberation teachings in the highest regard, even when I do not feel moved to practice them personally.

It is an undeniable fact that, *in practice*, there is a striking similarity between Hindu and Buddhist forms of Yoga. This similarity is quite remarkable when we consider Hindu and Buddhist Tantra-Yoga. Historically, Tantra (or Tantrism) has been something of a syncretistic spiritual movement, which has led to a blurring of practical and theoretical distinctions. In his groundbreaking work *Yoga: Immortality and Freedom*, Mircea Eliade called it a "pan-Indian vogue."[2]

Of course, Hindu and Buddhist forms of Yoga also have their unique features, but the common ground between the Tantric forms of these two great spiritual cultures is truly astonishing.

At the heart of both Hindu and Buddhist Tantric practice are (1) *guru-yoga* (focus on one's teacher), (2) visualization of and identification with a given deity, (3) mantra recitation, (4) knowledge and mastery of the currents (*nādī*) of subtle energy (*prāna*) as a prerequisite of enlightenment, and (5) "magical" transformative rituals.

Enlightened masters like Matsyendra, Goraksha, Jālandhara, Caurangi, and Virūpaksha are celebrated equally in traditional Buddhist and Hindu circles. In a number of instances, the Tantric deities are the same (e.g., Tārā, Bhairava, Mahākāla, Ganesha, Vaishravana) as are also mantras (e.g., *om*, *hūm, lam*, etc.).

Thus, rather than feeling confused, I feel a sense of exhilaration about the existence of so much common ground between the various schools of Hindu and Buddhist Tantra-Yoga. This is also why from the outset I emphasized the need for Yoga Research and Education Center, which I founded in 1996, to foster the dialogue between Hinduism and Buddhism as *spiritual* traditions as opposed to *religious* cultures (though religious/theological dialogue seems appropriate too).

Today when I read a Buddhist *Tantra* like the *Guhya-Samāja* or a Hindu *Tantra* like the *Kula-Arnava*, I am keenly aware of the many practical and theoretical/philosophical parallels (without, of course, glossing over differences). What is most important, my personal practice has benefited from studying not only Buddhist scriptures but also Hindu Yoga texts.

At the same time, however, I must admit that the "stages of the path" (Tibetan: *lam-rim*) teachings of the Gelugpa order and similar efforts among the other Tibetan Buddhist orders impress me as being unbelievably exhaustive. These teachings, which date back to Atīsha (c. 1000 C.E.) and were developed in detail by Je Tsongkhapa (the founder of the Gelugpas, c. 1400 C.E.), offer a systematic presentation of the key elements of the Tantric path into which any additional practice or idea can be helpfully located. The *lam-rim* teachings appear to be unique in the world, and thus far I have not come across anything comparable within the Hindu tradition.

The *lam-rim* teachings were developed on Indian soil but flourished in Tibet after Buddhism had vanished from India. To the outsider these teachings may seem like dry scholastic refinements, but one need only to delve into them a little bit to appreciate their immediate practical relevance. They cover every aspect of life that is in any way significant to spiritual practice. Hence they are of inestimable value to the serious practitioner who wants a clear road map to inner growth and liberation. Although there is nothing equivalent to the *lam-rim* teachings within the fold of Hinduism, many of the essential ideas of the *lam-rim* teachings can also be found in the various branches of Hindu Yoga. The reason for this commonality is our shared human constitution and the universal principles underlying the path of self-transformation and enlightenment.

The integrative teachings of Tantra drive home the point that we all suffer until we have succeeded in elevating ourselves beyond our karmic conditioning. Both our common experience of suffering and our shared potential for enlightenment should give us cause for much tolerance and compassion. Whether we are practitioners of Hindu or Buddhist Yoga—or indeed any other spiritual discipline—in order to enjoy the pinnacle of enlightenment, or liberation, we all must cross the artificial boundaries erected between one tradition (or conceptual universe) and another, as well as between ourselves and others. This sense of boundary crossing lies at the heart of Tantra.

❦ 16 ❦
Vajrayāna Buddhist Yoga

BUDDHISM COMES IN THREE vehicles (yāna), often called "scopes": Hīnayāna, Mahāyāna, and Vajrayāna. Hīnayāna holds high the ideal of liberation (nirvāna); Mahāyāna added to this the ideal of the bodhisattva, the
spiritual practitioner who aspires to nirvāna in order to benefit all sentient
beings; Vajrayāna,[1] or Tantric Buddhism, expanded this vision further by in-
sisting that, because suffering is rampant in the world, every effort should be
made to attain liberation as quickly as possible and by any means.

Today Vajrayāna is practiced exclusively in the form of Tibetan Buddhism, which, since the Chinese invasion of Tibet in 1959, has spread
throughout the world. Under the inspirational leadership of the Dalai Lama
and the Karmapa, the two best known and honored adepts of Tibetan Buddhism, the teachers (Tibetan: lama; Sanskrit: guru) of Vajrayāna have freely
shared their knowledge and wisdom through personal instruction and the
printed medium. Thousands of Westerners have taken refuge in the Buddha,
the Dharma, and the Sangha, received all kinds of initiations (abhisheka),
and are practicing the Tantric Yoga of Tibet more or less intensively.

Vajrayāna's heritage is traditionally traced back to the Buddha himself,
though its scriptures are historically of a later date. Its scriptural foundations
are the Prajnā-Pāramitā texts of Mahāyāna, the works of Nāgārjuna (c. 100
C.E.) and his disciples, and the Tantras and their commentaries, as well as
other independent writings by adepts. The doctrinal focus is on emptiness
(shūnya) and compassion (karunā) in the form of bodhicitta, the "enlightenment mind," or the mind suffused with the desire to attain liberation
speedily for the sake of all other beings. Vajrayāna practice revolves around
"Deity Yoga" (devatā-yoga) and Guru-Yoga (devotional practices relative to
one's teacher or teachers). The former is a sophisticated visualization practice in which the practitioner gradually merges with the visualized deity
or higher being. In contrast to Deity Yoga and Guru Yoga, the "formless
path" relies on recollecting the primordial condition of enlightenment. This
is the essence of mahā-mudrā (great seal) and dzog-chen (Tibetan: great

perfection). Garab Dorje, the master who first expounded the principles of *dzog-chen*, is said to have lived between the third century B.C.E. and the first century C.E.[2] He elucidated this advanced practice thus:

> If thoughts arise, remain present in that state;
> if no thoughts arise, remain present in that state;
> there is no difference in the presence in either state.[3]

Vajrayāna consists of numerous teaching lineages in the following four branches:

1. The Nyingma (Old School) traces itself back to Buddha Samanta-bhadra and Buddhas Vajradhāra and Vajrasattva (both emanations of Samantabhadra). The most important human teachers are Shāntarakshita (c. 800 C.E.), Padmasambhava (Guru Rinpoche, c. 800 C.E.), Vairocana (c. 850 C.E.), Longchen Rapjampa (1308–1363), and today's lineage holder Pema Norbu (Penor) Rinpoche (1932–   ). The Nyingmapas follow the old Tibetan translations of the Sanskrit *Tantras*.

2. The Sakya Order is named after the "gray earth" of the Tsang province where the original Sakya monastery was founded in 1073 C.E. This order looks upon the Indian adept Virūpa (ordination name: Dharmapāla) as its originator, while Könchok Gyalpo (1034–1102) is remembered as the founder of the monastery. The order is directed by the Khön family and in the past was closely associated with the Nyingmapas, until Könchok Gyalpo chose to follow the new translations of the *Tantras*, which were prepared during the Indian adept Atīsha's stay in Tibet. Great Sakya masters include Könchok Gyalpo's son Kunga Nyingpo (1092–1158), Drakpa Gyaltsen (1147–1216), Sakya Pandita (1182–1251), and Chögyal Phakpa (1235–1280). The present head of the Sakyapas is Sakya Trizin Ngawang Kenga (1945–   ). The Sakyapas use the *Hevajra-Tantra* as the doctrinal basis of their "Fruit and Path" (*lam dre*) system, according to which the path is inseparable from its results.

3. The Kagyu Order derives its name from the shortening of a phrase that means something like "the unbroken lineage of profound instruction in the four transmitted teachings [of *mahā-mudrā*, *tumo*, *ösel*, and *karma-mudrā*]." Its history began with the Indian adept Tilopa (988–1069), who is said to have received instruction directly from Buddha Vajradhāra. He was fol-lowed by Nāropa (1016–1100), Marpa the Translator (1012–1097), Milarepa (1040–1123), Gampopa (1079–1153), and a long line of great masters down to

the sixteenth Karmapa Ranjung Rigpe Dorjey (1924–1981), Kalu Rinpoche (1905–1989), and the seventeenth Karmapa Ogyen Drodul Trinley Dorje, who is in his early twenties. (The Chinese named a contender when Trinley Dorje fled to India.) The Kagyupas favor long solitary retreats, and an important practice are the Six Yogas of Nāropa, consisting of the Yoga of Inner Heat (*tumo*), the Yoga of the Illusory Body (*gyu lu*), Dream Yoga (*mi lam*), the Yoga of Clear Light (*ösel*), the Yoga of the Intermediate State (*bardo*), and the Yoga of Consciousness Transference (*phowa*). Another emphasis is the practice of *mahā-mudrā* (great seal), which involves realizing directly our own Buddha nature, and the meditative practice of *chöd* (Cutting Off), which consists in mentally offering up one's body piece by piece in order to overcome attachment to the physical form.

4. The Gelug (Virtuous) Order is the reformed order founded by Je Tsongkhapa (1357–1419), who in his lifetime already was venerated as a full *buddha*. His collected works, which are still considered fundamental for those wishing to advance in the study and practice of the Tantric path, comprise eighteen large volumes. The Gelugpas greatly emphasize doctrinal study and *dharma* debate. Gedun Drup (1391–1474), a direct disciple of Je Tsongkhapa, became the first Dalai Lama, who founded Tashilhunpo monastery in the Tsang province of Tibet. The greatest Gelugpa master of modern times was Phabongkha Dechen Nyingpo (1878–1941). Today, apart from the fourteenth Dalai Lama, the best known Gelugpa teacher is Lama Thubten Zopa (1946–   ), heart disciple of Lama Thubten Yeshe (1935–1984). Together with his teacher, Lama Zopa established in 1975 the Foundation for the Preservation of the Mahayana Tradition (FPMT).

Of the four branches of Tibetan Buddhism, the most numerous and influential is the Gelug order. The Tantric Yoga of Je Tsongkhapa unfolds in four levels of competence, generally referred to as "classes" of Tantra (Tibetan: *gyu*):

1. Kriyā-Tantra (Action Tantra): external rituals leading toward purification of body, speech, and mind.

2. Carya-Tantra (Performance Tantra): external rituals combined with meditation and visualization of particular deities.

3. Yoga-Tantra: meditation and visualization of oneself as a deity (Deity Yoga).

4. Anuttara-Yoga-Tantra (Highest Yoga Tantra): Deity Yoga combined with a high awareness and control of the subtle energetic currents (called

"winds," *vāyu*) of the body. This class of Tantra comprises the stage of generation and the stage of completion ending in actual Buddhahood. The latter has six levels, notably the creation of an "illusory body," which is necessary for the attainment of Buddhahood.

The practitioner is encouraged to practice Anuttara-Yoga-Tantra as soon as he or she has achieved adequate competence. In order to do so as efficiently as possible, the Gelugpas follow the *lam-rim* (stages of the path) teachings, which originated with Atīsha (982–1054) and were greatly developed by Je Tsongkhapa and others. These teachings map out the entire path in minute detail, so that practitioners are given all possible help in their efforts to grow and master all the aspects of their yogic training.

According to Je Tsongkhapa's magnificent *Lam-Rim Chen-Mo* (Extensive Exposition of the Stages of the Path), the path begins with various preliminary practices, notably taking refuge in the "three jewels," i.e., the Buddha, the Dharma, and the Sangha—the Enlightened one, the Teaching, and the Community of practitioners.

The practitioner also is expected to do prostrations, make offerings, and recite prayers and mantras, all of which are thought to purify the mind. Part of the preliminaries is Guru Yoga, the devotional focus on one's teacher and the lineage founder and other great masters. This practice continues also in subsequent stages. Next, the practitioner is asked to cultivate the Vajrasattva meditation and mantra, which deepen the purification process and lay the ground for *shamatha* meditation. An important part of the Gelug tradition is study, which must not be confused with mere theoretical learning; study is meant to clarify and strengthen one's motivation to realize Buddhahood via the *bodhisattva* ideal. The *bodhisattva* seeks to awaken *bodhicitta*, or the will toward enlightenment for the sake of others.

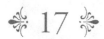

Introducing the Great Literary Heritage
of Hindu Yoga

As Westerners following the Yoga tradition from the East, it is crucial that we steep ourselves in the Yoga heritage. How else can we be sure that what we are doing is authentic Yoga? It will not do any good to use this or that meditation technique or engage in this or that physical practice without knowing their deeper purpose and philosophical underpinning. As part of our study of Yoga, it seems advisable that we become thoroughly acquainted with the literature of this age-old tradition. The good news is that many of the Yoga texts, originally composed in Sanskrit or one of the vernacular languages of India or Tibet, are available in English renderings. Ideally, the dedicated student should read every Yoga scripture available in English.

Looking at the entire literature of Hindu Yoga, which is the focus of the present essay, we can distinguish four broad historical categories (with other divisions being feasible): (1) Archaic Yoga—Vedic and non-Vedic teachings, (2) Preclassical Yoga—Upanishadic, and epic teachings, (3) Classical Yoga—Patanjali's eightfold path, and (4) Postclassical Yoga—nondualistic traditions subsequent to Patanjali.

ARCHAIC YOGA

The many scriptures of what can be called "Archaic Yoga" or "Vedic Yoga" comprise the four *Vedas*—*Rig-Veda*, *Yajur-Veda*, *Sāma-Veda*, and *Atharva-Veda*—and the ritual texts of the *Brāhmanas* and *Āranyakas*, which are based on these four hymnodies. Most scholars believe that the early Indic civilization also contained groups that did not have the *Vedas* at the core of their worldview. Sometimes the spiritual teachings of this non-Vedic cultural thread are grouped under the collective heading of *shramana*, or "ascetic/mendicant," and Gautama the Buddha and Vardhamāna Mahāvīra are generally regarded as belonging to one of those non-Vedic groups. Ethnic plurality—and hence we may surmise also cultural diversity—appears to have been present already in the ancient town of Mehrgarh, which has been dated back to the mid-seventh millennium B.C.E. However, we know of these *shramana* teachings in the Vedic era only indirectly through references in the *Vedas*. The *muni* (ecstatic sage) or *keshin* (long-haired ascetic) is often re-garded as representing a non-Vedic cultural stream and as standing in oppo-sition to the Vedic *rishi* (seer-bard). This aspect of early Indic cultural history is still little understood and deserves further investigation.

The *Rig-Veda*, which a growing number of scholars are now dating back to the third or fourth millennium B.C.E., is a truly amazing collection of hymns composed by seers (*rishi*) whose inner gaze penetrated beyond the visible (material) realm into the invisible (subtle) realms. For thousands of years this great work was faithfully transmitted by word of mouth, until it was written down in the fourteenth century. It required incredible feats of mem-ory to recall the hymns correctly—an art at which all ancient peoples seem to have excelled. Because the *Rig-Veda* represents the most sacred portion of the entire Hindu canon, the *brahmins* carefully guarded it from the eyes of the uninitiated. In fact, it was not until the nineteenth century that out-siders came to read it. By that time even the *brahmins* themselves had for-gotten the meaning of many of the archaic words and were largely ignorant of the deeper meaning of the more than 10,000 verses.

Through the efforts of modern scholarship, spearheaded by great Euro-pean scholars like Paul Deussen and Max Müller, the meaning of the *Rig-Veda* has been gradually recovered. This salvaging work is far from over. As a matter of fact, the deeper meaning of the *Rig-Veda* and the other Vedic hymnodies or "collections" (*samhitā*) is still largely lost to us. This was made clear by Sri Aurobindo, the father of modern Integral Yoga, who applied his own deep understanding of Yoga to the Vedic heritage. His book *On the Veda* is must reading. (Bibliographic references are appended to the pres-ent essay.)

PRECLASSICAL YOGA

The teachings of Preclassical Yoga succeeded the *Vedas* (c. 4500–2500 B.C.E.) but preceded the famous *Yoga-Sūtra* of Patanjali (c. 100–200 C.E.), which has come to be appreciated as the classical philosophical expression of Yoga. The texts of the preclassical era teach various versions of Sāmkhya-Yoga according to which the ultimate reality is single but manifests in successive levels of existence, ending with our familiar physical cosmos.

The idea is found already in the *Rig-Veda* but is developed more fully in the *Upanishads*. In these esoteric scriptures, we encounter for the first time a clear enunciation of the teachings of nondualism (*advaita*) combined with the doctrine of emanationism: The manifold universe emerges out of the transcendental Singularity in definite stages. This led, in due course, to the classical form of Sāmkhya (which is concerned with mapping the stages of this process of emanation and the various categories to which it gives rise). While the early *Upanishads*, such as the *Brihad-Āranyaka-*, *Chāndo-gya-*, and *Taittirīya-Upanishad*, do not yet use the term *yoga* in the later technical sense, they are of course completely familiar with the kind of spiritual discipline that it came to signify in later times.

The oldest work of this genre that knows the word *yoga* in its technical sense is the *Katha-Upanishad*, which belongs to the pre-Buddhist era. This text outlines the basic practices and ideas of Yoga. There are several reasonably reliable translations of this *Upanishad*, notably the readily available renderings by S. Radhakrishnan and R. E. Hume. Since this work, like so many of the Yoga and Vedānta scriptures, is at times rather obscure, students may also want to consult Krishna Prem's insightful book.

While working through the *Katha-Upanishad*, it serves to also study the *Shvetāshvatara-Upanishad* and the *Maitrāyanīya-Upanishad*, which are somewhat younger and thus show the next stage in the evolution of Yoga. Again the translations by Radhakrishnan and Hume are a good starting point.

The principal scripture of Preclassical Yoga is the widely read *Bha-gavad-Gītā*, which is the "New Testament" of Hinduism. Few people know that it is traditionally considered to be an *Upanishad*, that is, a secret doctrine that has been revealed, rather than authored by a human individual. Technically, the *Gītā* is an integral part of the *Mahābhārata*, which is one of India's two great national epics. Although translations of this beautiful text abound, some of the most popular ones leave much to be desired. I can recommend the renderings by Sarvepalli Radhakrishnan and Krishna Prem (who writes from a practitioner's point of view). For an excellent later (poetic and yogic) commentary on the *Gītā*, Jnānadeva's thirteenth-century *Jnāneshvarī* is a priceless gem. It was composed in the Marathi language and is available in a reliable and readable English translation by V. G. Pradhan. To really appreciate the *Gītā*, students should definitely ac-

quaint themselves with the broader cultural and historical background from which it emerged, and here my own book *Introduction to the Bhagavad-Gītā* may be found helpful.

Preclassical materials are also contained in other sections of the *Mahābhārata*, such as the *Moksha-Dharma* and the *Anu-Gītā*. Unfortunately, these sections are not readily accessible, though students may search out F. Edgerton's *The Beginnings of Indian Philosophy*, which contains excerpts from the *Moksha-Dharma*. This section and also the *Anu-Gītā* were translated with the rest of the epic by K. M. Ganguli and also by M. N. Dutt. Yogic materials are found especially in books 6, 12, and 13 of this mammoth work.

Like the *Mahābhārata*, the *Rāmāyana* epic also focuses on teachings revolving around the core value of *dharma*, or morality. In addition, it features yogic teachings under the name of *tapas*, "asceticism."

CLASSICAL YOGA

The teachings of Classical Yoga are codified in the short *Yoga-Sūtra* of Patanjali along with the various Sanskrit commentaries on this text. Classical Yoga is also known as *yoga-darshana*, or the philosophical system of Yoga. There are many paraphrases but only a few good translations of Patanjali's work, which is difficult to understand, because it presupposes a fair amount of knowledge about Indian thought and culture. Nevertheless, it can be very rewarding to carefully plow through this scripture. I have done so with students in a weekly class stretching over nine months, and they clearly benefited from this exercise, in terms of their understanding of both Patanjali's system and Yoga theory and practice in general.

A good, if technical, translation is that by James H. Wood, which also includes the two main Sanskrit commentaries by Vyāsa and Vācaspati Mishra. From a practical perspective, I can also recommend Bernard Bouanchaud's *The Essence of Yoga* and B. K. S. Iyengar's *Light on the Yoga Sūtras of Patañjali* and *Light on Aṣṭānga Yoga*. I myself have authored several books on Classical Yoga, which many years ago was my primary area of research. My rendering of Patanjali's text includes the transliterated Sanskrit text and word-by-word translation. For a scholarly study that makes a plea for a non-dualistic reading of the *Yoga-Sūtra*, I can recommend Ian Whicher's *The Integrity of the Yoga Darśana*.

Many Sanskrit commentaries have been written on the *Yoga-Sūtra*, all of which are rather technical. However, serious students may want to know that translations of two important Sanskrit commentaries are at long last available in English: the *Yoga-Vārttika* of Vijnāna Bikshu, which has been ably translated by T. S. Rukmani, and the *Yoga-Bhāshya-Vivarana* of Shankara Bhagavatpāda, which has been translated independently by Trevor Leggett and by T. S. Rukmani. The *Vivarana*, which some authorities attribute (probably wrongly) to the same Shankara who was the greatest proponent of Advaita (non-dualistic) Vedānta, is a fascinating text that contains many original ideas.

POSTCLASSICAL YOGA

Postclassical Yoga is embodied in a great many works from the following categories:

- The Tantric literature, which is vast and highly esoteric and includes the *Āgamas*, *Tantras*, and *Shāstras*, as well as the massive literature of Kashmiri Shaivism and Southern India's Shaiva Siddhānta, and the Tamil writings of the Siddhas. Of actual *Tantras*, Yoga practitioners should at least study the *Kula-Arnava-Tantra* and the fairly recent but significant *Mahānirvāna-Tantra*. An important work written in Tamil rather than Sanskrit is the *Tiru-Mantiram* of Tirumūlar, which exists in a somewhat poor English rendition.
- The *Purānas*, which are encyclopedic repositories of traditional wisdom, including everything from cosmology to philosophy to stories about kings and holy men. They contain many yogic legends and teachings. The following are especially important: the *Bhāgavata-Purāna* (also known as *Shrīmad-Bhāgavata*), *Shiva-Purāna*, and *Devī-Bhāgavata-Purāna* (a Tantric work).
- The so-called *Yoga-Upanishads* (some twenty texts), most of which were composed after 1000 C.E. and include three extensive works: the *Darshana-Upanishad*, *Yoga-Shikhā-Upanishad* and *Tejo-Bindu-Upanishad*.
- The texts of Hatha-Yoga, such as the *Goraksha-Samhitā*, *Hatha-Yoga-Pradīpikā*, *Hatha-Ratna-Avalī*, *Gheranda-Samhitā*, *Shiva-Samhitā*, *Yoga-Yājnavalkya*, *Yoga-Bīja*, *Yoga-Shāstra* of Dattātreya, *Sat-Karma-Samgraha*, and the *Shiva-Svarodaya*, which are all available in English.
- Vedāntic scriptures like the voluminous *Yoga-Vāsishtha*, which teaches Jnāna-Yoga, and its traditional abridgment, the *Laghu-Yoga-Vāsishtha*, both available in English renderings.
- The literature of the *bhakti-mārga* or devotional path, which is especially

prominent among the Vaishnavas (worshipers of Vishnu) and Shaivas (worshipers of Shiva). There is a considerable literature on *bhakti* in both Sanskrit and Tamil, as well as various vernacular languages. In particular, I can recommend Nārada's *Bhakti-Sūtra*, Shāndilya's *Bhakti-Sūtra*, and the extensive *Bhāgavata-Purāna*, which is a detailed (mythological) account of the birth, life, and death of the God-man Krishna, with many wonderful and inspiring stories of yogins and ascetics. This beautiful work contains the *Uddhāva-Gītā*, Krishna's final esoteric instruction to sage Uddhāva. Goddess worship from a Tantric viewpoint is the core of the *Devī-Bhāgavata-Purāna*, which should also be studied.

In addition, sincere Yoga students should also read and ponder the great yogic texts associated with the different schools of Buddhism and Jainism. To encounter the world of Yoga through its literature will challenge the practitioner in many ways: The texts, even in translation and with notes, are often difficult to comprehend and demand serious concentration and perseverance. Yet we do not have to become scholars, but our study (*svādhyāya*) will show us what it takes to be a real *yogin* and what magnificent tools Yoga puts at our disposal. It will also further our self-understanding and strengthen our commitment to practice. In his *Treasury of Good Advice* (1.6), Sakya Pāndita, who was one of the great scholar-adepts of Vajrayāna Buddhism, wrote:

> Even if one were to die first thing tomorrow, today one must study.
> Although one may not become a sage in this life, knowledge is firmly accumulated for future lives, just as secured assets can be used later.

RESOURCES

General

Daniélou, Alain. *Yoga: The Method of Re-Integration*. London: Christopher Johnson, 1949.

——. *The Gods of India: Hindu Polytheism*. New York: Inner Traditions International, 1985.

Dasgupta, Surendranath. *A History of Indian Philosophy*. Cambridge, Mass.: Cambridge University Press, 1952–55. 5 vols.

——. *Hindu Mysticism*. Delhi: Motilal Banarsidass, 1927.

Eliade, Mircea. *Yoga: Immortality and Freedom*. Princeton, N.J.: Princeton University Press, 1973.

——. *Patañjali and Yoga*. New York: Schocken Books, 1975.

Feuerstein, Georg. *The Yoga Tradition*. Prescott, Ariz.: Hohm Press, rev. ed., 2000.

——. *The Shambhala Encyclopedia of Yoga*. Boston: Shambhala Publications, 1997.

———. *Wholeness or Transcendence? Ancient Lessons for the Emerging Global Civilization.* Burdett, N.Y.: Larson, 1992.

———. *The Teachings of Yoga.* Boston: Shambhala Publications, 1997.

———, Subhash Kak, and David Frawley. *In Search of the Cradle of Civilization: New Light on Ancient India.* Wheaton, Ill.: Quest Books, 1995.

Rai, R. K. *Encyclopedia of Yoga.* Varanasi, India: Prachya Prakashan, 1975.

Varenne, Jean. *Yoga and the Hindu Tradition.* Chicago: University of Chicago Press, 1976.

Archaic Yoga

Vedas

Aurobindo. *On the Veda.* Pondicherry, India: Sri Aurobindo Ashram, 1976.

Bloomfield, Maurice. *The Religion of the Veda.* New York: Putnam's Sons, 1908.

———, trans. *Hymns from the Atharva Veda.* Delhi: Motilal Banarsidass, repr. 1964.

Chand, Devi, trans. *The Yajurveda.* New Delhi: Munshiram Manoharlal, 1998.

Dange, S. A. *Sexual Symbolism from the Vedic Ritual.* Delhi: Ajanta Books, 1979.

Frawley, David. *Gods, Sages and Kings: Vedic Secrets of Ancient Civilization.* Salt Lake City, Ut.: Passage Press, 1991.

———. *Wisdom of the Ancient Seers: Mantras of the Rig Veda.* Salt Lake City, Utah: Passage Press, 1992.

Gonda, Jan. *The Vision of the Vedic Poets.* The Hague: Mouton, 1963.

———. *Vedic Literature: Samhitās and Brāhmanas. A History of Indian Literature,* vol. 1, fasc. 1. Wiesbaden, Germany: Otto Harrasowitz, 1975.

Griffith, R., trans. *The Hymns of the Rig Veda.* Delhi: Motilal Banarsidass, repr. 1976. 2 vols.

Johnson, Willard. *Poetry and Speculation in the Rg Veda.* Berkeley: University of California Press, 1990.

Kak, Subhash. *The Astronomical Code of the Rgveda.* New Delhi: Aditya Prakashan, 1994.

Macdonell, A. A. *Vedic Mythology.* Varanasi, India: Indological Book House, repr. 1963. 2 vols.

Miller, Jeanine. *The Vedas: Harmony, Meditation and Fulfillment.* London: Rider, 1974.

———. *The Vision of Cosmic Order in the Vedas.* London: Routledge & Kegan Paul, 1985.

O'Flaherty, Wendy Doniger. *The Rig Veda.* New York: Penguin Books, 1981.

Panikkar, Raimundo. *The Vedic Experience—Mantramanjarī: An Anthology of the Vedas for Modern Man and Contemporary Celebration.* London: Darton, Longman & Todd, 1977.

Whitney, William David, trans. *Atharva Veda Samhitā.* Cambridge, Mass.: Harvard University Press, 1950. 2 vols.

Brāhmanas

Caland, W., trans. *Pañcavimśa-Brāhmana.* Calcutta: Asiatic Society of Bengal, 1931.

Eggeling, Julius, trans. The Śatapatha-Brāhmana According to the Text of the Mādh-yandina School. Delhi: Motilal Banarsidass, repr. 1993. 5 vols.

Haug, Martin, trans. *Aitareya Brahmanam of the Rigveda*. Delhi: Bharatiya, repr. 1976. 2 vols.

Keith, A. B., trans. *Rigveda Brāhmanas Translated*. Cambridge: Harvard University Press, 1920. Includes *Aitareya-* and *Kaushītaki-Brāhmana*.

Āranyakas

Keith, A. B., trans. *The Aitareya Āranyaka*. Delhi: Eastern Book Linkers, repr. 1995.

Preclassical Yoga

Upanishads

Deussen, Paul. *The Philosophy of the Upanishads*. New York: Dover, repr. 1966.

Hume, R. E. *The Thirteen Principal Upanishads*. Oxford, England: Oxford University Press, 1971.

Krishna Prem. *The Yoga of the Kathopanishad*. London: Watkins, 1955.

Radhakrishnan, Sarvepalli. *The Principal Upanishads*. Atlantic Highlands, N.J.: Humanities Press, 1978.

Mahābhārata and Rāmāyana

Bhaktipada, Swami. *Rama: The Illustrated Ramayana*. Moundsville, W. Va.: Palace Publishing, 1989.

Buck, W. *Mahabharata*. Berkeley: University of California Press, 1973. A condensed retelling.

Chinmayananda, Swami, trans. *Śrī Rāma Gītā*. Los Altos, Calif.: Chinmaya Publications West, 1986.

Dange, S. A. *Legends in the Mahābhārata*. Delhi: Motilal Banarsidass, 1969.

Dutt, M. N. *A Prose English Translation of the Mahabharata*. Calcutta: H. C. Dass, 1895–1905. 8 vols.

Edgerton, F. *The Beginnings of Indian Philosophy*. London: Allen & Unwin, 1965.

Ganguli, K. M. *The Mahābhārata*. 12 vols. A four-volume paperback edition was published by Munshiram Manoharlal in 1991.

Goldman, Robert P., et al., ed. and trans. *The Rāmāyana of Vālmīki*. Princeton, N.J.: Princeton University Press, 1984–96. 7 vols.

Hopkins, E. W. *Epic Mythology*. Delhi: Motilal Banarsidass, repr. 1974.

Richman, Paula. *Many Rāmāyanas: The Diversity of a Narrative Tradition in South Asia*. Berkeley: University of California Press, 1991.

Shastri, Hari Prasad, trans. *Ramayana of Valmiki*. London: Shanti Sadan, 1952-59. 3 vols.

Van Buitenen, J. A. B., trans. *The Mahābhārata*. Chicago: University of Chicago Press, 1973–78. 3 vols. Project in progress.

Bhagavad-Gītā

Aurobindo. *Essays on the Gita*. Pondicherry, India: Auromere, 1979.

Feuerstein, Georg. *Introduction to the Bhagavad-Gītā*. Wheaton, Ill.: Quest Books,

1983. A new edition of this book and the translation listed next is in progress and will be issued by Shambhala Publications probably in 2003.

———. *Bhagavad-Gītā: A Critical Rendering*. New Delhi: Arnold-Heinemann, 1981.

Krishna Prem. *The Yoga of the Bhagavad-Gita*. Harmondsworth, England: Penguin Books, 1973.

Pradhan, V. G. *Jnāneshvarī*. Albany, N.Y.: SUNY Press, 1986. [Marathi commentary on the *Gītā*]

Radhakrishnan, S. *The Bhagavadgītā*. San Francisco: Harper & Row, n.d.

Sharma, Arbind. *The Hindu Gītā: Ancient and Classical Interpretations of the Bhagavadgītā*. La Salle, Ill.: Open Court, 1986.

Zaehner, R. C. *The Bhagavad-Gītā*. Oxford, England: Oxford University Press, 1969.

Classical Yoga

Yoga-Sūtra and Its Commentaries

Bouanchaud, Bernard. *The Essence of Yoga: Reflections on the Yoga Sutras of Patanjali*. Portland, Ore.: Rudra Press, 1997.

Dasgupta, Surendranath. *A Study of Patanjali*. Calcutta: University of Calcutta, 1920.

———. *Yoga As Philosophy and Religion*. London: Kegan Paul, 1924.

———. *Yoga Philosophy in Relation to Other Systems of Indian Thought*. Calcutta: University of Calcutta, 1930.

Feuerstein, G., trans. *The Yoga-Sūtra: A New Translation and Commentary*. Folkstone, England: Dawson, 1981.

———. *The Yoga-Sūtra: An Exercise in the Methodology of Textual Analysis*. New Delhi: Arnold-Heinemann, 1979.

———. *The Philosophy of Classical Yoga*. Manchester, England: Manchester University Press, 1981.

Govindan, Marshall. *Kriya Yoga Sutras of Patanjali and the Siddhas*. Eastman, Quebec: Kriya Yoga Publications, 2000.

Iyengar, B. K. S., trans. *Light on the Yoga Sūtras of Patanjali*. San Francisco: HarperSanFrancisco, 1993.

———. *Light on Astānga Yoga*. Mumbai, India: YOG, 2000.

Leggett, Trevor, trans. The Complete Comentary by Śankara on the Yoga-Sūtra-s. London: Kegan Paul International, 1990.

Rukmani, T. S., trans. *Yogavārttika of Vijnānabhiksu*. New Dehli: Munshiram Manoharlal, 1981 and 1983. 4 vols.

———, trans. *Yogasūtrabhāṣyavivarana of Śankara*. New Delhi: Munshiram Manoharlal, 2001. 2 vols.

Whicher, Ian. *The Integrity of the Yoga Darśana: A Reconsideration of Classical Yoga*. Albany, N.Y.: SUNY Press, 1998.

Woods, J. H., trans. *Yoga System of Patañjali*. New Dehli: Motilal Banarsidass, 1977. Includes translations of the *Yoga-Bhāshya* and the *Tattva-Vaishāradī* commentaries.

Postclassical Yoga

Late Upanishads

Aiyar, K. Narayanasvami, trans. *Thirty Minor Upanishads, Including the Yoga Upanishads*. El Reno, Okla.: Santarasa Publications, repr. 1980.

Ayyangar, T. R. Srinivas, and G. Srinivasa Murti, trans. *The Yoga Upanisads*. Adyar, India: Adyar Library, 1952.

Varenne, Jean. *Yoga and the Hindu Tradition*. Chicago: University of Chicago Press, 1976.

Tantras

Avalon, Arthur [Sir John Woodroffe]. *Shakti and Shākta*. New York: Dover, 1978.

Basu, Manoranjan. *Fundamentals of the Philosophy of Tantras*. Calcutta: Mira Basu Publishers, 1986.

Bharati, Agehananda. *The Tantric Tradition*. London: Rider, 1965.

Bhattacharya, N. N. *History of the Tantric Religion*. New Delhi: Munshiram Manoharlal, 1974.

Brooks, Douglas Renfrew. *The Secret of the Three Cities*. Chicago and London: University of Chicago Press, 1990.

———. *Auspicious Wisdom: The Text and Traditions of Śrīvidyā Tantrism in South India*. Albany, N.Y.: SUNY Press, 1992.

Daniélou, Alain. *While the Gods Play: Shaiva Oracles and Predictions on the Cycles of History and the Destiny of Mankind*. Rochester, Vt.: Inner Traditions International, 1987.

———. *Shiva and Dionysus: The Religion of Nature and Eros*. New York: Inner Traditions International, 1984.

Dimock, E. C. *The Place of the Hidden Moon: Erotic Mysticism in the Vaiṣṇava Sahajiyā Cult of Bengal*. Chicago: University of Chicago Press, 1966.

Frawley, David. *Tantric Yoga and the Wisdom Goddesses*. Salt Lake City, Ut.: Passage Press, 1994.

Goswami, Syundar Shyam. *Layayoga*. Rochester, Vt.: Inner Traditions International, 1999.

Goudriaan, Teun, trans. *The Vīnāśikhātantra: A Śaiva Tantra of the Left Current*. Delhi: Motilal Banarsidass, 1985.

———, and Sanjukta Gupta. *Hindu Tantric and Śākta Literature*. Wiesbaden, Germany: Otto Harrassowitz, 1981.

Govindan, Marshall. *Thirumandiram: A Yoga Classic by Siddhar Thirumoolar*. Translated by B. Natarajan. Montreal: Babaji's Kriya Yoga and Publications, 1993.

Krishna, Gopi. *Living with Kundalini*. Boston and London: Shambhala Publications, 1993.

Magee, Michael, trans. *Kaulajnāna-nirnaya of the School of Matsyendranātha*. Varanasi, India: Prachya Prakashan, 1986.

Mishra, Kamalakar. *Kashmir Śaivism: The Central Philosophy of Tantrism*. Cambridge, Mass.: Rudra Press, 1993.

Mookerjee, Ajit. *Kundalini: The Arousal of the Inner Energy*. New York: Destiny Books, 1982.

———, and Madhu Khanna. *The Tantric Way: Art, Science, Ritual*. London: Thamas and Hudson, 1977.

Muller-Ortega, Paul Eduardo. *The Triadic Heart of Śiva: Kaula Tantricism of Abhinavagupta in the Non-Dual Śaivism of Kashmir*. Albany, N.Y.: SUNY Press, 1989.

Pandit, M. P., trans. *The Kulārnava Tantra*. Madras: Ganesh, 1973.

Rai, Ram Kumar, trans. *Kulārnava Tantra*. Varanasi, India: Prachya Prakashan, 1983.

Sannella, Lee. *The Kundalini Experience*. Lower Lake, Calif.: Integral Publishing, 1992.

Silburn, Lilian. *Kundalini: The Energy of the Depths*. Albany, N.Y.: SUNY Press, 1988.

Singh, Jaideva, trans. *Śiva Sūtras: The Yoga of Supreme Identity*. Delhi: Motilal Banarsidass, rev. 1980.

———, trans. *The Yoga of Delight, Wonder, and Astonishment*. Albany, N.Y.: SUNY Press, 1991. A rendering of the *Vijñāna-Bhairava*.

Tigunait, Rajmani. *Śaktism: The Power in Tantra*. Honesdale, Penn.: Himalayan International Institute, 1998.

White, David Gordon. *The Alchemical Body: Siddha Traditions in Medieval India*. Chicago and London: University of Chicago Press, 1996.

Zvelebil, Kamil V. *The Poets of the Powers*. Lower Lake, Calif.: Integral Publishing, 1993.

———. *The Siddha Quest for Immortality*. Oxford: Mandrake of Oxford, 1996.

Purāṇas

A Board of Scholars, trans. *The Linga Purāna*. Delhi: Motilal Banarsidass, 1973. 2 vols.

———, trans. *The Śiva Purāna*. Delhi: Motilal Banarsidass, 1969–70. 4 vols.

Banerjea, K. N. *Pauranic and Tantric Religion*. Calcutta: University of Calcutta, 1966.

Deshpande, N. A., trans. *The Padma Purāna*. Delhi: Motilal Banarsidass, 1988–90. 5 vols.

Gangadharan, N., trans. *The Agni Purāna*. Delhi: Motilal Banarsidass, 1984–87. 4 vols.

Goswami, C. L., trans. *Śrīmad Bhāgavata Mahāpurāna*. Gorakhpur, India: Gita Press, 1971. 2 vols.

Madhavananda, Swami, trans. *Uddhāva Gītā*. Calcutta, India: Advaita Ashrama, 1971.

Raghunathan, N. *Śrīmad Bhāgavatam*. Madras, India: Vighneswara Publishing House, 1976. 2 vols.

Tagare, G. V., trans. *The Bhāgavata Purāna*. Delhi: Motilal Banarsidass, 1976–78. 5 vols.

———, trans. *The Brahmānda Purāna*. Delhi: Motilal Banarsidass, 1983–84. 5 vols.

———, trans. *The Nārada Purāna*. Delhi: Motilal Banarsidass, 1980–83. 5 vols.

———, trans. *The Vāyu Purāna*. Delhi: Motilal Banarsidass, 1987–88. 2 vols.

Vijnanananda, Swami, trans. *The Śrīmad Devī Bhāgavatam*. New York: AMS Press, repr. 1974.

Wilson, H. H., trans. *The Vishnu Purāna: A System of Hindu Mythology and Tradition*. Calcutta: Punthi Pustak, repr. 1961.

Yoga-Vāsishta

Atreya, B. L. *The Yogavāsistha and Its Philosophy*. Moradabad, India: Darshana Printers, 3d ed., 1966

Narayanaswamy Aiyer, K., trans. *Laghu-Yoga-Vasishta*. Madras: Adyar Library and Research Center, 1975.

Kuvalayananda, Swami, and Swami Digambarji, trans. *Vāsishta Samhitā: Yoga Kānda*. Lonavla, India: Kaivalyadhama, 1969.

Mitra, Vihari Lal, trans. *The Yoga-Vāsishta-Mahārāmāyana*. Varanasi, India: Bharatiya Publishing House, 1976. 4 vols.

Venkatesananda, Swami, trans. *The Concise Yoga Vāsishta*. Albany, N.Y.: State University of New York Press, 1984.

Hatha-Yoga

Arya, Usharbudh. *Philosophy of Hatha Yoga*. Honesdale, Penn.: Himalayan International Institute, 1985.

Avalon, A. [Sir John Woodroffe]. *The Serpent Power*. New York: Dover, 1974.

Awashti, B. M., trans. *Yoga Bīja*. Dehli: Swami Keshwananda Yoga Institute, n.d.

——, and A. Sharma, *Yoga Śāstra of Dattātreya*. Dehli: Swami Keshawananda Yoga Institute, 1985.

Banerjea, A. K. *Philosophy of Goraknath with Goraksha-Vacana–Sangraha*. Gorakhpur, India: Mahant Dig Vijai Nath Trust, [1961].

Bernard, Theos. *Hatha Yoga: The Report of a Personal Experience*. London: Rider, 1968.

Briggs, George W. *Goraknāth and the Kānphata Yogīs*. Delhi: Motilal Banarsidass, repr. 1973.

Digamgarji, Swami, and M. L. Gharote, trans. *Gheranda Samhitā*. Lonavla, India: Kaivalyadhama, 1978.

—— and R. Kokaje, trans. *Hathayogapradīpikā of Svātmārāma*. Lonavla, India: Kaivalyadhama, 1970.

—— and S. A. Shukla, trans. *Gorakṣaśatakam*. Lonavla, India: Kaivalyadhama, 1958.

Feuerstein, Georg, trans. "Goraksha Paddhati" in *The Yoga Tradition*. Prescott, Ariz.: Hohm Press, rev. ed. 2001. 532–59.

——. "Advaya-Tāraka-Upanishad" in *The Yoga Tradition*. 427–31.

——. "Amrita-Nāda-Bindu-Upanishad" in *The Yoga Tradition*. 416–20.

——. "Kshurikā-Upanishad" in *The Yoga Tradition*. 434–37.

Harshe, R. G., trans. *Satkarmasangrahah*. Lonavla, India: Kaivalyadhama, 1970.

Iyangar, S., trans. *The Hathayogapradīpikā of Svātmārāma*.Madras, India: Adyar Library and Research Center, 1972.

Mohan, A. G., trans. *Yoga Yajñavalkya*. Madras: Ganesh & Co., 2000.

Rai, R. K., trans. *Shiva Svarodaya*. Varanasi, India: Prachya Parakashan, 1980.

Reddy, M. V., trans. *Hatharatnavalī*. Arthamuru, India: M. Ramakrishna Reddy, 1982.

Vasu, S. C., trans. *The Geranda Samhitā: A Treatise on Hatha Yoga*. London: Theosophical Publishing House, 1976.

——. *The Śiva Samhitā*. New Dehli, India: Oriental Books Reprint Corp., 1975.

Bhakti-Mārga

Hardy, Friedhelm. *Viraha-Bhakti: The Early History of Krsna Devotion in South India.* Delhi: Oxford University Press, 1983.

Harshananda, Swami, trans. *Śāndilya Bhakti Sūtras.* Prasaranga, India: University of Mysore, 1976.

Miller, Barbara Stoler, trans. *Love Song of the Dark Lord: Jayadeva's Gitagovinda.* New York: Columbia University Press, 1977.

Prem Prakash, trans. *The Yoga of Spiritual Devotion: A Modern Translation of the Narada Bhakti Sutras.* Rochester, Vt.: Inner Traditions International, 1998.

Tripurari, Swami. *Rasa: Love Relationships in Transcendence.* Eugene, Or.: Clarion Call, 1994.

Vivekananda, Swami. *Karma Yoga and Bhakti Yoga.* New York: Ramakrishna-Vivekananda Center, 1982.

❧ 18 ❧
Yoga Symbolism

YOGA IS STEEPED IN symbolism. Some symbols are shared between the great yogic traditions of Hinduism, Buddhism, and Jainism; others are unique to each. For Western students, this represents a particular challenge, as the meaning of the yogic symbols is seldom obvious. Basically, we can distinguish two kinds of symbolism: a spontaneous, "natural" symbolism and an artificial symbolism. Both arise from the higher mind (*buddhi*), which is the preferred mental organ of the Yoga adepts. The lower mind (*manas*) is logical and literal; the higher mind is translogical and metaphoric. The *buddhi* is an impersonal agency, which functions as the organ of wisdom and also acts as the depository of the deep symbols or archetypes. It has much in common with the concept of the universal unconscious in Jungian psychology. Unlike English, the German language makes a useful distinction between *Vernunft* and *Verstand*, which fairly accurately correspond to *buddhi* and *manas* respectively. The former is the fertile ground in which creativity, poetry, and symbolism flourish.

Natural symbolism is basic to all good poetry. When the poet calls Nature a "bloody tooth," we have an instance of natural symbolism. An example of artificial symbolism is the secret code of the *Tantras*, known as *sandhyā-bhāshya* or "twilight language," which is a construct of the logical mind under the inspiration of the *buddhi*.

The earliest manifestations of spontaneous symbolism can be seen in the poetry of the *Rig-Veda*, though this archaic work also contains numerous examples of artificial symbolism. Sometimes the two forms of symbolism are used conjointly; sometimes no clear distinction can be made. It took a great Yoga master — Sri Aurobindo — to draw our attention to the fact that the *Vedas* are laden with profound symbols most of which had escaped the notice of scholars or been misunderstood by them. In his book *On the Veda*, he writes:

> The [Rig-]Veda is a book of esoteric symbols, almost of spiritual formulae, which masks itself as a collection of ritual poems. The inner sense

is psychological, universal, impersonal; the ostensible significance and the figures which were meant to reveal to the initiates what they concealed from the ignorant, are to all appearance crudely concrete, intimately personal, loosely occasional and allusive. To this lax outer garb the Vedic poets are sometimes careful to give a clear and coherent form quite other than the strenuous inner soul of their meaning; their language then becomes a cunningly woven mask for hidden truths. More often they are negligent of the disguise which they use, and when they thus rise above their instrument, a literal and external translation gives either a bizarre, unconnected sequence of sentences or a form of thought and speech strange and remote to the uninitiated intelligence. It is only when the figures and symbols are made to suggest their concealed equivalents that there emerges out of the obscurity a transparent and well-linked though close and subtle sequence of spiritual, psychological and religious ideas.[1]

Aurobindo's orientation has yielded important new insights into the thought of the Vedic seers (*rishi*), who "saw" the truth. He showed a way out of the uninspiring scholarly perspective, with its insistence that the Vedic seers were "primitive" poets obsessed with natural phenomena like thunder, lightning, and rain. The one-dimensional "naturalistic" interpretations proffered by other translators missed out on the depth of the Vedic teachings. Thus Sūrya is not only the visible material Sun but also the psychological-spiritual principle of inner luminosity. Agni is not merely the physical fire that consumes the sacrificial offerings but the spiritual principle of purifying transformation. Parjanya does not only stand for rain but also the inner "irrigation" of grace. Soma is not merely the concoction the sacrificial priests poured into the fire but also (as in the later Tantric tradition) the magical inner substance that transmutes the body and the mind. The wealth prayed for in many hymns is not just material prosperity but spiritual riches. The cows mentioned over and over again in the hymns are not so much the biological animals but spiritual light. The Panis are not just human merchants but various forces of darkness. When Indra slew Vritra and released the floods, he not merely inaugurated the monsoon season but also unleashed the powers of life (or higher energies) within the psyche of the priest. For Indra also stands for the mind and Vritra for psychological restriction, or energetic blockage.

Aurobindo contributed in a major way to a thorough reappraisal of the meaning of the Vedic hymns, and his work encouraged a number of scholars to follow suit, including Jeanine Miller and David Frawley.[2]

There is also plenty of deliberate, artificial symbolism in the hymns. In fact, the figurative language of the *Rig-Veda* is extraordinarily rich, as Willard Johnson has demonstrated.[3] In special sacrificial symposia, the hymn composers met to share their poetic creations and stimulate each other's creativity and comprehension of the subtle realities of life. Thus many hymns are deliberately enigmatic, and often we can only guess at the solutions to their enigmas and allegorical riddles. Heinrich Zimmer reminded us:

> The myths and symbols of India resist intellectualization and reduction to fixed significations. Such treatments would only sterilize them of their magic.[4]

As Sadashiv Ambadas Dange has shown, sexual symbolism is very extensively used in the *Rig-Veda* and subsequently was greatly elaborated in the *Brāhmanas* (ritual texts).[5] In the *Rig-Veda*, for instance, the concept of *mithuna* ("coupling, "copulating") is applied to the symbolic coupling of Heaven and Earth, water and fire, the two Ashvins, day and night, etc. The Vedic sexual symbolism clearly foreshadows the Tantric heritage of medieval India. The famous hymn of Dīrghatamas ("Long Night") in the *Rig-Veda* (1.164) mentions in verse 35 that the *soma* libation is the semen of the virile stallion (i.e., Heaven); the womb belongs to Mother Earth. She gives birth to the solar year, or the sacrifice, or the sacrificial fire. Verse 16 of the same hymn mentions that the months of the year are said to be male, but the seer knows them to be female (i.e., receptive). Without the key to the symbolic language of the four *Vedas*, the extensive ritual literature of the *Brāhmanas* and *Āranyakas* remains largely incomprehensible.

We see a new kind of symbolism emerging in the *Mahābhārata* epic and the *Purānas*. Myths and allegories abound in these works, and often they are best explained from a yogic perspective. There are also riddles whose answers expectedly must be sought in the yogic environment of intense inner experimentation. A classic example is the two-level dialogue between two sages, Vandin and Ashtāvakra, which is found in the *Mahābhārata* (3.134). At the first level, which is obvious, it consists of cryptic statements, extending over various sets from one to thirteen units each. At the deeper level, according to the seventeenth-century commentator Nīlakantha, this dialogue revolves around the philosophical positions of the two sages.

For instance, Vandin states that "a *single* fire flames forth as many [sparks]" to which Ashtāvakra responds that "the *two* friends Indra and Agni roam [together]." Nīlakantha explains that Vandin means to say that the many senses are ruled by a single faculty, namely the higher mind (*buddhi*). Ashtāvakra, a stout adherent of Advaita Vedānta, counters by stating that in addition to the higher mind a second faculty is needed, namely transcendental Consciousness. In other words, the *buddhi* requires the Self, or ultimate Consciousness, in order to manifest the phenomenon of ordinary consciousness. And so on.

Number symbolism has always been important to the Indic mind. Already the *Rig-Veda* contains hymns that delight in numeric riddles. The Vedic seers (*rishi*) were veritable masters in the art of symbolism and riddles. Language, they felt, can point to the dark enigmas that the logical mind fails to fathom but that become clear in inspired vision. The Vedic penchant for symbolism and riddles continued in the post-Vedic era.

The entire *Mahābhārata*, for instance, appears to be constructed on the basis of the symbolic number 18, as I have explained in my *Introduction to the Bhagavad-Gītā*.[6] The war, which is the trigger of the epic's dramatic story and didactic passages, in all probability has historical roots, but it also has always been understood allegorically, as a moral and psychological struggle between good and evil forces both outside and within the human psyche. If the *Mahābhārata* revolves around the ideal of *dharma*, or moral virtue, the epic drama of the *Rāmāyana* is primarily concerned with the age-old ideals of truth and fidelity. The divinized figures of King Rāma and his beloved spouse Sītā have inspired countless generations in India.

A beautiful example of archetypal poetic symbolism is present in the well-known Krishna legend, as told in the *Bhāgavata-Purāna*: The Godman Krishna plays his magical flute and enchants all the female and male cowherds, who fall in love with him and become utterly self-forgetful in his company—a symbol of the human psyche yearning for the ultimate Reality. The love play (*līlā*) between Krishna and the cowherds is an apt description of the playful dynamics that occurs on the yogic path between the aspirant and the *guru*, who embodies the transcendental Principle.

Shiva's world-destroying dance is another potent symbol that can be understood both cosmologically and psychologically. From a yogic perspective, the dance disentangles all the mental webs by which we have imprisoned ourselves through our incessant karmic activities or volitions. Shiva, as Natarāja ("Lord of Dance"), is the destroyer of our delusions and illusions. He is an inner force that undermines our laboriously created conceptualizations of the world, so that we may see reality "as it is" (*yathā-bhūta*).

The Goddess Mohinī ("She who deludes") is thought to tempt us with misconceptions and delusional fantasies, so that only serious spiritual seek-ers can find their way to Reality. The elephant-headed, pot-bellied God Ganesha, again, is traditionally called upon to remove all such obstacles. Each deity represents a particular symbolic function whose depth we can plumb only when we delve into our own psyche by means of Yoga. The artistic representations of the numerous deities of Hinduism, Buddhism, and Jainism all are full of yogic symbolism. That symbolism is most promi-nent in the profound teachings of Tantra.

To appreciate this fact, we just need to look at the esoteric meaning of *hatha*—as in Hatha-Yoga, a branch of Tantra. The dictionary meaning of the term *hatha* is simply "force" or "power," and the commonly used ablative *hathāt* means "by force of." Esoterically, however, the syllables *ha* and *tha*—quite meaningless in themselves—are said to symbolize "Sun" and "Moon" respectively. Specifically, they refer to the *inner* luminaries: the "sun" or solar energy coursing through the right energetic pathway (i.e., the *pingalā-nādī*) and the "moon" or lunar energy traveling through the left pathway (i.e., the *idā-nādī*). Hatha-Yoga utilizes these two currents—corresponding to the sympathetic and parasympathetic nervous systems respectively—in order to achieve a psychoenergetic balance and mental tranquillity.

When this energetic harmony is achieved, the central channel (i.e., the *sushumnā-nādī*) is activated. As soon as the life force (*prāna*) flows into and up the central channel, it awakens the serpent power (*kundalinī-shakti*) and pulls it into the central channel as well. Thereafter the *kundalinī* rises to the crown of the head, leading to a sublime state of mind-transcending unified consciousness (or *nirvikalpa-samādhi*, "formless ecstasy"). The symbolism of Kundalinī-Yoga is very intricate. Tantra also operates with an artificial "twilight" language that is intelligible only to initiates. For instance, the widely used term *padma* ("lotus") may signify the vagina, while *vajra* ("thunderbolt") may represent the penis. It all depends on the context, and this is one reason why the *Tantras* are so difficult to translate; another rea-son is that they often deal with yogic experiences or intricate ritual practices unfamiliar to the uninitiated translator.

No systematic study of the incredibly vast and rich symbolism found in the scriptures of India has yet been undertaken, though it would be a most worthwhile—if challenging— task. Students, especially those dealing with Tantra, must sensitize themselves to the symbolic dimension so as not to fall prey to false literalism, which can lead to dogmatism and misapplication of the teachings.

PART TWO

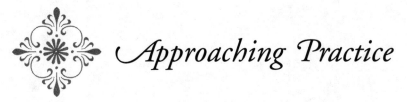 *Approaching Practice*

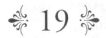

Approaching Spiritual Practice

WHEN PEOPLE DISCOVER that there is such a thing as spirituality, they understandably feel as excited as did Columbus upon setting eyes on the shores of America. Spirituality affords them a broader vista than they ever considered possible. They suddenly realize that conventional society is designed—partly consciously but for the most part quite unconsciously—to prevent us from seeing our full potential as human beings. Conventional life primarily revolves around the pursuit of rather limited goals: physical comfort, material possessions, sex, emotional gratification, mental stimulation, and power.

According to Hinduism, there are four legitimate pursuits to which we can dedicate our time and energy: (1) *artha*—material welfare, (2) *kāma*—physical, emotional, and intellectual satisfaction, (3) *dharma*—morality (notably, justice), and (4) *moksha*—spiritual fulfillment.

Much, if not most, of conventional life falls into the categories of *artha* and *kāma*. Our civilization has invented countless ways to keep our attention focused on comfort and pleasure. Every year billions of dollars are spent in advertising to make sure that we keep up our consumption of material goods, whether we need them or not, and that we strive for a "comfortable" life.

Dharma is pursued in a much more limited way. Our moral standards appear to be at an all-time low, which is in keeping with the Indic notion of the *kali-yuga* or dark age, which is expected to prevail upon Earth for many millennia more. By comparison, the contemporary New Age belief in the imminent upliftment of humankind, by magical *fiat* and without any effort at all, appears like a mere whimsical hope. We must acknowledge that American society in particular suffers from widespread injustice in the legal system and that litigation has become a way of life.

If moral integrity is not high on our list of priorities, spiritual aspiration is almost entirely absent from our lives. Few people really understand what spirituality is, and fewer still actively pursue a spiritual path. The situation is somewhat different in India. With the exception of the Western-educated élite, the traditional value of liberation (*moksha*) is still allowed a certain space in people's belief system. They are at least aware of this great ideal in India's past and among today's renouncers of worldly life, even though they themselves may not feel ready to pursue it. There is a sense of awe about yogis and wandering *sadhus*, who are still a visible element of Hindu society. Admittedly, however, even the native population of India—with the exception of spiritual practitioners of one type or another—has only an inadequate understanding of the yogic lifestyle and often fails to distinguish genuine adepts from impostors. It is also true that in view of the increasing modernization, the traditional reverence for the sacred is gradually being eroded to the detriment of Indic society.

When a Western seeker encounters spirituality, he or she must come to terms with the four core pursuits of material welfare, physical-emotional-intellectual satisfaction, and moral integrity. Central to spiritual practice are self-inspection and self-understanding. We must be willing to examine our habit patterns: how we act and react in all kinds of situations. Then we must be willing and able to also understand what we see about ourselves. The next step is to eliminate those habit patterns that are not conducive to further spiritual growth and replace them with positive habit patterns.

Newcomers to spiritual life often do not realize that spiritual practice requires consistent self-application, that is, a measure of effort. They tend to assume that their peep beyond the walls of conventional life is sufficient in itself. But to see a boat is not the same as rowing it to the other shore. Intellectualizing spiritual life is less than helpful.

But even when neophytes actually take up a course of spiritual practices (*sādhana*), they still sooner or later encounter the fire test of an ordinary daily routine. Then the challenge is to renew one's spiritual practice every day. Otherwise boredom sets in, which undermines the will to transform oneself.

Neophytes feed on their own initial zest, always looking for the next "spiritual" hit—a nice meditation, a spectacular vision, a sign from God, or a compliment from the teacher or fellow student. Little do they suspect that this "honeymoon period" is about to be tested. Typically, the teacher ignores them or instead of sweet compliments utters sharp criticisms. Their fellow students or relatives tell them that they are fully deluded, while others might disparage them for their new way of life. Few pass beyond this stage to go on to regular (unspectacular) daily practice. Many get quickly discouraged when the emotional highs become scarce and they are beginning to confront the stark reality of their own confusion, negativity, or presently limited capacity for spiritual life.

The next hurdle is the recognition that we have many deeply ingrained habit patterns that take time—a lot of time—to change. At first the typical neophyte is sure that he or she has a tremendous capacity and will grow more quickly than others. Then the sobering realization dawns that the degree of self-transformation is equal to the effort made.

If neophytes have persisted thus far, they will almost inevitably encounter doubt (*samshaya*)—doubt about their own capacity; doubt about their teacher; doubt about the efficacy of the teaching. It is not far from the truth to say that practitioners who do not befriend doubt are bound to become self-deluded. If there really is no doubt or self-delusion, then they are quite simply enlightened.

Another obstacle, not often identified, is the fact that practitioners' karmic tendencies (read unconscious or semiconscious habit patterns) are magnified because awareness is enhanced through regular practice. This can be likened to a bright searchlight shining deep into the well of the mind. In the depth of the unconscious reside all kinds of unpleasant realities that get flushed out by steady application to self-inspection and self-understanding. At times, the unconscious materials that drift into the conscious mind seem overwhelming, and then it becomes clear that spiritual life is a form of brinkmanship. The Indic tradition speaks of the razor-edged path.

Gradually spiritual practitioners learn to overcome their intrinsic materialism (i.e., constantly thinking in terms of the visible reality only). There is a progressive loosening of the ego knot or "self-contraction" (*ātma-samkoca*) by which the ordinary individual anxiously seeks to hold everything together. Spiritual practitioners learn to be humorous about everything, including themselves. Life is seen from a new perspective: as a strange play in which we are willy-nilly involved and which we can either misunderstand and suffer or understand and transcend even while being fully engaged in its drama.

Practitioners must prevail over spiritual materialism—the false sense of accumulating "higher" experiences. They can realize inner freedom only to the extent that even the goal of liberation is renounced. Liberation, or enlightenment, is not a thing to be attained or acquired. It is living in the moment from the most profound understanding and without egoic attachment to anything.

Those who parade their extraordinary spiritual accomplishments in front of others are possibly the least illumined of all. They merely substitute material commodities for "spiritual" merchandise. The Indic heritage knows of many adepts who after years of intense practice achieved a high state of consciousness or astounding paranormal ability only to promptly plunge from grace. The higher the adept's elevation, the steeper the drop into oblivion and misery. Therefore the authorities of Yoga ever admonish practitioners to be circumspect, to keep their attainments to themselves, to focus on the cultivation of moral integrity, understanding, self-transcendence, and not least service to others.

It was a great Western adept—Omraam Mikhaël Aïvanhov (1900–1986) —who periodically reminded his disciples that all beginnings are charged with particular potency and that therefore we must enter new beginnings with the utmost care and best understanding we can muster. This is especially true of the beginning of spiritual life.

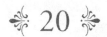

The Twelve Steps of Spiritual Recovery

In RECENT YEARS, much has been said and written about addiction to alcohol, tobacco, drugs, food, sex, and relationships. We can now appreciate how widespread a phenomenon addiction really is. In my book *Sacred Sexuality*,[1] I made the point that ordinary life itself can be considered a form of addiction, because we are habituated to its dominant state of consciousness.

That state of consciousness revolves around the dichotomy between ego and world. We naturally and habitually experience ourselves as separate from everything and everyone else. This split between subject and object is the basis of perception. However, this dichotomy is particularly marked in what the Swiss cultural philosopher Jean Gebser called the "rational consciousness," which is the ruling structure of consciousness in our Western civilization. As he explained in *The Ever-Present Origin*,[2] the rational consciousness is divisive, atomizing, and ultimately destructive. It is the deficient form of the mental structure of consciousness, which emerged around 500 B.C.E., during what Karl Jaspers named the "axial age."[3]

The rational consciousness has perverted the natural perceptual dynamics between the experiencing subject and the experienced object into a sweeping ideology, which is now overshadowing not only science and technology but all branches of our culture and all aspects of our personal lives. This, in turn, has sharpened the opposition between ego and world to the point where we experience ourselves as estranged from the world we live in.

Because of this alienation we are sick at heart, and our world is in pieces. We can usefully compare this state of affairs to the problematic and troubled life of addicts. By calling the strongly ingrained habit of dualistic perception of ego and world an addiction, we admit to ourselves that this state, though common and widely reinforced in our Western culture, is by no means natural.

First of all, when we deny that there is anything wrong with our "ordinary" state, we engage in collective self-denial. Addicts always tend to live in a state of denial. They refuse to admit that they have a serious drinking problem or a problem with drugs. They do everything to maintain the illusion that all is well with them. By labeling our ordinary state, the consensus consciousness, as "normal" we dismiss and disempower all other states of consciousness. This is clearly shown in the fact that we call them "altered" states, meaning that they are "merely" modifications of the ordinary waking state to which we ascribe "normalcy." Sometimes they are collectively and pejoratively referred to as "irrational" states of consciousness, which suggests of course that the rational consciousness is the supreme standard of judgment.

Second, our insistence on seeing ego and world in stark opposition engenders isolation and fear. Addicts chronically suffer from both these negative experiences. In order to maintain their state of illusion about themselves, they have to cut themselves off from others, and this inevitably creates fear. Similarly, our own alienation is attendant with fear—both the fear of interference from the outside world, of unwanted feedback from others, and the realistic fear that one's life has gone out of control.

Third, in our addiction to the rational consciousness and its countless props we believe the myth that we are really powerless to do anything about it. Addicts typically feel disempowered. The object to which they are addicted seems to them bigger and more powerful than their will. Similarly, stuck as we are in the lopsided worldview spawned by the rational consciousness, which tends to discredit other forms and states of consciousness, we do not believe that there is anything we can do about our situation. As addicts of the rational consciousness we do not believe in a universe that is inherently benign. We refuse to consider that the world we live in is actually comprised of the kinds of dimensions of reality that religions and spiritual traditions talk about. We disallow ourselves the possibility of inner or spiritual growth, because our view of human potential is limited to the capacities of the rational mind, which is viewed as the finest product of evolution.

Fourth, like the typical addict, we tend to weave all kinds of explanatory tales to justify our present condition to ourselves and to each other. In this category belongs the "everybody thinks so" attitude, which is modeled not on the few exceptional men and women who can see farther than the rest, but on the lowest common denominator of understanding and living: a flagrant perversion of the democratic ideal. In other words, through word magic we engage in an act of massive repression by which we deny ourselves the opportunity to grow; we deny ourselves access to those forms and states of consciousness that our rational consciousness forces us to deny and belittle. Thus our experiential repertoire remains limited, even truncated.

Fifth, addicts tend to be inflexible, dogmatic, and arrogant about defending their position, and we addicts of the rational consciousness are subject to the same mood. Because we have entrenched ourselves in an untenable position, in which the rational ego rules supreme, we meet any challenge to our unviable approach to life with haughty intransigence. We need to be right, because our entire worldview and life-style are at stake.

And yet, sixth, like true addicts, those of us who are transfixed in the rational consciousness are deeply suffering our mood of separation, self-centeredness, and self-fragmentation. All life, observed Gautama the Buddha, is suffering. But there is suffering and then there is suffering. It appears that whenever we take the presumed independence of the human personality too seriously, cutting ourselves off from other beings and regarding the world as an enemy to be conquered, we become our own source of suffering. This suffering is superimposed on any adversity and pain we may experience as part of our human adventure on this planet. It is a psychological malaise from which we can recover only when we stop pinching ourselves.

Our addiction to the "normal" rational consciousness is so potent that we cannot easily shake this habit even when we have realized that our habit of egoic self-encapsulation is artificial and self-inflicted and resting on a denial of the essential interconnectedness and interdependence of everything. This universal interlinking, or what the Czech indologist Adolf Jánaček called the "panplectal principle,"[4] has been unceasingly proclaimed by generations of mystics and spiritual visionaries who have experienced the unbroken unity and wholeness of the cosmos.

From this much broader, multidimensional perspective of the world, ordinary life is based on an impoverished and even distorted view of reality. When Freud spoke of the psychopathology of everyday life, he caught a glimpse of this fact.[5] Only he did not look deeply enough, or he would have seen that the dichotomic rational consciousness itself is the root of our malaise. For it is the rational consciousness that creates the unhealthy split of the ego from the id, or consciousness from the unconscious. Freud's work was a first effort within modern rationalistic psychology to reintegrate the unconscious with the conscious part of the human psyche and culture. However, it was still largely subject to the constraints and prejudices of the rational consciousness itself. Thus, most significantly, Freud was unable to move beyond his concept of the unconscious as a dumping ground and so could never appreciate the rich texturing of other forms and states of consciousness and philosophies based on experiences of "nonordinary" reality.

When Gebser stated in *The Ever-Present Origin* that the present-day crisis is a crisis of consciousness, he meant that it is a crisis of the rational consciousness. Freud was as yet unable to see this, but some of his students, notably C. G. Jung,[6] took the next step. In doing so, they created a first tentative bridge between psychology and spirituality.

Spiritual life can be regarded as a course of gradual recovery from the addiction to the peculiar type of awareness that splits everything into subject and object. This primary addiction is the seedbed from which arise all secondary addictions. These latter are possible only because the ego is confronted by objects, which it tries to control or by which it is, or feels, controlled.

To be more specific, the secondary addictions are all substitutes for the bliss that is the essence of the experience of transparency, which is at the heart of the integral consciousness, as defined by Gebser. This experience of transparency reveals the archaic interconnectedness and simultaneity of all beings and things without disowning, displacing, or distorting the cognitive realizations characteristic of the magical, mythical, and mental structures of consciousness.

The secondary addictions are desperate, if mistaken, attempts to remove the primary addiction, which is our addiction to self-conscious experience, revolving around the division between subject (mind) and object (world). They are mistaken because instead of removing the primary addiction, they fortify it and thus also aggravate the sense of isolation and powerlessness experienced by the faltering rational personality. The British novelist Aldous Huxley saw this very clearly. He said:

> The urge to transcend self-conscious selfhood is, as I have said, a principal appetite of the soul. When, for whatever reason, men and women fail to transcend themselves by means of worship, good works, and spiritual exercises, they are apt to resort to religion's chemical surrogates alcohol and "goof-pills" in the modern West, alcohol and opium in the East, hashish in the Mohammedan world, alcohol and marijuana in Central America, alcohol and coca in the Andes, alcohol and the barbiturates in the more up-to-date regions of South America.[7]

Huxley did not even mention workaholism and sex as two widely used substitutes for the realization of originary bliss. He spoke, however, of some people's fascination with, and fatal attraction to, precious stones. This passion for gems, Huxley observed, is anchored in the fact that they "bear a faint resemblance to the glowing marvels seen with the inner eye of the visionary."[8] But deeper still than such splendid visions is, to use Gebser's terms, the transcendental "light" of the undivided Origin itself.[9]

Realizing that "light" through voluntary self-transcendence is the ultimate form of healing both the person and the planet. That is the purpose of authentic spirituality. Spiritual life can usefully be pictured as a progressive recovery from the addiction of ordinary life, which is inherently schizoid and hence lacking in fullness and bliss. The well-known twelve-step program of recovery used in the literature on addiction also can serve as a convenient model for the spiritual process. Spiritual recovery is an uncovering of the spiritual dimension, whether we call it transcendental Self, God, Goddess, or the Ultimate—the dimension that is ordinarily covered up by the self-divided ego-personality, especially when it comes under the influence of the rational consciousness.

Here are the twelve steps of spiritual recovery:

1. We admit the fact that our ordinary human condition, based on the dualistic perception of life, is a stubborn habit that we normally conceal from ourselves through denial.

2. We begin to look and ask for guidance in our effort to cultivate a new outlook that embraces the spiritual vision of the interconnectedness of all existence. The means of doing so are varied from supportive spiritual environments to uplifting books.

3. We initiate positive changes in our behavior, which affirm that new outlook. It is not enough to read and talk about spiritual principles. Spirituality is intrinsically a practical affair.

4. We practice self-understanding; that is, we accept conscious responsibility for noticing our automatic programs and where they fall short of our new understanding of life.

5. We make a commitment to undergoing the catharsis, or purification, necessary to change our old cognitive and emotional patterns and stabilize the new outlook and disposition, replacing the egoic habit of splitting everything into irreconcilable opposites with an integrative attitude.

6. We learn to be flexible and open to life so that we can continue to learn and grow on the basis of our new outlook.

7. We practice humility in the midst of our endeavors to mature spiritually. In this way we avoid the danger of psychic inflation.

8. We assume responsibility for what we have understood about life and the principles of spiritual recovery, applying our understanding to all our relationships so that we can be a benign influence in the world.

9. Guided by our new outlook, we work on the integration of our multiply divided psyche.

10. We cultivate real self-discipline in all matters, great and small.

11. We increasingly practice spiritual communion, which opens us to that dimension of existence where we are all connected. Through such communion and through continued growth in self-understanding, we become transparent to ourselves.

12. We open ourselves to the possibility of bliss, the breakthrough of the transcendental reality into our consciousness, whereby the ego principle is unhinged and we fully recover our spiritual identity. Through this awakening the world becomes transparent to us and we are made whole.

❧ 21 ❧
Happiness, Well-Being, and Reality

IN SEARCH OF WHOLENESS, HEALTH, AND HAPPINESS

No one likes to suffer.[1] Everyone is seeking to maximize happiness and minimize unhappiness. Therefore, the pursuit of happiness was written into the American Constitution as a basic human right. However, the Constitution does not offer a clear explanation of what happiness is. Nor does it tell us how to realize happiness.

What, then, is happiness? First of all, we must note that happiness is often confused with pleasure. From the fountains of pleasure, noted the Roman poet and philosopher Lucretius in *De Rerum Natura* (On the Nature of Things), there arises something of bitterness that torments us amid the flowers themselves. Or, as another poet put it, even the sweetest rose has its thorns. The particular sting of pleasure is that it is short-lived. Hence we often hunt after a pleasurable repetition, and in the process run the risk of becoming addicted. Pleasure is inherently addictive, precisely because it is not completely fulfilling. However much the pleasure, we always hunger for more. This can lead to extreme situations, such as in the case of a drug addict who forgoes everything—including propriety and sanity—in order to acquire the substance that gives him pleasure.

Happiness, on the other hand, is deep, full, and enduring. It is satisfying in itself. Therefore it gives us peace and tranquillity. Whereas suffering follows in the wake of pleasure, either because the pleasure has ended or because its pursuit has led to painful imbalances, happiness has no untoward repercussions. It gives rise to harmony. The American philosopher George Santayana wrote in *Little Essays,* "Happiness is the only sanction of life; where happiness fails, existence remains a mad and lamentable experiment."[2]

Happiness ends all sorrow; it concludes our frantic search for the next injection of pleasure. The person who is happy does not look for greater

95

happiness. But pleasure always spurs us on to experience greater pleasure. It drives us, and in driving us it enslaves us. Happiness, however, sets us free. It is freedom.

When we are happy we are whole. The pleasure-seeker is feeling incomplete and therefore is looking for completion, except his or her search is focused on external means that can never bring true happiness. If pleasure were the same as happiness, our Western consumer society, which provides unparalleled access to pleasures of all kinds, would produce the happiest human beings on earth. Instead, our society is filled with desperate and emotionally disturbed and spiritually unfulfilled individuals. In fact, many mental health authorities think it is the sickest society ever to exist on this planet. According to a recent poll, more than one-third of the American population is thought to suffer from one or the other mental illness—from chronic depression to schizophrenia. This is a scary figure, but not surprising when we look at our contemporary lifestyle of work, pressure, haste, drivenness, and consumerism.

As long as we are spiritually fragmented, we must expect to also be physically, emotionally, and mentally unfit. Spiritual wholeness and psychosomatic well-being go hand in hand. Millions suffer from chronic diseases that are the result of emotional disturbance and wrong attitudes to life, expressed in unwholesome habits.

TRUE PHILOSOPHY AS THE PATH TO HAPPINESS

Clearly, when we speak of wholeness, well-being, and happiness we inevitably touch on issues that exceed psychology, medicine, or morality and that reach into the realm of philosophy. Let us define philosophy—the "love of wisdom"—as the systematic concern with the Big Questions: those questions that demand answers of *why* rather than *how* something is the way it is. In particular, philosophy is the study of the meaning of human existence.

The kind of philosophy that we have in mind is not of the academic variety, which exercises the logical mind without necessarily aiming at providing practical guidance in life. We understand philosophy as a practical activity in which both the intellect and the heart (intuition) are employed in order to generate living wisdom that can fruitfully be applied in daily life. The purpose of such philosophy is to show us the path to wholeness, well-being, and happiness.

This type of philosophy is at the heart of the spiritual traditions of the world. It is therefore also an important aspect of Buddhism, which is a tradition that is making inroads in the West. Buddhism can be understood as a pathway to ultimate wholeness, well-being, and happiness. But what do we mean by "ultimate"? To answer this question, we must first consider the nature of reality, because our understanding of happiness depends on our understanding of reality. From the Buddhist perspective, happiness is not merely momentary pleasure but abiding joy. Similarly, wholeness is not merely psychological integration but a comprehensive state of spiritual freedom. And well-being is not merely physical health or even psychological health but the irrevocable realization of a dimension of existence, or reality, that transcends all suffering. We call it the dimension of the spirit, or our intrinsic Buddha nature.

REALITY IS REALLY IMPORTANT

That we are alive is an undeniable fact. Beyond this, we can say few things that one or the other person might not wish to contest. But in order to communicate with one another, we must resort to language, however limited and limiting it may be.

One of the long-standing arguments has been over the nature of reality. What is real and what is unreal or illusory? The answer is by no means clear to everyone. But it is important how we respond to this question, because it determines how we relate to ourselves and to other people and situations. Reality, or our understanding of it, matters. It "really" is important for us all.

Ask yourself: How real am I as a human being? This question is worthy of our most careful consideration. How real are your perceptions? One moment you seem to recognize a person a long distance away, the next you realize it is merely a tree trunk.

Or, more significantly, for years you perceived someone as your greatest adversary only to discover that he or she has been quietly supportive of you, without the slightest trace of enmity. Or you perceived a situation as a golden opportunity only to be profoundly disappointed by it.

How real are your feelings? At first you felt deeply in love with someone; then, before you knew it, you felt out of love. Or at one point you considered yourself really badly off, but then you heard someone else's story and you realized that you were much better off. Or you had a terrible hangover and thought you were really sick, but then you went on a boat and learned that there are degrees of sickness and that one can get a whole lot sicker.

How real is the world around you? Is it really around you? Or do you really only know it indirectly through nerve impulses traveling from your skin to your brain where they get translated into feelings and thoughts? Or is there something altogether different happening?

What is reality anyway? How real is real? Now, you don't have to become a professional philosopher to answer these questions. In fact, professional philosophers often do not offer satisfying answers that can be used in daily life. For meaningful answers we can more profitably look to the spiritual geniuses who have explored both inner and outer reality.

One such spiritual genius was Gautama the Buddha, whose enlightenment under the *bodhi* tree 2,500 years ago planted the seed for the world religion of Buddhism. But "religion" is the wrong word to describe Buddhism. Buddhism is essentially a spiritual path containing within itself a whole range of approaches. They are all founded in a practical understanding of what reality is, and how we may relate to it appropriately and fruitfully.

The Buddha (Awakened one) has not supplied us with a ready-made definition of reality, as this would merely captivate our intellect and leave our emotional being untouched. Instead he gave us a comprehensive understanding of reality, which, when we have assimilated it, is convincing to the mind and satisfying to the heart, thus stimulating us to appropriate action. For the purposes of the present discussion, however, I would like to offer the following working definition of reality: Reality is that which is when the mind does not introduce any distortions.

REALITY IS REALITY IS REALITY

The American writer Gertrude Stein wrote, "A rose is a rose is a rose." This was not meant to be a definition, of course. But it is a very powerful statement nonetheless. Above all, it is a pronouncement that stops us in our tracks, rather like a Zen *koan*. When we ponder reality, we make the same experience. Reality is reality is reality. We cannot say more about it. Whatever we could say about it would be mind-made, and we have already said that it is the mind that is responsible for distorting reality. Even saying that is almost already too much.

But when we know the mind's tricky nature, we can perhaps get away with making some statements about reality that will not be misleading. At least some of the great realizers chose not to be silent. In opting to communicate, however, they necessarily had to resort to language: to express the seemingly inexpressible in words. Thus, according to the Mahāyāna *Sūtras*, the Buddha himself spoke of Reality as Suchness (*tathatā*), Thusness (*tathātva*), Emptiness (*shūnyatā*), All-Knowledge (*sarva-jnāta*), Limit of Existence (*bhūta-koti*), Transcendence (*para*), Body of Reality (*dharma-kāya*), Root of Reality (*dharma-dhātu*), Realness (*dharmatā*), Thus-Gone (*tathā-gata*), Mind Only (*citta-mātra*), Enlightenment (*bodhi*), and Extinction (*nirvāna*).

REALITY AND WELL-BEING

Why is it so important that we apprehend Reality? To put it in a nutshell: As long as we are attuned to Reality, we are well and whole. The moment we are out of sync with Reality, we suffer. No one wants to suffer—even masochists seek pleasure in pain—but suffering is very much a part of human experience. Why? Because, with few exceptions, people are confused about reality and are largely out of sync with it—so much so that many are not even aware of it. Unless they are struck by disaster or are suffering from an illness, they might not even be aware that they are suffering in a more fundamental sense. When asked, they will tell you that they are as happy "as can be expected" and "grateful to be alive." They don't seem to be in touch with the black hole in their hearts, which does not allow them to really trust or love anyone. Nor are they aware of their low-energy relationship to life, which makes them passive and merely reactive. Or else they are so frenetic that they cannot ever sit still and ask themselves why they are rushing through life; what it is they are trying to escape.

MIND: A HALL OF MIRRORS

Why is it so difficult to be attuned to reality? Because of the distorting mirror of the finite human mind, or consciousness, depending on the filters of our brain. We are unable to perceive Reality as it truly is. Therefore we are also unable to live in accordance with Reality. Our view of things determines our action. If our view is mistaken, our actions are inappropriate. From a spiritual perspective, wrong view leads to actions that are conducive to more wrong view and unhappiness, keeping us trapped in this vicious circle. This is what is known as *karma*. *Karma* is the concatenation of action and reaction, or cause and effect, rooted in wrong view or ignorance.

Ignorance is the condition of the unenlightened mind, the mind that perceives Reality as other than what it is in itself. Upon enlightenment, ignorance is lifted and the distorting quality of the mental mirror is also removed. The enlightened being realizes Reality as it is (*yathā bhūta*). Enlightenment and Reality are of the same essential quality. No experience is involved, for experience depends on an object that is outside of oneself. The realization called enlightenment is unmediated. It does not depend on the intervention of the finite mind. The enlightened being *is* Reality. Therefore the enlightened being is as indescribable as Reality itself.

The enlightened being is essentially happy because the whole karmic cycle has been transcended. For actions based in true knowledge, or enlightenment, are nonbinding and conducive to happiness. *Nirvāna* is not a dull state of unconsciousness. But neither is it consciousness in the conventional sense. The Buddha himself avoided as much as possible to squeeze it into limited linguistic categories, and he refused to speculate about metaphysics. Out of compassion for those still lacking his supreme realization, however, he did occasionally make statements about *nirvāna* that help us understand that it is highly desirable. Over the centuries, teachers following the Buddha's footsteps have likewise—and more frequently—allowed themselves to speak of the ultimate realization in more concrete terms for the benefit of their disciples. Their words are of course only signposts. When we forget that, we slip into making an ideology out of the spiritual path, and ideologies by definition do not bring us closer to Reality. As the Zen masters made it clear in dramatic language: When we see the Buddha on the road, we must kill him. Even the desire for enlightenment must ultimately be jettisoned along with all our preconceptions of it. Only Reality itself is liberating.

❧ 22 ❧
The Quest for Happiness

IT IS A SIGN OF HEALTH and sanity to seek happiness. The founding fathers of the United States acknowledged this indirectly when, on July 4, 1776, they declared the "Pursuit of Happiness" one of the "inalienable rights." Happiness has been called the American dream. But it is the dream of all peoples and races, so long as their vital powers are unsapped. Only an enervated individual or group will choose unhappiness, pain, or suffering over joy and delight.

I am not merely talking about pleasure or amusement when I mention happiness or joy. I do mean bliss, ecstasy, rapture, felicity—what the sages of India call *ānanda*. Could it be a sign of our times that so much attention, energy, time, and money are invested in the contemplation of disaster, misfortune, crime, war, conflict, trouble, and violence of one kind or another? We read about all kinds of adversities in the papers, see them on TV, hear about them on the radio, and gossip about them with our friends and coworkers. It seems we are intent on bombarding each other with bad news. Somehow it keeps the adrenaline going, and we do tend to confuse stress with aliveness.

Then, suddenly, for one reason or another, we come to a halt and ask ourselves: Am I happy? Am I happy living like this, doing what I am doing? The fact is, we would not be asking ourselves these questions if we were not experiencing unhappiness. We may be blessed (or cursed, as the case may be) with material plenty, and yet we may be deeply disturbed. Why? Most of the time, we do not have an answer for our distress. Sometimes we imagine that if the right job turned up or the right man or woman came along, all would be well with us. Or we feel that a glass of bourbon or a nice long holiday might fix it all. But we are only fooling ourselves. The glass will be empty, and our vacation will come to an end, as indeed will everything else. Sooner or later, the same feeling of unfulfillment or unhappiness will undoubtedly surface again.

There are many people who would claim that they are generally happy.

But are they really happy? Blissfully happy? Ecstatically happy? Happy even when things around them seem to come apart at the seams? Or does their happiness depend on external circumstances or internal conditions? Can they remain blissful when their son has just totaled their car? Or when they learn from their accountant that they owe back taxes?

It is natural enough for feelings of anger or frustration to appear under such circumstances. The question is whether we can feel *beyond* these negative emotions and continue to be a loving presence? If we can honestly say Yes, then we are in a state that has traditionally been celebrated as a highly positive spiritual accomplishment; maybe not yet enlightenment or Self-realization but reasonably close to it.

But let us assume we are not so fortunate. What can we do to become happy? The short answer is: nothing! In fact, the more actively we seek out happiness, the less likely we are to find it. The reason for this is that all forms of seeking pertain to the finite, egoic consciousness (our everyday identity), whereas true, permanent happiness is the unconditional Reality itself, which transcends the ego. So—all we can hope to accomplish through our search for happiness is pleasurable experiences, and we already know that they do not last.

When I say we can do nothing to *become* happy, this is only half the truth. It would be unfortunate if happiness were to elude us forever. But, happily, it does not. It is accessible to us: We must simply *be* happy in every moment. I learned this secret from one of my teachers, and I do not think I would ever have discovered it on my own. It sounds so simple and even paradoxical. Yet it is really profound wisdom. We cannot *become* happy; we can always only *be* happy.

Most people have experienced moments of joy or delight at one time or another in their lives. That means we know what happiness feels like . . . what we experience when our whole body radiates with joyous energy and we feel like embracing everyone and everything. In those precious moments, we are in touch with something more real than our ordinary self or the world that our ordinary self experiences. Our ego is temporarily suspended, and our consciousness and energy are stepped up manifold. There is simply an overwhelming feeling of happiness, of blissfulness, which has the quality of love. We can always remember, with our whole body, those occasions of extraordinary joy. Whenever we center ourselves, whenever we are fully present *as* the whole body, we get in touch with the larger Reality in which we are immersed. And that larger Reality is neither depressed nor problematical. Then our energy starts to flow more freely, and we feel a deep sense of security, intuiting that our true identity is untouched by any conflict or pain.

To remember to be present as the body is a skill that can be learned. To *be* presently happy rather than to seek to *become* happy is an open option for all of us—in every single moment. We can either lose ourselves in fear, anger, sorrow, lust, jealousy, pride, self-complacency, and all the other diverse egoic states, or we can feel through to the great pool of bliss that lies beyond them.

Happiness is our birthright. But we must claim it.

❧ 23 ❧
Spiritual Discipline

DISCIPLINE—THAT IS, the disciplining of the mind—is a fundamental prerequisite of spiritual growth. There are those who think that spiritual awakening, or enlightenment, is spontaneous and does not call for any action on our part. Some even regard all effort as an obstacle to enlightenment, but this does not constitute the whole truth. While it is true that the great sages all have testified that enlightenment is our innate condition, they also have always emphasized the need for proper preparation. If some practitioners, such as Ramana Maharshi, have attained enlightenment apparently without effort, we must assume that they prepared for that auspicious moment over many lifetimes. This is the traditional explanation of their instant awakening. Without the notion of rebirth, however, we are left with only one other explanation, namely that their enlightenment was simply a random occurrence; that they "lucked out." If we were to accept this, we would also have to assume that spiritual effort is a waste of time. In that case, we could live as we will and hope for the best. But this is exactly what most people have opted to do, and their individual destiny is no secret to us: Instead of being free, they suffer from much unhappiness.

Irrespective of the metaphysical debate about the nature of enlightenment and how it is realized, it is an undeniable fact that we grow spiritually—in our awareness and capacity for self-transcendence and happiness —by virtue of our application to spiritual values and ideals. Here *application* means translating ideals or values into daily practice. This is what the Sanskrit concept of *sādhana*, or spiritual discipline, is all about. The word is derived from the verbal root *sādh* meaning "to accomplish." The same root also yields the words *siddhi* (accomplishment or perfection) and *siddha* (accomplished one or adept). Accomplishment comes at various levels, and the ultimate accomplishment is understood to be enlightenment. A *siddha* is usually an adept who has attained enlightenment. A person practicing a spiritual discipline is called a *sādhaka* if male or a *sādhikā* if female.

Spiritual practice is first and foremost mind training, that is, the disciplining of those aspects of our inner life that prevent us from realizing our innate enlightenment. What are those aspects?

The most important blockage is our ignorance (*avidyā*) of Reality as it truly is: that is, our basic spiritual blindness, which not only prevents us from seeing Reality but actually distorts it. That distortion is expressed in the illusion that we are separate from everyone and everything else. This is a function of *asmitā* ("I-am-ness") or *ahamkāra* ("I-maker"), the ego-personality, which makes an island of each of us in the midst of a supposedly hostile world in which we have to struggle for survival. All this can also be summed up as "delusion" (*moha*).

Part of *moha* is the notion that *thinking* about enlightenment is sufficient for realizing it. Not a few Western practitioners have fallen prey to this error, because they failed to understand the distinction between intellectual comprehension and true understanding. The former remains on the abstract theoretical level, whereas the latter represents the influx of wisdom into the mind, which brings about genuine inner transformation followed by appropriate practical changes in our behavior. For instance, we might have understood that we are mostly sleepwalking through life; yet, this understanding in itself will not awaken us. We also must practice self-awareness or self-remembering in every moment. Or, to give another example, we might recognize that we are unhappy and tend to mistakenly seek happiness by external means; however, this recognition in itself is not enough to bring us happiness; we also must cease wresting happiness from people and things and take the appropriate steps to uncover our inner happiness.

Ignorance of our true nature (which is eternally free, blissful, and luminous) and the false sense of self arising from it also create in us a basic mood of fear (*bhaya*). This fear can be articulated in the form of fear of another, fear of change, fear of the unknown, fear of death, and so on. Fear undermines our innate happiness and freedom. It can also prevent us from taking the leap into spiritual practice.

Another result of our fundamental ignorance and self-centeredness is a grasping attitude toward life: greed (*lobha*). We pile up things around us to conceal our sense of inadequacy and our fear and to bolster up our false sense of being an independent self or ego-personality. Like fear, greed comes in many forms, including what could be called "spiritual consumerism" —the widespread attitude of accumulating teachers and teachings as if they were valuable collectibles. Since spiritual life is based on genuine self-transcendence and consistent self-discipline, it cannot be "bought."

Spiritual consumerism equips us to come into possession of counterfeit spirituality only, which is never conducive to true happiness and freedom.

Spiritual ignorance and self-centeredness also manifest in anger (*krodha*), a particularly negative emotion that is destructive of oneself and others. In a spiritual context, anger shows its face in the choleric rejection of actual self-discipline as well as the teachers and teachings standing for such a discipline. The ego-personality by tendency does not want to change or be interfered with. But all of spiritual practice is designed to break down the walls of the ego, so that the light of the Self (*ātman*) may enter and reintegrate the human being with the rest of the universe.

Over the millennia, the great masters of Yoga have developed numerous systems of mind training that serve the purpose of illumination, or enlightenment (*bodha*). All are meant to remove ignorance, self-centeredness, self-delusion, greed, anger, and other similar obstacles to enlightenment. Whatever the system, each calls for two things: steady practice (*abhyāsa*) on the one side and dispassion (*vairāgya*) on the other. Practice, or consistent discipline, has the purpose of penetrating the ego-illusion and thus revealing Reality, while dispassion is the means whereby we can rid ourselves of undesirable ballast that stands in the way of realizing true freedom and happiness. Together practice and dispassion propel us onward to enlightenment. Step by step we realize our true nature by shedding everything that cloaks Reality. But we must actually take those steps. Thinking alone will not get us there. Only the organ of wisdom—*buddhi*—has the power to transform us so that our true nature can shine forth. As the masters of Yoga assure us, we are always already enlightened, but this must become our immediate and continuous apperception. And that realization flowers through spiritual discipline.

❧ 24 ❧
Life Is an Earthquake

THE DEVASTATING EARTHQUAKE in Turkey in 1999, with its numerous af-
tershocks, was a vivid reminder that there can be no perfect security and
safety in life. However, one suspects that many, if not most, people do not
consider this important lesson in its full depth but simply get on with their
lives as soon as the immediate danger is over. They dress their wounds, clear
the debris, lend their neighbors a helping hand, and then return to their
jobs and routines — back to business as usual. Perhaps only those who are hit
the hardest by a calamity begin to question life more seriously.

"Why me?" they might ask. "Why is life filled with hardship and pain?
Why doesn't there seem to be any divine justice?" Such questions have been
asked since time immemorial whenever people have had to face serious
difficulties, injury, loss, and especially death. It seems that suffering stimu-
lates metaphysical inquiry.

If such questioning does not happen more seriously in our own time, it
is because our civilization is highly secularized. We tend to feel ill at ease
with metaphysics and look down on traditional wisdom, which could provide meaningful answers to our existential questions. Under the pressure of
the dominant secular mindset, people are apt to suppress the questions that
arise naturally within them in the course of life's vicissitudes. All too often
we allow ourselves to be distracted by the countless forms of entertainment
offered by TV and the other media. Even reading about the suffering of
earthquake victims can become a morbid entertainment that merely buries
one's own suffering and questioning.

Yet, it is important that we question life. For without profound questioning, we will find no deep answers and solutions to our problems. This is
best illustrated in the early life of Gautama the Buddha. He was born hand-
some and wealthy, heir to a small kingdom in northern India. Legend has it
that he lived a completely sheltered life, dedicated to the pursuit of pleasure. Then, one day, the reality of life caught up with the delicate prince.
While on an outing, as scriptural tradition tells us, Gautama encountered a

man bent over by age, a sick person, and a corpse. These encounters shook him so deeply that, at the age of twenty-nine, Gautama renounced his inheritance and adopted the life of a wandering ascetic in search of peace and tranquillity. After six years of struggle, punctuated by fierce asceticism, he discovered the "middle way" to true wisdom. After his spontaneous enlightenment at the age of thirty-five, Gautama the Buddha expressed his principal insights thus:

> Birth is suffering. Old age is suffering. Illness is suffering. Death is suffering. Grief, lamentation, pain, affliction, and despair are suffering. To be united with what is unloved or to be separated from what is loved is suffering. Not to obtain what is longed for is suffering. In short, the five aggregates [of human existence] are suffering.[1]

This is so because life is impermanent and filled with constant change. Death puts a final limit on everything. This is indeed the stark reality of the human condition. The Bulgarian adept Omraam Mikhaël Aïvanhov put it this way:

> Generally speaking, people cling to life on earth because they do not know that there is another, better life elsewhere; they are ready to commit every kind of crime to ensure their survival in this world. In this way they pile up countless debts, and some day they are going to have to honor those debts. But a disciple sees things quite differently. He says to himself: "Life on earth is a drudgery. We are hemmed in and limited, trodden underfoot, tormented and abused in every way."[2]

If we close our eyes to this truth, we do so to our own detriment. At the same time, however, we must not succumb to gloom, which would be mere self-indulgence. That is why, in Aïvanhov's words, the disciple must accept the conditions into which he or she is born, while striving to transcend them and attain inner freedom. Thus the spiritual traditions seek to foster in us an awareness of life's impermanence while at the same time reminding us of our true nature, the higher Self, which eternally abides beyond the conditional realms. Only when we make that connection to the Self, or the ultimate Reality, can we make sense of the human situation. Otherwise it must seem like a dreadful business, without meaning or mercy.

The great spiritual masters of the world also have taught us that conditional existence is governed by the law of cause and effect, or *karma*. This allows us to get a proper perspective on the occurrence of pain and suffering in our lives. Whatever happens to us is because of our previous intentions, thoughts, and actions, which set in motion unstoppable cosmic ripples. As Aïvanhov expressed it:

> Nature has succeeded in registering everything and this is what moral law is based upon: the memory of nature. Yes, memory, nature has a memory that never forgets, and so much the worse for the person who does not take this memory into consideration! It goes on anyhow, registering his jangling thoughts and inner turmoil until the day when he can stand no more, he is overcome and gives up. No one can avoid this law, no one has ever been powerful enough to succeed in escaping it. . . .[3]

If we want to avoid future suffering, we must change our present motivation, thoughts, and actions, so that we may reap a more benign destiny. If we dedicate ourselves solely to the realization of higher ideals, like compassion, generosity, and patience, we will ultimately reap the fruit of enlightenment, or spiritual liberation.

The spiritual path is a long road. But it is a road all of us must travel sooner or later. As we cultivate those higher ideals, we will find our lives becoming so much simpler, happier, and more meaningful. It is then that we can begin to enjoy life's beauty without romanticizing it. From that higher viewpoint, even earthquakes, terrible as they are, cannot threaten our inner peace and harmony. We simply do what is necessary, all the while remembering that we are one with everything and therefore cannot possibly be subject to any loss. In our true nature we are one, immortal, changeless, free, and blissful.

❧ 25 ❧
Samsāra Means Running Around in Circles

THE SAGES OF INDIA coined an excellent term for the kind of situation that we find ourselves in so long as we are not enlightened, or liberated. They speak of *samsāra*, which literally means "confluence"—the flowing together of the conditions that shape our finite lives. Another, more descriptive translation of this term is "running around in circles." For this is exactly what is occurring at the level of conditional existence, which is our current state. Countless beings endlessly repeat themselves; that is, they duplicate their karmic patterning over and over again.

Samsāra, then, is congealed behavior—habit. More precisely, it is the sum total of the habits of all beings and things. Even a piece of rock can be said to be subject to a habit pattern. Unlike the behavior of a human being, which can be varied and occasionally even surprising, a rock's behavior is largely static and totally predictable. It is behavior nonetheless, unless we insist on restricting the use of this term only to animate or sentient beings.

While we expect the behavior of an inanimate thing like a rock to be completely predictable, we consider stasis—or rigidity—among our fellow humans as neurotic and undesirable. Yet rigidity is a matter of degree, and we can witness a wide range of responsiveness in members of the human species. Some individuals are more rigid and predictable than others. Some behave like clockwork, others are out of control. The people of the Prussian town of Königsberg were able to set their watches after their famous townsman Immanuel Kant, who went for his afternoon constitutional at exactly the same time every day. But even those people who are out of control or "crazy," are in many ways still quite predictable, because their behavior too is merely karmic self-replication.

And this is the crux of the matter: All of us are prone to repeat ourselves endlessly. There is a marked lethargy in the human psyche, and resistance to change is deep seated in us. We all seem to fear change, and with some people this fear is so overwhelming that it paralyzes them. Others conceal their fear by behaving "as if" they were free of it; they challenge themselves, even at the risk of their own life. Yet, they may be daredevils only in certain areas, while in others they are dominated by the kind of arrested development that springs from fear. For instance, a person can be utterly heroic and self-transcending while scaling the most treacherous mountain on earth, but down below in the valley, their fear-bound conservatism is locking them into self-defeating karmic patterns of emotional dependence, sexual obsession, moral rigidity, or neurotic avoidance of anything that challenges their subjective picture of the world. At the peak, way above the timberline, they sense a freedom that escapes them in the valley. But that freedom can only be illusory so long as the mental habit patterns impelling the mountaineer to seek the adventure of the climb are still intact. True freedom dawns when the karmic tendencies that create the ego-personality in the first place are transcended.

Thus *spiritual* self-transcendence is true heroism—hence one of the appellations by which adepts are known in India is *vīra*, or "hero." Self-transcendence alone terminates the self-repeating loop that the Indic sages call *samsāra*. The freedom that the liberated being realizes is the unmappable landscape of the Spirit (*ātman, purusha*) itself. That freedom is *nirvāna*—the wind-still condition, the state of perfect tranquillity that no conditional event of *samsāra* can undermine. Hence the liberated being who is still immersed in the finite realm of existence is not intimidated by *samsāra*. There is no fear of change. Nor is there any fear of death, which, from the ordinary human perspective, represents the ultimate transition. For the liberated being, *samsāra* is a complete non-event. In fact, the liberated awareness does not even operate with the kind of dualism implicit in the conceptual distinction between *nirvāna* and *samsāra*. On the contrary, as the Mahāyāna Buddhist master Nāgārjuna pointed out so vigorously, *nirvāna* is *samsāra* and *samsāra* is *nirvāna*.

This grand spiritual realization entails the recognition that even while we are afraid of change and death and are troubled by the vicissitudes of *samsāra*, we are immersed in the freedom of the Spirit, or transcendental Reality. For the Spirit, which is devoid of any trace of suffering, is our inalienable nature. We are simply ignorant of this deep truth and consequently deem ourselves to be finite beings who are destined to suffer and die. In other words, it is our ignorance (*avidyā*) of our true nature that is responsible for our misidentification with a particular body-mind. In actuality, according to Yoga, our true identity is the Spirit, which is the same super-conscious Reality in every being and thing.

As soon as we take our first breath in a human body, this illusion is created and becomes more overpowering as the brain/mind is educated to function ever more in human ways. In the end, we might even come to the conclusion that there is no reality beyond the body-mind, and that consciousness is a function of the brain. The testimony of all great spiritual masters, however, is otherwise: What we conventionally call consciousness (*citta*) is merely the borrowed light of a sublime radiance that exceeds the physical and mental levels of existence. It is indeed largely dependent on brain functions, which, in turn, are dependent on the body's biochemistry. But Awareness—or Supraconsciousness (*cit*)—requires for its existence no neurons, chemicals, or atomic and subatomic particles. It is, in fact, that in which all matter and thought arises and vanishes in every moment.

That verity is glimpsed in higher states of ecstasy (*samādhi*) and fully realized upon enlightenment (*bodhi*), which is a permanent identity shift: Instead of experiencing ourselves as a specific individuated being, we realize our true nature as the superconscious substratum of all individuated beings and their perceived environments.

Upon enlightenment, we cease to run around in circles. On the contrary, we stand at the still point, the axle hole (*kha*) of the great samsaric wheel, which continues to whirl round and round at dizzying speed for all those who are as yet unenlightened. Our own bodies, which are crystallized karmic residue, continue to live out their destiny (which is inevitable death), but "we"—as Spirit—are completely unaffected by the bodily processes and experiences.

According to some schools of Yoga, the enlightened being's supraconscious radiance gradually transforms and transubstantiates the physical body itself and creates a "body of light" or superconductive body (*ativāhika-deha*). This nonphysical vehicle defies the laws of Nature and is endowed with all kinds of extraordinary capacities. It is really an extension of the enlightened being's unfettered mind, which has pierced the veil of illusion (*māyā*) and is perfectly attuned to the ultimate Reality. This superconductive body allows the liberated one to remain in the conditional realms and serve the awakening of others, without becoming subject to decay and death, which is the inexorable fate of ordinary bodies.

26

Spiritual Friendship

THE SPIRITUAL PATH has often been compared to a razor's edge. One moment of inattention and years of steadfast practice can be undone instantly by a sudden resurgence of old patterns of thought and behavior. Therefore traditional Yoga authorities have long recommended that sincere practitioners should cultivate the friendship of like-minded and like-hearted people, who uphold the highest ideals of the spiritual path.

As social creatures, much of our thinking and doing is influenced by our social environment. The popular saying "Birds of a feather flock together" captures the situation well. Worldly friends produce in us worldly thoughts and intentions, whereas spiritual friends uplift our mind and heart. How can we tell a worldly from a spiritual friend? A worldly friend's mind revolves around money, work, sex, pleasure, success, etc. His or her speech will be coarse, uninspiring, repetitive, divisive, idle, and hurtful. There will be little silence and likely even anxiety about silence. The worldly person replicates the noise of our social environment and thus contributes to it.

> Just as *kusha* grass wrapped around rotting fish
> Will soon begin to smell the same,
> A person who associates with bad friends, in time,
> Will certainly come to resemble them.[1]

The action to be taken is obvious:

> Shun unvirtuous friends who have bad characters,
> cynical outlooks, and prejudice,
> Believe their own view to be the best, are boastful,
> and disparage others.[2]

The *Dhamma-Pāda* (78) declares:

Avoid evil-doers as friends. Do not befriend low people. Take virtuous people for friends and associate with the best.

In the *Khagga-Visāna-Sutta* (24) of the *Sutta-Nipāta*, we read:

One should associate with a friend who is learned, knows the teaching, has acquired and cultivates knowledge, has understood the meaning of things and has removed his doubts.

The *Hiri-Sutta* (3) states:

He who is constantly anxious and conflicted and always looks for flaws is not a friend. He who cannot be alienated from one by others, like a son from his father's heart, is indeed a friend.

Conventional friendship consolidates our conventional view of life, which is a flat perspective by contrast with the deep and unobstructed view inspired by spiritual friendship. Conventional friendship springs from and reinforces *samsāra*. Spiritual friendship is rooted in and promotes *nirvāna*.

Beware also of *dharma* friends who bring worldliness to their spiritual practice. Their talk about spiritual matters is an occasion to brag, belittle others, or gain advantage—in other words, to cherish themselves. Their words are apparently about the path, but their mind is firmly entrenched in worldly matters. They are pretenders. Better to associate with a silent friend who is firmly on the path than a talkative friend who follows the pathways of the ego.

Sat-sanga means "association with the virtuous or real." Usually this refers to keeping the company of an adept, who embodies spiritual values, that is, connects us with that which is true, real, or virtuous (*sat*).

In Buddhism, the word *sangha* or "community" suggests the same: the mutually beneficial association of those who follow the Buddha's teachings (*dharma*). Members of the Sangha are by definition refuge holders, that is, they have sincerely taken refuge in the "three jewels" (*tri-ratna*): the Buddha, the Dharma, and the Sangha. Taking refuge implies that we not merely believe in the "three jewels" but actively endeavor to follow in the footsteps of the Buddha and other great masters who have attained liberation or at least higher realizations by virtue of their own practice of the Buddha's teachings.

The greatest spiritual friend is one's *guru* (Sanskrit) or *lama* (Tibetan). Some Buddhist schools consider him or her the fourth worthy object of refuge. He or she only has one's best interest in mind, namely one's ultimate freedom and happiness. The Buddhists call such a one *kalyana-mitra* or "beautiful friend." He or she is "beautiful" because of his or her capacity and intent to beautify or ennoble others.

Taking refuge in the Buddha, the Dharma, and the Sangha is said to dispel all fear. Taking refuge in anyone or anything else does not have the same effect. It may postpone fear but cannot remove it altogether, because they do not lead us to our true nature, which is the Buddha nature beyond all possible worldly destinies. The *Udāna-Varga* (25.5) declares:

> People degenerate by relying on those inferior to themselves.
> By relying on equals, they stay the same.
> By relying on those superior, they attain excellence.
> Thus rely on those who are superior to yourself.[3]

Instead of "making" friends, practitioners of Yoga would do better to cultivate unlimited friendliness (*maitrī*): They become a friend for all beings, having their highest good at heart. With this outlook, one has the whole universe as one's friend.

❧ 27 ❧
The Guru: Dispeller of Darkness

THERE IS AN ANCIENT Upanishadic prayer that captures the essence of all Yoga practice:

> From the unreal lead us to the Real.
> From darkness lead us to the Light.
> From death lead us to Immortality.

This prayerful request is addressed to the Divine, but it could just as well be addressed to the guru. According to an esoteric explanation, the Sanskrit word guru denotes "dispeller of darkness." If the guru is fully realized, or enlightened, he or she is in fact a bringer of Light. As such the guru is traditionally considered to be an embodiment of the ultimate Reality.

For us Westerners this is very difficult to grasp and even more difficult to accept. When we stand before a guru—a sad-guru or true master—we tend to see only the bodily person in front of us. In other words, we only see with our eyes, and hence we do not see deeply enough. We are spiritually blind. Our physical sight can actually prove an impediment when it comes to divining a true teacher. We can develop a profound (spiritual) relationship to him or her only when we come to fully understand that the realized sage is, in consciousness, always and irrevocably identical with the ultimate Reality.

Understandably, the many would-be masters who nowadays peddle their wares on the open market and compete for disciples do not inspire much faith and confidence in us. I have met a fair number of spiritual teachers in my life, and exceedingly few have struck me as having achieved more than skill in meditation, psychospiritual healing, lecturing, or the "party tricks" of paranormal abilities—all of which can also be acquired by completely unspiritual rogues. Realized beings of the caliber of a Ramana Maharshi (whom I would have dearly loved to meet), the sixteenth Karmapa Rangjung Rigpe Dorje (who died shortly before I was to meet him), or Garchen Rinpoche (from whom I received the mahā-mudrā initiation) are few and far between.

We can say something about the spiritual stature of a person not only from their life but also from the manner they depart our material world. The death of truly great beings is said to be attended by auspicious omens. Thus when Bhagavan Ramana left his body at 8:47 P.M., a meteor trailed across the sky from the north-east heading toward the peak of Arunachala, Ramana's beloved mountain. During the cremation ceremony of the sixteenth Karmapa (1924–1981), a giant rainbow surrounded the Sun on a clear, bright day. In her book *Daughter of Fire*, the Russian-born Sufi master Irina Tweedie describes how when her own guru dropped his mortal coil an unusual rainbow appeared, which had her teacher's specific color missing.

There is a traditional piece of wisdom that states that teachers can take their disciples only as far as they themselves have traveled. To put it differently, some teachers will be able to boost our 20-watt light to perhaps 200 or 2,000 watts or maybe even to twenty kilowatts. This would certainly bring us a little closer to the "luminosity" of enlightenment, but to be close does not mean to be there. Some teachers are inclined to forget this, and many students are anyway not motivated sufficiently to go all the way and to look for a *sad-guru*, a teacher of the True, who can take them safely the whole route.

Not a few students think they can make it on their own. They are merely deceiving themselves. I had a period in my own life when I fostered this mistaken view and as a consequence ran into more cul-de-sacs than I care to remember. The irony is that I cannot even plead ignorance about the traditional function of the *sad-guru*: I had read all the texts and studied many of them in depth. But disappointments with teachers along the path can easily color our perspective. Fortunately, many years ago, I came to believe very firmly that a spiritual teacher is essential. And if we really want to go the whole way, we must prepare ourselves for the eventuality of an encounter with a genuine guru. A well-known traditional saying has it that when the disciple is ready the guru will appear. I feel that this is as true today as it was millennia ago. The *sad-guru* is the gate, and *sat-sanga* or "true relationship" to such a teacher is the key.

✵ 28 ✵
The Guru Function: Broadcasting Reality

PREAMBLE

There are many types of spiritual teachers, all differing in their spiritual maturity, intellectual capacity, learning, personal complexity, and style of teaching. To simplify, most teachers are just one or two steps ahead of the neophyte. Yet, while their spiritual attainments may be quite modest, they can still be helpful to seekers, providing they remain humble, honest, and alert. It is all too easy for up-and-coming teachers to commit the egocentric error of wanting to play master.

Then there are those who have advanced farther on the ladder of self-transcendence and enlightenment. Naturally, they can be of immense help to seekers, who need guidance, confirmation, and occasional encouragement. Because of their inner attainments, such teachers also display the curious psychophysical effect of "spiritual contagion." This effect, which enhances the quality of the disciple's being and consciousness is particularly pronounced in the case of an enlightened master. Hence such teachers have always been highly valued in the esoteric traditions of the world.

Some adepts, like Ramana Maharshi or Faquir Chand, become teachers by default, because people seek out their company and spiritual help, though they themselves would be content to live in solitude. Others choose to have a few disciples whom they can instruct in a more intimate way. Yet others, like Gautama the Buddha, set out to create a whole new path and community.

A few teachers prefer to be informal with their disciples, while most others insist on formality. There are teachers who interfere only minimally in the day-to-day living of their disciples, and then there are teachers who prescribe and enforce a strict lifestyle. Some teachers are quiet and ordinary, while others, like Bhagwan Rajneesh (alias "Osho") or Sathya Sai Baba, prefer a more flamboyant style of self-presentation. Some adepts, like Ramana Maharshi, choose relative silence as a means of communicating with their disciples; others, like Jiddu Krishnamurti, are forever eloquent, believing that knowledge can somehow point the way to enlightenment. Some teachers refuse to call themselves teachers, because they feel they have nothing to teach; their teaching consists in their merely being present. And so on.

Psychologist Guy Claxton, a former disciple of Bhagwan Rajneesh, has found the image of the guru as teacher somewhat misleading. He offers these comments:

> The most helpful metaphor is . . . that of a physician or therapist: enlightened Masters are, we might say, the Ultimate Therapists, for they focus their benign attention not on problems but on the very root from which the problems spring, the problem-sufferer and solver himself. The Master deploys his therapeutic tricks to one end: that of the exposure and dissolution of the fallacious self. His art is a subtle one because the illusions cannot be excised with a scalpel, dispersed with massage, or quelled with drugs. He has to work at one remove by knocking away familiar props and habits, and sustaining the seeker's courage and resolve through the fall. Only thus can the organism cure itself. His techniques resemble those of the demolition expert, setting strategically placed charges to blow up the established super-structure of the ego, so that the ground may be exposed. Yet he has to work on each case individually, dismantling and challenging in the right sequence and at the right speed, using whatever the patient brings as his raw material for the work of the moment.[1]

Claxton mentions other guises, "metaphors," that the guru assumes to deal with the disciple: guide, sergeant-major, cartographer, con man, fisherman, sophist, and magician. The multiple functions and roles of the authentic adept have two primary purposes. The first is to penetrate and eventually dissolve the egoic armor of the disciple, to "kill" the phenomenon that calls itself "disciple."

The second major function of the guru is to act as a transmitter of Reality by magnifying the disciple's intuition of his or her true identity. Both objectives are the intent of all spiritual teachers. However, only fully enlightened adepts combine in themselves what the Mahāyāna Buddhist scriptures call the wisdom (*prajnā*) and the compassion (*karunā*) necessary to rouse others from the slumber of the unenlightened state. In the ancient *Rig-Veda* (10.32.7) of the Hindus, the guru is likened to a person familiar with a particular terrain who undertakes to guide a foreign traveler. Teachers who have yet to realize full enlightenment can guide others only part of the way.

But the accomplished adept, who is known in India as a *siddha*, is able to illumine the entire path for the seeker.

Such fully enlightened adepts are a rarity. Whether or not they feel called to teach others, their mere presence in the world is traditionally held to have an impact on everything. All enlightened masters, or realizers, are thought and felt to radiate the numinous. They are focal points of the sacred. *They broadcast Reality.* Because they are, in consciousness, one with the ultimate Reality, they cannot help but irradiate their environment with the light of that Reality. This spiritual "field effect" apparently extends to all creatures and things, but is particularly felt by those who are in close proximity to the adept or who are sensitive to his spiritual transmission. The natural "aura" of the enlightened being, which has a transformative effect, obliges the world to engage in involuntary spiritual practice *(sādhana).* The contemporary American adept Adi Da (Da Free John) once remarked about this phenomenon that "even the walls" participate in this process. How literally he meant this statement is apparent from the following account by one of his students:

> In the summer of 1982, I found myself unexpectedly in the personal company of my guru. I saw him enter into what everyone believed to be the condition of unqualified *samādhi* or ecstasy. All present were instantly overtaken by a powerful meditative mood. As we later confirmed to each other, everyone had the subjective sensation of the room seemingly flying apart with everything and everybody in it. *Everyone reported distinctly hearing the wooden walls and ceiling beams crackle.* There was also the sensation of a strange but distinct pressure upon the whole body, notably the front. This incident left me puzzled and excited for a long time. For me, it was a demonstration of the subtle forces that are in operation around the adept.[2]

The same student also had this to report:

> Whenever I would sit in meditation or *darshana*[3] with my guru, my body felt as if it had been exposed to a high dose of radiation. For days and weeks afterwards, my entire chest would burn or radiate. The focus of this sensation was toward the right side of my heart. This feeling intensified whenever I would meditate on my own. Associated with this physical symptom was an unusual emotional rawness. I felt ripped open, utterly vulnerable in my emotions. It seemed to me that my teacher had "relo-

cated" the center of my attention from the brain to the heart, where it belongs. Through my guru's grace, my heart has been awakened.[4]

Guy Claxton comments:

> By sitting in the Master's presence, aware of him without thought or judgment, the seeker begins to imbibe and manifest the same quality of clarity and stillness. There is, as Zen says, a direct transmission outside the scriptures, heart to heart. The Master is a queen bee around which the community of seekers—in Buddhism the sangha—gathers to drink his essence.[5]

The spiritual "presence" of the teacher is felt as a force impinging on the body. Both Bhagwan Rajneesh and Swami Muktananda, who achieved world renown in the 1970s and 1980s, delighted in demonstrating their ability to manipulate and project this force both with individual students and in large gatherings. I believe that this was a large part of their spectacular attraction.

However, a teacher need not be enlightened to muster this kind of psychophysical energy. I myself have had an interesting experience of this phenomenon. While still living in England, I meditated periodically under the guidance of Irina Tweedie,[6] a Sufi teacher. After one session in particular, I felt my entire body and being suffused with energy. It so happened that about the same time a neighbor of mine had found out that I was a meditator and wanted to learn meditation from me. As I had not been authorized to teach meditation, I politely refused. Almost every time we would run into each other, he would ask again, quite seriously, about it.

After a half dozen requests, I finally agreed to show him what to do. I specified a day and a time. To my surprise, when he arrived at my home, he was dressed in his Sunday best. He later told me that he had prepared himself as if he were going to church. I asked him to make himself comfortable on a chair while I settled down on a sofa opposite him. I began to explain to him how to relax the body as a precondition for meditation.

I had barely uttered a few sentences when I felt a rush of psychophysical energy seemingly enter my body from behind and explode out toward him. My speech became slurred and my eyelids got heavy, but I kept my eyes focused on him. As the wave of energy hit him, he visibly jerked back, looking at me fearfully. Then a second wave passed through me to him, and again he startled. By the time a third rush of energy reached him, he was in deep meditation. I felt a force field connecting our bodies, and while I stayed in meditation, he too remained meditating.

We talked about the experience later, and he confirmed my own sense of what had happened. At first he had felt terror at possibly being hypnotized by me; then when the second wave of energy penetrated him, he again felt pushed back by it but started to yield to it. The third time he simply let go, allowing the energy to do its work in his body-mind. He had never meditated before. I was as surprised about this effect as he was. The same energy transfer occurred subsequently every time we got together for meditation. At one point it became clear to me that he needed to make certain changes in his life before he could benefit from further sessions.

Fortunately since I did not consider myself a guru or even a meditation teacher, I also did not interpret this experience as something I myself was generating. Rather, I regarded it as a gift (*prasāda*) and advised my neighbor to do the same. Having had this experience, however, and also having on numerous occasions been the recipient of such energy transmission, I can readily see why some teachers might attribute special significance to this ability. The same holds true of mystical experiences. It is all too easy to read into them more than is warranted. It is also easy to see how disciples can become addicted to the "hit" of spiritual transmission from a guru and how they might confuse that ability with enlightenment, wisdom, and compassion.

True Gurus, False Gurus, Crazy Gurus

There are many teachers, like lamps in house after house, but hard to find, O Devī, is the teacher who lights up all like the Sun.

Many are the teachers who rob the disciple of his wealth, but rare is the teacher who removes the disciple's affliction.

He is the [true] teacher by whose very contact there flows the supreme bliss (*ānanda*). The intelligent man should choose such a one as his teacher and none other.[7]

These stanzas are found in the *Kula-Arnava-Tantra*, a Sanskrit work on Hindu esotericism dating from the eleventh century C.E. They are spoken by God Shiva, the Lord of *yogins*, to his divine spouse Devī. But his words were intended for human ears, and they are as relevant today as they were a millennium ago, if not more so. Evidently, there are true and false spiritual teachers, or gurus. Very likely, there are many who fall between these two categories; they are neither completely white nor entirely black but come in different shades of gray.

How can one tell the genuine master from the fraudulent opportunist, whose paradoxical behavior and holy folly simply conceal wanton inconsistency? The question is pressing but by no means new. It has been asked again and again over the millennia, and for two reasons. First, because there is no easy answer and, second, because the chaff is never far from the wheat; darkness is never far from light.

There are not a few gurus who profess to be, or are portrayed by their followers as being, if not *the* World Teacher, then at least fully enlightened masters. The question of authenticity naturally rears its head. Who would deny that there are, in the words of Idries Shah, "phonies" among today's crop of spiritual teachers? In addition to the fakes, there are also the self-deluded. In most other cases, I daresay, the claim to enlightenment falls far short of reality, though no intentional deception may be at work. The temporary experience of *unio mystica,* or ecstatic unification, is often confused with enlightenment. Also, some practitioners mistake the peculiar "witnessing" state for transcendental realization.

The existence of fake gurus, or gurus who are less than they claim or pretend to be, is certainly deplorable, but their fraudulence or weakness should not induce us to discard the figure of the spiritual guide as a whole. Psychologist John Welwood, who has given these issues considerable thought, observes:

> To discount all spiritual masters because of the behavior of charlatans or misguided teachers is as unprofitable as refusing to use money because there are counterfeit bills in circulation. The abuse of authority is hardly any reason to reject authority where it is appropriate, useful, and legitimate. It is possible that in the present age of cultural upheaval, declining morality, family instability, and global chaos, the world's great spiritual masters may be among humanity's most precious assets. Glossing over important distinctions between genuine and counterfeit masters may only contribute further to the confusion of our age, and retard the growth and transformation that may be necessary for humanity to survive and prosper.[8]

In view of the sophistication displayed by some of the more successful counterfeit gurus, the question of authenticity is an urgent one. We sense something of this problem in the Biblical story of Jesus' asking his disciples to state who they thought he was, in contrast to the public opinion. Several centuries earlier, as recorded in the *Bhagavad-Gītā* (11.54–72), the warrior-mystic Arjuna asked his theophanic guru, Krishna, about the signs by which one may recognize a truly enlightened being. How, Arjuna inquired, does the one who is "steadied in gnosis" *(sthita-prajnā)* speak, sit, and move about? Krishna responds by speaking of the God-realizer's psychological characteristics—notably his ego-freedom, inner peace, and detachment. This is the approach taken in most of the Sanskrit literature. Thus, the *Uddhava-Gītā* (6.8.11–12), which is one of the many "imitation" *Gītās*, contains these stanzas:

> The sage (*vidvas*), though abiding in a body, does not [really] abide in a body rather like one who has awakened from a dream. The fool, however, though not abiding in the body, nevertheless abides in the body like one seeing a dream.

> Thus unattached while reclining, sitting, walking, bathing, seeing, touching, smelling, eating, and hearing, etc., the sage is not bound by the "qualities" [of Nature] in any [of his actions]; although abiding in Nature, he is unattached, like sky, Sun, and wind.

But how can we judge whether a teacher is truly unattached, beyond egoism, and above the play of Nature's forces? Again John Welwood makes a most valuable point:

> We cannot rely on descriptions of external behaviors alone to distinguish between genuine and problematic spiritual teachers. Developing criteria for judging a teacher's genuineness by examining external behavior alone would, for one thing, neglect the context—both interpersonal and intrapersonal—from which the behavior draws its meaning; and for another, it would tend to identify one particular model of a spiritual teacher as being ideal or exclusively valid, which would be as great a fallacy as elevating a single mode of psychotherapy to a similar position.[9]

Welwood further notes that therapists have very dissimilar personalities and employ many different styles of therapy, and, we might add, are varyingly competent. They are found to help some but not necessarily all of their clients. Similarly, not every guru is good for every disciple. The relationship between master and student is one key. The other, as Welwood points out, is the source of a teacher's authority. In the case of an awakened adept, that source is his or her enlightened attunement to Reality itself. In all other cases, which are the overriding majority, the teacher is authorized by a lesser competence.

The trouble is that an unenlightened teacher may present himself or herself as a fully awakened adept and dupe credulous devotees. The history of spirituality is full of questionable individuals of this kind. Scandals of rogue teachers have made the headlines repeatedly in recent years.

What lessons can we learn from all of this? First, the seeker must understand that spiritual teachers represent different levels of personal attainment and that enlightenment is rare indeed. Second, the seeker must acknowledge that, being a seeker rather than a master, he or she is not properly qualified to pronounce *final* judgment about any teacher's level of spiritual attainment. The editors of the widely read volume *Spiritual Choices* proffer this excellent advice:

> It is impossible for one who is lodged in mundane consciousness to evaluate definitively the competence of any guide to transformation and transcendence, without having already attained to an equal degree of transcendence. No number of "objective" criteria for assessment can remove this "Catch-22" dilemma. Therefore the choice of a guide, path, or group will remain in some sense a subjective matter. Subjectivity, however, has many modes, from self-deluding emotionality to penetrating, illuminative intuition. Perhaps the first job of the seeker would best be to refine that primary guide, one's own subjectivity.[10]

Ram Dass (Richard Alpert), who has functioned on both sides of the fence (as a devotee of Neem Karoli Baba and as a teacher in his own right), has made the following complementary observation:

> Some people fear becoming involved with a teacher. They fear the possible impurities in the teacher, fear being exploited, used, or entrapped. In truth we are only ever entrapped by our own desires and clingings. If you want only liberation, then all teachers will be useful vehicles for you. They cannot hurt you at all.[11]

This is true only ideally. In practice, the problem is that in many cases students do not know themselves sufficiently to be conscious of their deeper motivations. Therefore they may feel attracted precisely to the kind of teacher who shares their own "impurities" — such as hunger for power — and hence have every reason to fear him or her. It seems that only the truly innocent are protected. Although they too are by no means immune to painful experiences with teachers, at least they will emerge hale and whole, having been sustained by their own purity of intention.

Accepting the fact that our appraisal of a teacher is always subjective so long as we have not ourselves attained his or her level of spiritual accomplishment, there is at least one important criterion that we can look for in a guru: Does he or she genuinely promote disciples' personal and spiritual growth, or does he or she obviously or ever so subtly undermine their maturation? Would-be disciples should take a careful, levelheaded look at the community of students around their prospective guru. They should especially scrutinize those who are closer to the guru than most. Are they merely sorry imitations or clones of their teacher, or do they come across as mature men and women? The Bulgarian spiritual teacher Omraam Mikhaël Aïvanhov, who died in 1986, made this to-the-point observation:

> Everybody has his own path, his mission, and even if you take your Master as a model, you must always develop in the way that suits your own nature. You have to sing the part which has been given to you, aware of the notes, the beat and the rhythm; you have to sing it with your voice which is certainly not that of your Master, but that is not important. The one really important thing is to sing your part perfectly.[12]

The question of a teacher's authenticity can be answered only when we see the gestalt of his or her work with disciples. It is not important whether a teacher can go in and out of mystical states at will, or whether he or she can perform all kinds of paranormal feats, or whether he or she can jolt the disciple's nervous system through the transmission of life force, and so forth. It does not even make any difference whether a teacher has a splendid lineage or tradition to fall back upon, or whether he or she enjoys a large following. What really matters is whether a guru, in effect, works the miracle of spiritual transformation in others. As Saint Matthew reminds us:

> Ye shall know them by their fruits . . . every good tree bringeth forth good fruit; but a corrupt tree bringeth forth evil fruit.

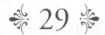

Understanding the Guru

Preamble

The traditional role of the guru, or spiritual teacher, is not widely understood in the West, even by those professing to practice Yoga or some other Eastern tradition entailing discipleship. In the following I will endeavor to shed some light on it, utilizing traditional statements found in the rich Sanskrit literature of Hindu, Buddhist, and Jaina Yoga. Many, if not most, of my observations also apply to the Sufi *zaddik*, the Christian *spiritual director*, the Hebrew *rabbi*, the Muslim *shaykh*.

In considering the guru, we inevitably look upon him (or her) from the outside. We can do so through the eyes of either a disciple or an impartial onlooker. In the latter case, the question is necessarily: How impartial are we or, more fundamentally, how impartial can we be? What cultural and personal (psychological) blinders color our view? To state the obvious, conventional folk have always had their problems with spiritual teachers. The neglect or even oppression of the Hebrew prophets and the Christian mystics is well known to historians. Mohammed, founder of Islam, was badly treated by his own people. So was Jesus of Nazareth. So was Baha'ullah, founder of the Baha'i faith. Gautama the Buddha survived a murderous plot against him by his own cousin. His older contemporary Vardhamana Mahāvīra, founder of Jainism, was ill treated in his younger years as well. Socrates, an early European guru, was forced to drink the poison cup, as his philosophical wisdom was felt to corrupt the youth and thus threaten the very fabric of Athenean society.

The Guru as Initiator

Yoga is an initiatory tradition, which means it revolves around the communication of esoteric or spiritual knowledge from a qualified teacher to an initiated disciple. The knowledge that is being transmitted is not merely of an intellectual variety but has the special quality of liberating or illuminating wisdom (Sanskrit: *vidyā* or *prajnā*).

Through initiation (Sanskrit: *dīkshā*), the seeker is transformed into a disciple. A major function of the guru is to serve as a vehicle for this process. As initiator, the guru voluntarily assumes the tremendous responsibility of assisting the disciple's birth into the spiritual dimension. Hence the Sanskrit texts compare the guru to a mother and a father. Like one's parents, the initiatory guru makes a deep spiritual connection with the initiate, which is thought to endure beyond the present lifetime.

Initiation occurs at various levels and through various means. In most instances it consists of a formal ritual in which the guru transmits a portion of his spiritual power (*shakti*) awakened through a mantra that is whispered into the disciple's left ear. But great adepts can initiate by a mere touch or glance or even simply by visualizing the disciple. Sri Ramakrishna, the great nineteenth-century master, placed his foot on Swami Vivekananda's chest and promptly plunged his young disciple into a deep state of formless ecstasy (*nirvikalpa-samādhi*).

THE GURU AS TRANSMITTER

According to Indic Yoga, the guru is a teacher who not merely instructs or communicates information, as does the preceptor (*ācārya*). Rather the guru transmits wisdom and, by his very nature, reveals—to whatever degree—the spiritual Reality. If the guru is fully enlightened, or liberated, his every word, gesture, and mere presence is held to express and manifest the Spirit. He or she is then a veritable beacon of Reality. Transmission in such a case is spontaneous and continuous. Like the Sun, to which the *sad-guru* or teacher of the Real is often compared, he or she constantly transmits the liberating "energy" of the transcendental Being.

In Yoga, with adepts who are not yet fully liberated, transmission is largely but not exclusively based on the teacher's will and effort. Many schools also admit of an element of divine grace (*prasāda*) entering into the configuration for which the teacher serves as a temporal vehicle.

Thus the traditional teacher plays a crucial role in the life of the disciple. As the Sanskrit word *guru* (meaning literally "weighty") suggests, he or she is a true "heavyweight" in spiritual matters.

The Guru as Guide

Apart from triggering and even constantly reinvigorating the spiritual process in a disciple, the guru also serves as a guide along the path. This occurs primarily through verbal instruction but also by being a living example on the spiritual path. Since the path to liberation includes many formidable hurdles, a disciple is clearly in need of guidance. The written teachings, which form the precious heritage of a given lineage of adepts, are a powerful beacon along the way. But they typically require explanations, or an oral commentary, to yield their deeper meaning. By virtue of the oral transmission received from his or her own teacher or teachers and also in light of his or her own experience and realization, the guru is able to make the written teachings come alive for the disciple. This is an invaluable gift.

The Guru as Illuminator

Tradition explains the term *guru* as being composed of the two syllables *gu* and *ru*; the former is taken to represent darkness, while the latter is said to stand for its removal. Thus the guru is a dispeller of spiritual darkness, that is, he or she restores sight to those who are blind to their true nature, the Spirit. If we compare the ego to a black hole from which no light can escape, the guru is like the radiant sun: an ever-lustrous being that illumines every dark niche in the disciple's mind and character.

This illuminating function depends on the degree of the guru's own realization. As tradition tells us, if the guru's enlightenment is merely nominal, so is his or her capacity to enlighten others. Therefore it behooves the prospective disciple to look closely at a teacher before committing to discipleship.

The Unconventional Nature of the Guru

Spiritual teachers, by their very nature, swim against the stream of conventional values and pursuits. They are not interested in acquiring and accumulating material wealth or in competing in the marketplace, or in pleasing egos. They are not even about morality. Typically, their message is of a radical nature, asking that we live consciously, inspect our motives, transcend our egoic passions, overcome our intellectual blindness, live peacefully with our fellow humans, and, finally, realize the deepest core of human nature, the Spirit. For those wishing to devote their time and energy to the pursuit of conventional life, this kind of message is revolutionary, subversive, and profoundly disturbing.

DISCIPLESHIP

In order to benefit from the guru's transmission of liberating wisdom, one must enter into the kind of intense transformative relationship with the guru that is known as *discipleship*. This involves a deep commitment to self-transformation, submission to a course of discipline by which the mind is tricked out of its conventional habit patterns, and a loving regard for the guru, who must be viewed not as an individual but essentially as a cosmic function. That function is designed to obliterate the illusion of discipleship.

Thus the spiritual process between guru and disciple is of a highly paradoxical nature: In order to open to the guru's transmission and allow it to work the miracle of transformation in us, we must assume the role of the disciple and hence deem the guru as external to ourselves. Yet the guru's transmission stems from the Spirit itself, which is not separate from us, since it is our very own ultimate identity. The whole spiritual path shares in this paradox. The reason, Yoga tells us, is that while we are inherently free, we do not at present realize this in every moment. Instead we consider ourselves conditioned by all kinds of limiting factors. This turns us into seekers. The search ends when we fully and in every moment live in and as the Spirit, which is truly indivisible whole, whereas the so-called *individual* is in fact a fragmented being conjured by the illusion of the ego.

The guru is the ultimate ego buster. Even while the guru has immense sympathy for the disciple who still thinks of himself as a finite island unto himself—an illusion that is fraught with suffering (*duhkha*)—the guru constantly and patiently attempts to draw the disciple out of himself and into the supra-individual and universal Self. In this task the guru is governed by wisdom (*prajnā*) and compassion (*karunā*), which are themselves supra-individual capacities that are oriented toward the Spirit rather than the finite human personality.

AUTHORITY OF THE GURU

These two capacities, which come alive in the guru by virtue of his or her own spiritual realization, give the guru the necessary authority in his labor of love of transmitting Reality. If a guru were merely compassionate, he or she would not be able to skillfully guide the disciple out of illusion. For the disciple would inevitably interpret the guru's compassion as love for the disciple as he or she is now. However, the guru loves the disciple in his or her true nature—as the Self (*ātman, purusha*), or Buddha nature, which at present is obscured by all sorts of misconceptions. If the guru were merely wise but lacking in compassion, most likely the disciple would become crushed under the demand for self-transformation. So long as a teacher is not fully realized, an imbalanced approach in transmission is always possible. At least some of the problems between contemporary teachers and disciples can be explained as due to an inadequate integration of wisdom and compassion on the part of the teacher. Disciples by their very nature are prone to misconceptions, projections, illusions, and delusions that prevent or delay a constructive relationship with the guru. Therefore the guru is primarily responsible for providing a viable avenue of self-transcending discipline for the disciple.

DISCOVERING THE INNER GURU

It is part of the disciple's self-understanding that he or she must ultimately transcend the external guru and discover the guru as a spiritual function or principle within. In their hurry for enlightenment, Western disciples all too often discard the external guru prematurely, leading them to the risk of further self-delusion. They then readily make the claim of being their own guru. However, short of ultimate realization, the only inner guru accessible to the average individual is the self, or ego. Since Yoga recognizes the ego-self as the cause of unenlightenment, the guidance of the ego cannot possibly lead to the highest realization. Instead of being a dispeller of spiritual ignorance, the ego as guru merely pushes the disciple into deeper ignorance, confusion, and ultimately despair. Thus, until the disciple is mature enough to discover and properly respond to the *guru* principle within, he or she should clearly practice *guru-yoga* in regard to an external teacher.

❈ 30 ❈
Holy Madness

SPIRITUAL LIFE AS REVERSAL

Since time immemorial the spiritual path has been understood as running counter to conventional views and behavior and even as undermining consensual reality. Spiritual or sacred life is inherently founded on a most profound reversal of conventional values and attitudes, or what in Tantra is known as *parāvritti*, meaning "turnabout" or "reversal." This revolutionary orientation is well captured in the archaic symbol of the Tree of Life, as described in the *Bhagavad-Gītā* (15.1–3). Its branches are pointing to the ground and its roots are extending into infinity up above. This is of course exactly what practitioners of Hatha-Yoga seek to emulate in the various inversion postures (*viparīta-karanī*), notably the headstand (*shīrsha-āsana*).

When we examine the great spiritual traditions of the world, we find that they have often deliberately cultivated unconventionality. This has given rise to what is termed "holy madness," which describes a spiritual style of life or teaching involving deliberate shock tactics that are designed to startle the ordinary person and, hopefully, shock him or her into a more accurate perception of reality. In Tibetan Buddhism, this orientation is also known as "crazy wisdom."

The phenomenon of holy madness is at home in Buddhism and Hinduism as much as in Sufism and Christianity, as well as in tribal religions. It always revolves around the figure of a saint, sage, or holy person. He or she typically instructs in, or gives testimony to, the sacred Reality by giving expression to the alternative values by which that Reality may be realized. Such an individual is a trickster, clown, breaker of taboos, master of disguise, and lover of the element of surprise.

FOOLS FOR CHRIST'S SAKE

In Christianity it was the apostle Paul who first acted out the role of the fool (Greek: *moros*). He was aware that Jesus himself had been accused by his enemies of both madness and demonic possession, and yet had triumphed over them all. So, Paul advised his fellow Christians by all means to cultivate the foolishness of spiritual life in order to avoid the temptation of thinking they have found wisdom in the world. Paul's advice was later followed with great enthusiasm by the desert fathers of the third and fourth centuries. They threw themselves completely at the mercy of the Divine, living lives of utter simplicity—a mad thing to do in the eyes of the world. These vocational *idiota*, as they were called, came to be known as "Fools for Christ's Sake." However, these self-effacing anchorites were anything but idiots, and some of them even had a background of great learning and worldly fame. They inspired generations of spiritual radicals within the Church.

Thus, in the sixth century, two well-bred young adults—Theophilius and Maria—traveled from place to place in the guise of a comedian and a prostitute. Their theatrical performances probably earned them more rough handling than cheers. No one recognized them as spiritual seekers until one day John of Ephesus found them absorbed in deep prayer. They had voluntarily chosen a life of eccentricity and hardship, so that they could grow nearer to God.

Similarly, the tenth-century saint Andrew, a teacher of the famous Epiphanius, adopted the life of a seemingly insane beggar. He roamed the streets naked and slept under the open sky in the company of wild dogs. Three centuries later, the respected Italian notary Jacopone da Todi made a spectacle of himself by crawling about naked in the marketplace, with a saddle strapped to his back. Contrary to the opinion of his outraged contemporaries, he had not gone mad but merely wanted to bring ridicule upon himself. Like his predecessors in the art of self-degradation, he hoped to demean himself, so that he might be uplifted spiritually.

Perhaps the best-known Fool for Christ's Sake is Saint Francis of Assisi. As a young man he renounced his family and considerable inheritance and took up the trying life of a spiritual pilgrim. He too began his religious vocation by stripping off all his clothes in front of a large crowd that had gathered in the public square of his hometown. Henceforth he lived in great poverty but with a heart full of praise for the Divine.

Of the forty-two canonized saints who lived as fools, no fewer than thirty-six belong to the Russian Orthodox Church. In Russia, the holy fool was called *yurodivy* (plural: *yurodivye*). The best known of Russia's fools was Saint Basil, who roamed the streets of sixteenth-century Moscow as a naked vagrant. He freely mixed with criminals and prostitutes, shed tears of sorrow at the dwellings of sinners, and pelted the hypocrites who vilified him with stones. Although the fools vanished from Russian (and also Western European) culture after the seventeenth century, they continued to figure in Russian literature, making their most notable literary appearance in Dostoyevsky's *The Idiot*.

MUSLIM FOOLS

Turning to the religious heritage of Islam, we encounter the fool in Sufism, which is Islam's mystical tradition. The delightfully quixotic figure of Mullah Nasrudin is a literary invention that captures some of the traits of the Sufi fool. Islam portrays the holy fool as a traveler on the "path of blame." The Sufi madcaps are known as *majzubs*, God-intoxicated mystics who are, as Pir Vilayat Inayat Khan once put it, always traumatic and unpredictable. Like their Christian counterparts, the Sufi fools courted blame and mockery with their eccentric behavior in order to intensify their spiritual commitment. But, unlike the Fools for Christ's Sake, their eccentricity did not always manifest in the practice of poverty and meekness. Occasionally, the *majzubs*—especially among India's Muslims—also demonstrated their holy madness by apparently indulging in gluttony and pride.

Thus, in the eleventh century, the *majzub* Abu Sa'id was the focus of constant gossip because of his erratic and "irreligious" behavior. Not only did he frequently hold sumptuous feasts, he also would sometimes wear the characteristic woolen garments of a Sufi, only to appear in expensive silk gowns on other occasions. When the local sultan had him officially investigated, Abu Sa'id promptly responded by holding another one of his feasts. The investigating committee quickly arrived at the conclusion that they were dealing not with a sybaritic impostor but a formidable spiritual teacher. All charges against him were dropped.

However, not all *majzubs* fared quite so well with the authorities. In the seventeenth century, Sarmad, who refused to wear any clothes, was executed under Emperor Aurangzeb. When the executioner tried to blindfold him, Sarmad smiled at him, saying: "Come in whatever garb you choose, I recognize you well." We also remember the horrible fate of the Sufi mystic Hallaj, who was crucified for proclaiming his perfect oneness with God.

Within Islam, which is fiercely monotheistic, any such claim is utterly heretical and punishable by death.

TIBETAN CRAZY WISDOM

Hallaj would have caused little stir among the Hindus and the Buddhists, who are quite familiar with extreme mystical utterances. For instance, the great dictum of Northern (or Mahāyāna) Buddhism is that the ultimate Reality (spoken of as "extinction," or *nirvāna*) is coessential with the phenomenal reality (called *samsāra*). This statement makes little sense from the perspective of the ordinary mind, which operates in the realm of dualities. It is, however, perfectly cogent from the point of view of enlightenment.

This identity of transcendence and immanence is the bread and butter of the Buddhist madcap who, in Tibet, is known as *myonpa*. The crazy adept takes his stand in that metaphysical truth and uses it to perplex and frustrate the ordinary mind of his disciples and, as is sometimes the case, of "innocent" bystanders.

One of the best-known crazy adepts of the Himalayan countries is Drukpa Kunley, who lived in the fifteenth century. Although Drukpa Kunley was an actual person, many of the stories told about him belong, at least in part, to the realm of legend and hagiolatry. Nevertheless, the outrageous exploits ascribed to him and other crazy-wisdom adepts convey quite well the flavor of Tibetan-style holy folly.

After his enlightenment, Drukpa Kunley divested himself of his monastic robes and became an itinerant "clown," achieving considerable renown for his ability to drink massive amounts of Tibetan beer and seduce the ladies. However, it is clear from the stories told about him that he was quite selective in his choice of women. He delighted in rejecting easy or conceited women, however pretty, but spared no efforts to win the heart of those in whom he saw great spiritual potential.

According to one legend, Drukpa Kunley once met a young Buddhist nun on her way into town. He quickly convinced her that she should let him make love to her, and she shyly submitted to the adept's advances. Then both went their own way. In due course, the nun gave birth. When the abbot discovered that the father of the child was Drukpa Kunley, he announced that no sin had been committed. The other young nuns became quite envious, wanting to experience sexual pleasure as well. A year later, the monastery was filled with babies—all said to have been fathered by the irrepressible Drukpa Kunley.

When Drukpa Kunley heard of his multiple fatherhood, he visited the monastery, and had all the young mothers assembled. Then he announced that he would be willing to care for any children that were truly his own, but all the others would have to be sacrificed to the Goddess. Then he grabbed hold of the child he knew to be his son and, invoking the Goddess, hurled him a great distance. There was a deafening thunder clap and the child was unharmed. Witnessing this procedure first with horror and then fear, the other nuns, who had falsely accused the adept of fatherhood, fled with their illegitimate babies.

Drukpa Kunley's countless sexual adventures were all initiatory occasions. He was a true Tantric, for whom sex is a vehicle of spiritual transformation. Followers of the left-hand path of Tantrism use sex as a sacrament and as a means of self-transformation and spiritual transmission.

How would our Western society react to radical teachers like Drukpa Kunley? In trying to answer this question, we need not idly speculate because we have the case of the late Lama Chögyam Trungpa, whose sexual encounters with his students made the headlines not too many years ago. Some of his students are still in recoil from his particular brand of crazy wisdom. We also have the case of the American-born adept Adi Da (Da Free John), who once declared himself to be a modern Drukpa Kunley, though who, by comparison with the legendary original, is relatively tame. Still, Adi Da also has more than once attracted media attention because of his Tantra-style teaching.

In the view of the adepts of Tantrism, asceticism and sexuality are by no means incompatible. Rejecting puritanism, they argue instead that unless we rediscover the sacred in our bodies, we will not discover it at all. I happen to believe they are right, though there is definitely room for questioning their approach.

THE SHOCK THERAPY OF ZEN MASTERS

In China and Japan, Mahāyāna Buddhism assumed the distinctive shape of Ch'an, better known by its Japanese name Zen. While the Zen tradition has become famous for its ideal of balance and harmony, it has harbored some of the most radically nonconformist minds in the premodern world. The Sudden School of Zen is associated in our minds with the shock tactics used by the Zen master to jar the student out of "consensus trance."

Thus, the ninth-century master Lin-chi (Rinzai) instructed his disciples to slay everything that stood in their way of enlightenment, not least the

Buddha himself. In his school, physical beatings, shouting, and agonizing paradoxical responses from the master were and still are a common occurrence. The Japanese teacher Gutei responded to all questions in the same manner: he simply raised one finger. When one of his students was once asked by a visitor to explain Gutei's teaching, the student likewise raised one finger. When Gutei heard of the incident, he sliced off the student's finger. Screaming with pain, the young man ran off. Gutei called after him, and when the disciple glanced back, the master gave him his famous single-finger gesture. Legend has it that this stopped the young man's mind completely, and he experienced sudden enlightenment.

We may surmise that in that moment the student was able to heartily laugh at himself. Zen acknowledges laughter as a sign of freedom and authenticity. The seventh-century Chinese madcap Han-shan, who was too eccentric for the monasteries of his time and was constantly evicted, achieved fame for his uproarious laughter. Likewise, the fierce expression on Bodhidharma's face is a put-on. It conceals huge laughter.

Hindu Dropouts

Hindu civilization has produced a type of holy fool who tends to be far more radical than his or her Christian and Muslim equivalents. India's brand of holy madness is embodied in the figure of the *avadhūta*. This Sanskrit word means literally "one who has cast off," meaning one who has abandoned all worldly concerns.

The *avadhūta* is a perfect renouncer: He is typically without home, family, job, obligations, or goals, and lives at the margins of human society. Ascetics of all kinds, who have dropped out of the social game, have existed in India for thousands of years. The *avadhūtas* have specifically been associated with the cult around the semilegendary God-man Dattātreya.

According to one story, the ascetic Dattātreya immersed himself in a lake and reappeared years later in the company of a beautiful maiden. His disciples were astonished but their faith in him remained unshaken. Dattātreya then started to consume wine with the girl, presumably as a prelude to making love with her. Even this serious breach of Hindu custom, we are told, failed to raise the slightest doubt in his disciples. They thus passed the ascetic's test of their faith.

The Hindu *avadhūta* is apt to resort to any measures to drive home a spiritual lesson, which can be risky at times, both for the holy fool and his or her audience. Most often, however, the fool's antics are simply odd, endangering no one. The contemporary adept Nityananda, teacher of the late Swami Muktananda, once besmeared himself from head to toe with excrement. His disciples were utterly embarrassed by his unseemly behavior, and finally convinced him to have himself scrubbed clean. Nityananda was prone to behave in unconventional ways, but his disciples were completely puzzled by this particular bizarre episode. Then some of the disciples confessed to having wondered whether Nityananda's sublime indifference extended to accepting excrement if it were offered to him. The following morning the culprits lined up to ask the *avadhūta's* forgiveness.

While most *avadhūta*, ancient and modern, have chosen a life of abject poverty, we know of some whose spiritual eccentricity took them in the opposite direction. Thus, the modern *avadhūta* Narayan Maharaj, who died in 1945, lived a truly regal existence. His disciples treated him as a living image of the Divine, pampering, decorating, and worshipping his body in the extreme. We can understand this curious practice better when we recall that holiness and sacred power have been integrally connected throughout history.

GURU WORSHIP

The saintly person has always been venerated as a receptacle of sacred power, as a connecting link between the ordinary world and the hidden dimension of the spirit, or the Divine. This belief is in fact fundamental to the Hindu and Buddhist tradition of *guru-yoga*—a yogic approach that makes the teacher, or guru, the principal focus of the disciple's attention.

The underlying idea is that by bonding with the teacher, the disciple is progressively drawn into the teacher's state of being. The West has, in recent years, learned something about this esoteric process of contagion largely through such popular spiritual figures as Swami Muktananda and Bhagwan Rajneesh (alias "Osho"), who were keen "transmitters." Both teachers have, alas, also demonstrated how sacred authority and spiritual power can become associated with questionable practices leading to accusations of moral corruption.

HOLY MADNESS AND INSANITY

Eccentrics have always been subject to ridicule by mainstream society, while more serious divergence from the social norm has predictably led to accusations of insanity. The holy madmen of the East, including the Fools for Christ's Sake, occasionally anticipated society's classification and condemnation. They called themselves "mad." From the perspective of the ordinary mind, the traditional approaches to the sacred can indeed look not only odd or bizarre but quite insane. This is especially true today where there is a much sharper distinction between the sacred and the profane than in the past. We apply the label "oddball," and worse, to the person who voluntarily renounces the luxuries of our consumer society—who refuses to own property, abstains from alcohol and meat, hugs trees, and marches in protest of war or nuclear power stations. If, on top of that, we find out that he or she has visions, we are quite ready to call the psychiatrist.

It is true that when we look at crazy adepts like Drukpa Kunley or Nityananda, we see phenomenal feats of renunciation. But we also see behavior that, certainly in the eyes of a psychiatrist, at times borders on the neurotic, if not psychotic. Some of these holy fools have in fact wondered about their own sanity. The saintly Ramakrishna, teacher of the world-famous Swami Vivekananda, is a case in point. For a period of time he ceremonially worshipped his own genitals, and on other occasions he installed himself on the altar of the temple where he served as head priest.

Such behavior is certainly not "normal." Nor is sitting on garbage heaps or sexually fondling women and girls, as has been reported of several contemporary Hindu adepts. When the *avadhūta* proclaims himself mad, should we take him at his word? Insanity is a loaded concept, and clinical textbooks notwithstanding, there is no consensus among psychiatrists about what it is exactly. We also know, certainly since Thomas Szasz's incisive writings, that the label "insane" has frequently been used as an ideological weapon by which nonconformists can effectively be stigmatized and silenced.

Psychotics tend to be dysfunctional individuals who, moreover, can be potentially dangerous to their surroundings. Now, judged by ordinary standards, many of the world's holy fools fit the description of a dysfunctional human being. They do not care to make sense. By their own admission, they are dangerous to the average individual who bases his or her life on rationality, order, predictability, and stability.

Yet, the holy fools are filled with a higher purpose, which belies the charge of insanity. When we examine their eccentric lives more closely, we find that they do make sense. Their madness is a self-chosen form of saying No to the ways of the world, which appear mad to them. It is, of course, always possible that a particular holy fool is not only metaphorically mad but shows actual signs of neurosis or psychosis. Religion, like politics, has always offered sanctuary to unstable individuals.

In my view, the history of holy madness does indeed include fools who were not merely God seekers but also suffering from mental instability. I also believe that this fact does not necessarily diminish their saintliness, though it puts it in perspective.

Regardless of their personal problems and the questionable moral status of some of their actions, the holy fools are a constant reminder that our perception of reality is largely a matter of choice, and that our choices are not necessarily the best we can make. Their challenge may be passive, as in the case of the Fools for Christ's Sake, or it may come as a deliberate onslaught, as with that archenemy of conventionality Drukpa Kunley.

Holy fools stop us in our tracks, which is exactly their intention. They confront us with alternative values and attitudes and thus with an alternative definition of reality. They have always been only reluctantly accommodated by their own cultures, however tolerant their fellow citizens may have been toward religious eccentrics. Yet, the fact that they have persisted in many different societies and religious communities throughout the ages may indicate that they have an integral social function to fulfill. Perhaps, their dissenting voices need to be heard for the good of the conforming majority. I believe that our era is the poorer for its dearth of holy fools.

❧ 31 ❧

Grace Has a Place in Yoga

WHEN MOST PEOPLE think of Yoga, they think of personal effort rather than grace. But since its earliest beginnings, Yoga has included in its understanding of the spiritual process the element of grace (*prasāda*), or divine intervention. As Swami Niranjanananda of the Bihar School of Yoga observed, "Self effort is the first step in the experience of grace."[1] Grace is in fact an integral component of all the many schools of Yoga that conceive of the ultimate Reality in personal terms. The classic path of this orientation is Bhakti-Yoga, which was given expression already in the 5,000-year-old *Rig-Veda* (3.59.2):

> Whosoever is in Your grace is neither slain nor conquered; and distress does not reach him either from afar or near.

Over two millennia later, the anonymous composer of the *Shvetāsh-vatara-Upanishad* (3.20b) declared:

> Free from grief one beholds, through the grace of the Creator, that [transcendental Being] as action-free (*akratu*), as majestic, and as the Lord (*īsha*).

Patanjali, the compiler of the *Yoga-Sūtra*, likewise did not fail to mention the role of the Lord (*īshvara*), who instructed the Yoga masters of yore. In aphorism 1.23, he names *īshvara-pranidhāna* as one of the principal means of self-transcendence leading to liberation. Vyāsa, in his *Yoga-Bhāshya* (1.23), explains *pranidhāna* as a kind of devotion (*bhakti*). In his valuable commentary on Patanjali's aphorism 1.23, B. K. S. Iyengar states:

> Through surrender the aspirant's ego is effaced, and the grace of the Lord pours down upon him like torrential rain.[2]

Devotion to the ultimate Being and grace form the nucleus of the spiritual practice mapped out in the *Bhāgavata-Purāna* (a ninth-century work). This scripture, held sacred by the Vaishnavas, has served many generations of sages and writers as the foundation for their own inspired writings.

The medieval Shaivas and Shāktas, too, included grace in their philosophy. If it did not correspond to an actual experience, why would untold generations of *yogins*, sages, and saints have sought it out so eagerly?

There are of course several ways of looking at grace. We could, for instance, see it as a function of our own stock of good karma. According to the age-old teaching of karma—the moral law of causation—we reap what we sow. Thus our good thoughts, our positive emotions or dispositions, and our morally sound actions create good karma for us. In other words, we are our own source of grace.

I believe that most of the experiences we attribute to "grace" are simply good karma manifesting for us, without the involvement of any other agent. However, I also believe that there are occasions when an apparently objective agency—residing in the subtle or even the transcendental dimensions of existence—favors us in some way. Tradition, moreover, speaks of the *guru's* grace and reminds us that the true teacher (*sad-guru*) is never far from the ultimate Reality. In other words, his or her grace is divine grace.

Sincere Yoga practitioners, especially those resorting to prayer, are likely to encounter graceful interventions more frequently than others. To quote Swami Niranjanananda again, "In order to be the recipient [of grace] one has to go through self effort."[3]

This very recognition lies behind Patanjali's recommendation to practice *īshvara-pranidhāna*, which broadly can be translated as a "positive regard for a higher principle." More narrowly, we can understand it as devotion to the Lord (*īshvara*), whom Patanjali considers to be a special kind of *purusha*, or transcendental Spirit. However we may conceptualize the ultimate Being, there is always room in our practice for opening to grace.

As part of this, Western Yoga practitioners, instead of relying exclusively on postures, breath control, and meditation, might also want to include the beneficial traditional practice of prayer (*prārthanā*).

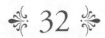

32

Tapas, or Voluntary Self-Change

ACCORDING TO HINDU mythology, the Divine Being, in order to create the universe voluntarily underwent intense self-discipline. This cosmic Yoga caused the Divine Being to sweat, thus producing out of its pores the cosmos with its countless beings and things. The process of voluntary self-limitation and self-challenge bears the name *tapas* in Sanskrit, which means literally "heat" or "glow."

The ancient sages (*rishi*) pointed to the Solar Being as the primary practitioner of *tapas* and in fact as the originator of Yoga. Often Westerners think of Patanjali as the "Father of Yoga," but this honorific title rightly belongs to Hiranyagarbha (Golden Germ/Womb). Even though in bygone ages, there may well have been a teacher by that name, Hiranyagarbha first and foremost denotes the Sun. In the *Bhagavad-Gītā* (4.1), the Sun—called Vivasvat—is referred to as the primordial teacher of ancient Yoga. The Sun necessarily also was the first teacher of *tapas*, since *tapas* is at the heart of all yogic disciplines. Indeed, before the word *yoga* was used in its technical meaning of "spiritual discipline," the term *tapas* enjoyed wide currency. Subsequently, it acquired more the connotation of "asceticism" or "austerity."

Tapas is any practice that pushes the mind against its own limits, and the key ingredient of *tapas* is endurance. Thus in the archaic *Rig-Veda* (10.136), the long-haired ascetic or *keshin* is said to "endure" the world, to "endure" fire, and to "endure" poison.[1] The *keshin* is a type of renouncer, a proto-*yogin*, who is a "wind-girt" (naked?) companion of the wild God Rudra (Howler). He is said to "ascend" the wind in a God-intoxicated state and to fly through space, looking down upon all things. But the name *keshin* harbors a deeper meaning, for it also can refer to the Sun whose "long hair" is made up of the countless rays that emanate from the solar orb and reach far into the cosmos and bestow life on Earth. This is again a reminder that the archaic Yoga of the *Vedas* revolves around the Solar Spirit, who selflessly feeds all beings with his/her/its compassionate warmth.

The early name for the *yogin* is *tapasvin*, the practitioner of *tapas* or voluntary self-challenge. The *tapasvin* lives always at the edge. He deliberately challenges his body and mind, applying formidable will power to whatever practice he vows to undertake. He may choose to stand stock-still under India's hot sun for hours on end, surrounded by a wall of heat from four fires lit close by. Or he may resolve to sit naked in solitary meditation on a wind-swept mountain peak in below-zero temperatures. Or he may opt to incessantly chant a divine name, forfeiting sleep for a specified number of days. The possibilities for *tapas* are endless.

Tapas begins with temporarily or permanently denying ourselves a particular desire—having a satisfying cup of coffee, piece of chocolate, or casual sex. Instead of instant gratification, we choose postponement. Then, gradually, postponement can be stepped up to become complete renunciation of a desire. This kind of challenge to our habit patterns causes a certain degree of frustration in us. We begin to "stew in our own juices," and this generates psychic energy that can be used to power the process of self-transformation. As we become increasingly able to gain control over our impulses, we experience the delight behind creative self-frustration. We see that we are growing and that self-denial need not necessarily be negative.

The *Bhagavad-Gītā* (17.14–16) speaks of three kinds of austerity or *tapas*: Austerity of body, speech, and mind. Austerity of the body includes purity, rectitude, chastity, nonharming, and making offerings to higher beings, sages, brahmins (the custodians of the spiritual legacy of India), and honored teachers. Austerity of speech encompasses speaking kind, truthful, and beneficial words that give no offense, as well as the regular practice of recitation (*svādhyāya*) of the sacred lore. Austerity of the mind consists of serenity, gentleness, silence, self-restraint, and pure emotions.

According to the *Bhagavad-Gītā* (17.17), a rounded spiritual practice entails all three kinds of penance, and it is practiced with great faith (*shraddhā*) and without expectation of reward. Such *tapas* is informed primarily by the quality of *sattva*, which stands for the principle of lucidity in the inner and outer world. The kind of austerity that has a predominance of the quality of *rajas*, the principle of dynamism in Nature, tends to be practiced with an ulterior motive, such as gaining respect, honor, or reverence, or for the sake of selfish display. Because of this, it also tends to be unstable and of short duration. When the quality of *tamas*, standing for the principle of inertia, characterizes the practice of austerity, it leads to foolish self-torture or injury to others.

Sattva, rajas, and *tamas* are the three primary constituents of Nature (*prakriti*). All created things, including the human psyche or mind, are a composite of these three factors called *gunas*. Since *tapas* depends on the mind of the Yoga practitioner, it is colored by these three, as they manifest in a particular individual. Depending on the quality of a practitioner's *tapas,* he or she will harvest the corresponding results. Unless the practice of austerity has a strong *sattva* ingredient, these results can range from physical pain and anguish to a complete failure of the spiritual process.

For instance, if a person practices *tapas* in order to acquire paranormal abilities (*siddhi*) that will impress or overpower others, he or she consolidates rather than transcends the ego and thus becomes diverted from the path. If, again, a practitioner confuses the balanced self-challenge of genuine *tapas* with merely painful penance, springing from sheer ignorance and a subconscious masochism, he or she is bound to reap only pain and suffering that will undermine his or her physical health, possibly contributing to emotional instability or even mental illness.

Two and a half thousand years ago, Gautama, the founder of Buddhism, learned the important difference between genuine (i.e., self-transcending) *tapas* and misconceived penance. For six long years he pushed himself until his bodily frame became emaciated and was close to collapse, but still without yielding the longed-for spiritual freedom. Then his inner wisdom led him to take the middle path (*madhya-mārga*) beyond damaging extremes. Gautama abandoned his severe, self-destructive *tapas* and nourished his body properly. His fellow ascetics, who had always looked to him for inspiration, thought he had returned to a worldly life and shunned him. Later, after Gautama's spiritual awakening, their paths crossed again and his radiance was so impressive that they could not help but bow to him with utmost respect.

Genuine *tapas* makes us shine like the Sun. Then we can be a source of warmth, comfort, and strength for others.

❦ 33 ❦
The Art of Purification

THE PHILOSOPHY OF PURITY

There are many ways of looking at the yogic or spiritual life. It has been viewed as a path, a journey, or a ladder to the ultimate Reality. It has also been considered a lifelong discipline, the culture of harmony, the right management of one's energies, or the endeavor to go beyond the "little self" (the ego-identity). Here I propose to examine the yogic life as a comprehensive endeavor at self-purification (*ātma-shuddhi*).

All spiritual traditions regard our ordinary human condition as somehow flawed or corrupt, as falling short of the unsurpassable perfection or wholeness of Reality. As a process of transformation, Yoga endeavors to re-form or, in the words of the Christian mystic Meister Eckhart, even "super-form" the spiritual practitioner. The old Adam has to die before the new super-formed being can emerge—the being who is reintegrated with the Whole.

Not surprisingly, this transmutation of the human personality is also often couched in terms of self-sacrifice. In gnostic language, the "lower" reality must be surrendered, so that the "higher" or divine Reality can become manifest in our lives. For this to be possible, the spiritual practitioner must somehow locate and emulate that higher Reality. He or she must find the "Heaven" within, whether by experiential communion or mystical union with the Divine or by an act of faith in which a connection with the Divine is simply assumed until this becomes an actual experience. Spiritual discipline (*sādhana*), then, is a matter of constantly "remembering" the Divine, the transcendental Self, or Buddha nature.

There can be no such transformation without catharsis, without shedding all those aspects of one's being that block our immediate apperception of Reality. Traditions like Yoga and Vedānta can be understood as programs of progressive "detoxification" of the body-mind, which clears the inner eye so that we can see what is always in front of us—the omnipresent Reality, the Divine. So long as our emotional and cognitive system is toxic or impure, that inner eye remains veiled, and all we see is the world of multiplicity devoid of unity. The modern gnostic teacher Mikhaël Aïvanhov remarked about this:

> Not so many years ago, when people's homes were still lit by oil lamps, the glass chimneys had to be cleaned every evening. All combustion produces wastes, and the oil in these lamps deposited a film of soot on the inside of the glass, so that, even if the flame was lit, the lamp gave no light unless the glass was cleaned. The same phenomenon occurs in each one of us, for life is combustion. All our thoughts, feelings and acts, all our manifestations, are the result of combustion. Now it is obvious that in order to produce the flame, the energy which animates us, something has to burn and that burning necessarily entails waste products which then have to be eliminated. Just as the lamp fails to light up the house if its glass is coated with soot . . . similarly, if a man fails to purify himself he will sink deeper and deeper into the cold and dark and end by losing life itself.[1]

To use another metaphor, Yoga is like an oxygen tank resting at the bottom of a deep and murky pool. Using the tank, we can safely float to the surface. As we ascend, we note that the water gets visibly clearer—the water being a symbol for one's own body-mind. We are immersed in the Divine, but we realize this only when we actively work on purifying our vision.

In his *Yoga-Sūtra* (3.55), Patanjali proffers this important definition of spiritual liberation, the goal of the yogic path:

> [The condition of] transcendental "aloneness" (*kaivalya*) [is attained] when the essence-of-mind (*sattva*) and Self are equal in purity.

The philosophy behind this statement is as follows. The transcendental Subject or Spirit (*purusha*) is inherently pure, perfect. The human mind, which Patanjali here calls *sattva*, is not. By purifying the mind until it becomes as transparent as a mirror, it approximates the eternal purity of the Self, reflecting the Self's natural "luminosity" and thus assuming the appearance of luminosity itself. In fact, enlightenment is when the mind, or consciousness, reflects the Self's innate luster without obstruction. This reflected luminosity registers even in the body, and then we speak of "transfiguration," as it occurred in the case of Moses, the prophet Elijah, and not least Jesus of Nazareth.

YOGIC TECHNIQUES OF PHYSICAL DETOXIFICATION

The most common Sanskrit term for "purification" is *shodhana*, and for the condition of "purity" it is *shuddhi or shauca*, the latter typically being applied to physical cleanliness. Let us begin with Classical Yoga, which is encoded in Patanjali's *Yoga-Sūtra*—a work that probably dates back to the second century C.E. From the *Yoga-Sūtra* (1.43), we learn that "through asceticism (*tapas*), owing to the dwindling of impurity, perfection of the body and the sense organs" is gained.

The practice of *tapas* traditionally includes such exercises as fasting for prolonged periods, standing or sitting stock-still, observing complete silence, or voluntarily exposing oneself to extreme heat or cold, hunger or thirst. These ascetic techniques, which are a part of Patanjali's *kriyā-yoga*, have the purpose of steeling the will and cultivating the innate potential of the body-mind. Bodily "perfection," we are told in the *Yoga-Sūtra* (3.46), consists in a pleasing physical form, gracefulness, and adamantine robustness.

The ideal of bodily perfection became a prominent theme in the period after Patanjali, especially in the schools of Hatha-Yoga, which has the avowed goal of creating an indestructible "divine body" (*divya-deha*). In the *Yoga-Bīja* (51-52), a medieval Sanskrit scripture, we read:

> The body [fashioned through] Yoga is exceedingly strong. Even the deities cannot acquire [such a durable body]. [The *yogin* endowed with such a body] enjoys various supernatural powers and is free from bondage to the body. The body [fashioned through Yoga] is like the sky; even purer than the sky.

To create such a superbody, the *yogin* begins by purifying the physical body. The *Gheranda-Samhitā*, a seventeenth-century manual of Hatha-Yoga, lists a large number of such purificatory practices. These are meant to "temper" the body through the "fire of Yoga." Purification is, first of all, accomplished through the "six acts" (*shat-karma*). These six acts comprise:

1. Basic cleansing techniques (*dhauti*), which include such practices as dental care, cleansing of the stomach by different means, and rectal cleansing
2. Water enema and dry enema (*vasti*)
3. Nasal cleansing (*neti*) by means of a thin thread

4. Rotation of the vertical abdominal muscles (*naulī*), which is thought to cleanse the stomach and intestines
5. Steady gazing (*trāṭaka*), which is held to purify the eyes
6. "Skull luster" (*kapāla-bhāti*), a form of breathing exercise that is thought to "brighten up" the whole head.

The *Brihad-Yogi-Yājnavalkya*, a medieval work, contains detailed instructions for the ritual of bathing (*snāna*), and other scriptures mention still further purificatory practices. All these techniques—some of which are quite dangerous when practiced without expert supervision—are said to cure a variety of diseases. The same claim is made for the different postures (*āsana*) and methods of breath control (*prāṇāyāma*). The daily ritual bathing, the *Brihad-Yogi-Yājnavalkya* (7.118 ff.) states, is best done in the early morning in a river connected to the ocean or in the ocean itself. Hot water is said to be useless. Bathing produces mental calm, removes negative emotions, and increases a person's well-being, vitality, and beauty.

This scripture further mentions that practitioners who are unable to take their ritual bath because of weakness or time constraints should purify themselves by means of *mantra* recitation. This is called "mantric bath" (*mantra-snāna*).

Two important yogic means of self-purification are fasting (*upavāsa*) and dieting (*āhāra*). Fasting has long been known as a highly efficient way of inducing an altered state of consciousness. Abstinence from food changes the chemical composition of the blood, which inevitably has an effect on the mind. But fasting has to be undertaken from the right inner disposition to bear spiritual fruit. Gandhi, who constantly experimented with fasting and strict dieting, observed:

> I am convinced that I greatly benefited by it both physically and morally. But I know that it does not necessarily follow that fasting and similar disciplines would have the same effect for all.
>
> Fasting can help to curb animal passion, only if it is undertaken with a view to self-restraint . . . if physical fasting is not accompanied by mental fasting, it is bound to end in hypocrisy and disaster.[2]

Already the more than three-thousand-year-old *Chāndogya-Upanishad* (7.26.2) notes the close connection between dietary purity and purity of being:

When food is pure, being (*sattva*) is pure. When one's being is pure, memory/mindfulness (*smriti*) is stable. On attaining [such] memory/mindfulness, all knots [at the heart] are released.

Swami Sivananda of Rishikesh, a twentieth-century master, reiterated ancient wisdom when he wrote:

Mind is formed out of the subtlest portion of food. If the food is impure, the mind also becomes impure. This is the dictum of sages and psychologists.[3]

In other words, food is not merely an aggregate of chemical compounds but contains the quintessence of organic matter, which is the life energy (*prāna*). While all types of food can be considered a form *of prāna*, however, they are not equally beneficial. Some kinds of food prove more or less toxic to the human system. The Yoga practitioner is therefore very circumspect about his or her nutrition. The *Bhagavad-Gītā* (18.8f.) categorizes food according to the model of the three types of primary constituents or *gunas* — *sattva*, *rajas*, and *tamas*. *Sattva* is elevating; *rajas* is aggravating; and *tamas* is sluggish.

Foods that promote life, lucidity (*sattva*), strength, health, happiness, and satisfaction and that are savory, rich in oil, firm, and heart[-gladdening] are agreeable to the *sattva*-natured [person].

Foods that are pungent, sour, salty, spicy, sharp, harsh, and burning are desired by the *rajas*-natured [person]. They cause pain, grief, and disease.

And [food] that is spoiled, tasteless, putrid, stale, left over, and unclean, is food agreeable to the *tamas*-natured [person].

Not all yogic authorities are in agreement over what constitutes a good diet. They all, however, emphasize the importance of dietary restraint (called *mita-āhāra*), or moderate eating.

From a yogic point of view, illness is the result of an imbalance in the circulation of the life force. Health must be restored before one can proceed to the higher yogic practices of breath control, sensory withdrawal, concentration, and meditation. Dieting is a key practice in this endeavor of harmonizing the body. Ecstasy (*samādhi*), the final stage of the path of Yoga, is explained as perfect inner balance—a balance that is hard to come by without a healthy body.

The single most important Hatha-Yoga technique of purification is a particular type of breath control that is performed by breathing alternately through the left and the right nostril. This practice is intended to remove all obstructions from the network of subtle channels through which the life force circulates, thus making proper breath control and deep concentration possible. In the ordinary person, state the scriptures of Hatha-Yoga, the circulation of the life force is obstructed. The technique of alternate breathing is known as *nādī-shodhana*.

When the subtle conduits (*nādī*)—or arcs of the life energy—are completely purified, the life force can circulate freely in the body, and it becomes amenable to voluntary control. Already Patanjali noted in his *Yoga-Sūtra* (2.52) that breath control has the effect of removing the "covering" (*āvarana*) that prevents one's inner light to manifest clearly.

The objective of Hatha-Yoga is to conduct the life force along the body's central axis to the crown of the head. This flow of *prāna* through the central conduit—called *sushumnā-nādī*—is thought to awaken the full psychospiritual potential of the body. This potential is better known as the "serpent power" (*kundalinī-shakti*).

When the *kundalinī* is awakened from its dormant state in the lowest center (*cakra*) at the base of the spine, it rushes up to the crown center. This ascent is accompanied by a variety of psychic and somatic phenomena. These include visionary states and, when the *kundalinī* reaches the top center, ecstatic transcendence into the formless Reality, which is inherently inconceivable and blissful. As the *kundalinī* force is active in the crown center, the rest of the body is gradually depleted of energy. This curious effect is explained as the progressive purification of the five elements (*bhūta*) constituting the physical body—earth, water, fire, air, and ether. The Sanskrit term for this process is *bhūta-shuddhi*.

Purification of the body not only leads to health and inner balance but also affects the way in which a person perceives the world. This is clearly indicated in Patanjali's *Yoga-Sūtra* (2.40), which states:

> Through purity [the *yogin* gains] a desire to protect his own limbs [and a desire for] noncontamination by others.

The decisive phrase *sva-anga-jugupsā* has often been translated as "disgust toward one's own body," but this is not at all in the spirit of Yoga.

Jugupsā is more appropriately rendered as "desire to protect." The adept is eager to protect his body against contamination by others. This is combined with an inner distance from one's own physical vehicle through sustained witnessing. This attitude is an important antidote against the kind of body narcissism to which Hatha-Yoga, like other systems of body culture, can give rise. Patanjali's aphorism reminds us that the real work is to be accomplished on the spiritual level. Then, as he puts it, the "Seer"—the transcendental Self—will truly shine forth. However, it makes sense to want to enjoy Self-realization in a healthy body, which is the ideal of Hatha-Yoga. This desire need not even be a selfish one, for we could probably serve others more effectively in a healthy body, perhaps even a body endowed with all kinds of extraordinary capabilities (*siddhi*).

YOGIC TECHNIQUES OF MENTAL CATHARSIS

Bodily *and* moral purity is fundamental to our physical and mental health. Hence Patanjali's eight-limbed yogic path begins with the ten rules of *yama* and *niyama*, which regulate the social life of Yoga practitioners as well as their relationship to their own body-minds and to the Divine (*īshvara*). Moral and physical purity create the necessary basis for the higher practices of Yoga, which aim at cleansing the mirror of the mind more directly.

Mental purification is accomplished by means of sensory inhibition (*pratyāhāra*), concentration (*dhāranā*), meditation (*dhyāna*), and ecstatic self-transcendence (*samādhi*). In his *Viveka-Cudāmani* (vs. 77), the famous Vedānta master Shankara characterizes objects (*vishaya*) as "poison" (*visha*), because they tarnish consciousness by distracting it from its real task, which is to mirror reality. Our attention is constantly pulled outward by objects, and this externalization of our consciousness prevents us from truly being ourselves. "When the mind pursues the roving senses," states the *Bhagavad-Gītā* (2.67), "it carries away wisdom (*prajna*), even as the wind [carries away] a ship on water."

Sense perceptions pollute our inner environment, keeping our mind in a state of turmoil. We are forever hoping for experiences that will make us happy and whole, but our desire for happiness can never be satisfied by external experiences. "Whatever pleasures spring from contact [with sense objects], they are only sources of suffering," declares the *Bhagavad-Gītā* (5.22). To find true happiness and peace, we need to unclutter our mind and remain still. The fatal consequences of focusing on objects rather than the ultimate Subject, the Self, are described very well in that ancient Yoga scripture (2.62–63):

When a man contemplates objects, attachment to them is produced. From attachment springs desire [for further contact with the objects] and from desire comes anger (when that desire is frustrated].

From anger arises confusion, from confusion [comes] failure of memory; from failure of memory [arises] the loss of wisdom *(buddhi)*; upon the loss of wisdom, [a person] perishes.

Emotional confusion *(sammoha)* profoundly upsets our cognitive faculties: We lose our sense of direction, purpose, and identity. The Sanskrit word for this state is *smriti-bhramsha* or "failure of memory/mindfulness." When we fail to "recollect" ourselves, wisdom *(buddhi)* cannot shine forth. But without wisdom, we, as members of the species *Homo sapiens,* are doomed to forfeit not only our status as human beings but our very life. Spiritual ignorance is binding and ultimately ruinous. Wisdom can set us free. In Shankara's *Ātma-Bodha* (vs. 16), we read:

Even though the Self is all-pervading, it does not shine in everything. It shines only in the organ-of-wisdom *(buddhi)*, like a reflection in a clear medium [such as water or a mirror].

The "organ of wisdom," which is often called the "higher mind," is predominantly composed of *sattva,* the lucidity factor of the cosmos. There is a family resemblance between the *sattva* and the Self, and this curious affinity makes it possible for the Self's radiant presence to manifest itself to human beings.

The discipline of sensory restraint is crucial to the emergence of wisdom or gnosis. Without it, concentration and meditation are impossible. Both these techniques have the purpose of vacating the inner space so that the "light" of the Self can manifest in full. Concentration is generally defined in the yogic scriptures as the "binding" of attention to a single focus. Meditation is the process of deepening that unfolds on the basis of such concentrated attention. It reveals more and more "subtle" aspects of one's chosen focus, whether it be a visualized deity or other "prop," a *mantra,* or a locus within one's body.

Ultimately, the knowledge gained in meditation is considered superior to the knowledge or experiences derived through contact with sense objects. Yet they too must be transcended. Meditation fulfills itself when the meditative consciousness is utterly vacated but lucid. At that point, a significant switch occurs in our awareness. All of a sudden we are fused with the object of contemplation. This is the much-desired state of ecstasy (*samādhi*) in which subject and object are merged and all opposites coincide. In this condition, we bask in the peace and happiness that are an integral part of our authentic nature, the transcendental Self.

However, even in the condition of *samādhi* spontaneous insights (*prajnā*) intrude, which are in the final analysis also "impurities." Hence they must likewise be transcended until we have fully recovered our identity as the Self in the extraordinary condition of transconceptual ecstasy (*nirvikalpa-samādhi*). Alas, this ecstatic state is only temporary, and before long our ordinary ego-centric awareness reconstitutes itself. Fortunately, *nirvikalpa-samādhi* (which is also known as *asamprajnāta-samādhi* in Classical Yoga) leaves a strong "aftertaste," which can then guide us in our further spiritual adventure.

The remaining challenge is to realize our higher or true nature in the midst of daily life. This is the ideal of "spontaneous ecstasy" (*sahaja-samādhi*), which is stable and permanent. This sublime condition of enlightenment is the same as "living liberation," about which Shankara says in his *Viveka-Cudāmani* (vs. 438):

> He who never has the thought of "I" with regard to the body and the senses and the thought of "this" in respect of something different to the "That" [i.e., Reality] is regarded as a [being] who is liberated in life (*jīvan-mukta*).

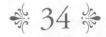

34

Obstacles on the Path
According to Patanjali

General

The yogic process, running counter to the externalizing tendency of the ordinary human mind, does not necessarily unfold smoothly. As already the *Bhagavad-Gītā* (6.6) recognizes, the self can be the Self's worst enemy.[1] Patanjali, in his *Yoga-Sūtra* (1.30), mentions no fewer than nine hindrances (*antarāya*) that may arise in the course of the yogic discipline:

> Sickness, apathy, doubt, heedlessness, sloth, dissipation, false vision, nonattainment of the stages [of Yoga] and instability [in those stages] are the distractions of consciousness; these are the obstacles.

These can all be understood as self-inflicted limitations, which retard or even negate the yogic process. They also can be seen as expressions of the unconscious, foiling the great yogic opus and thereby preserving the status quo of the unenlightened personality, the unredeemed self. Even when the desire for liberation (*mumukshutva*) is present, an aspirant is still subject to the antithetical forces of Nature (*prakriti*) governing his or her psyche. Seemingly accidental occurrences, like illness, that frustrate yogic progress are, in the final analysis, due to the fruition of the karmic deposits (*karma-āshaya*) and are thus self-induced.

It is significant that Patanjali characterizes the nine hindrances as "distractions of consciousness" (*citta-vikshepa*). They are disturbances, or dysfunctions, as is well captured in the word *vikshepa*, which derives from the prefix *vi-* ("dis-") and the verbal root *kship* meaning "to throw" or "to cast." The *vikshepas* scatter the *yogin's* mental focus and hence stand in the way of his or her sustained effort to cultivate single-mindedness or "one-pointedness" (*ekāgratā*).

According to the *Yoga-Bhāshya* (1.1), the stages or levels (*bhūmi*) of mental activity are the following five:

1. Restless (*kshipta*) or agitated, because of an overwhelming preponderance of *rajas*, the dynamic psychocosmic principle; in Shankara Bhagavatpāda's *Yoga-Bhāshya-Vivarana* it is compared to an overfull granary that bursts open

2. Deluded (*mūdha*) or infatuated, because of a surfeit of *tamas*, the psychocosmic principle of inertia, which ousts the important facility of discernment (*viveka*)

3. Distracted (*vikshipta*) or merely intermittently stable, because *sattva*, the psychocosmic principle of lucidity, is periodically present

4. One-pointed (*ekāgra*) or focused, as a result of the growing presence of *sattva* over *rajas* and *tamas*

5. Restricted (*niruddha*) or controlled, as a result of a preeminence of *sattva*, which is explained by Shankara Bhāgavatpāda as a thought-free state

The first three levels are typical of the state of mind that the ordinary individual experiences. Only the last two describe the quality of the *yogin's* consciousness.

The *Yoga-Bhāshya* (1.30) explains that the distractions can occur only so long as one of the five types of mental "fluctuations" (*vritti*) is present. In other words, the mind must either perceive, misperceive, imagine, remember, or be asleep. However, when these mental activities have been restricted (*niruddha*), then the obstacles mentioned by Patanjali can obviously not be effective. That is to say, a *yogin* may be ill but be quite undisturbed by his illness, as was the case with the well-known twentieth-century sage Ramana Maharshi of Tiruvannamalai, who, toward the end of his life, suffered from cancer. The disease must have caused him considerable pain, yet he remained serene and occasionally even joked about his pain-wrecked body and the doctor's concern about him.

So, it could be said that the obstacles are hindrances only so long as they affect the activities of the mind. In his *Yoga-Bhāshya-Vivarana* (1.30), Shankara Bhagavatpāda explains the word *antarāya* thus: "They move toward or create an interval, gap, or break—hence [they are called] obstacles." An "interval" (*antara*) is a disruption of the natural continuity of apperception by the Self (*purusha*), which is a mere witness (*sākshin*). In other words, it is a moment in which the Self is eclipsed, and a person loses himself or herself in the stream of arising thoughts, feelings, and sensations. Hence in the *Tattva-Vaishāradī* (1.30), Vācaspati Mishra states that the obstacles are specifically "obstacles to Yoga" (*yoga-antarāya*) and "distractions relative to the consciousness checked by Yoga." In his *Yoga-Bhāshya* (1.30), Vyāsa speaks of "opponents of Yoga" (*yoga-pratipaksha*), "obstacles to Yoga" (*yoga-antarāya*), and "blemishes of Yoga" (*yoga-mala*). Shankara Bhagavatpāda's *Vivarana* (1.30) states that they are equally injurious (*tulya-pratyanīka*), because they engender states of mind (rather than help transcend the mind itself). According to Nāgojī Bhatta's *Vritti*, these nine are produced by *rajas* and *tamas* and lead to a "state of multiple fluctuations" (*aneka-vrittitva*) of consciousness. The *Mani-Prabhā* declares: "They distract the mind and make it fall from Yoga." This is echoed in the *Yoga-Sudhākara-Candrikā*, which speaks of them as "obstructions" (*vighna*).

What are the nine obstacles in detail? In the following, I will use the statements found in the various Sanskrit commentaries on the *Yoga-Sūtra* to shed light on this question.

ILLNESS (*Vyādhi*)

Vyādhi is left undefined by the author of the *Yoga-Sūtra*, but the word has the simple meaning of "disease," "illness," "sickness," or "disorder." It is derived from the prefixes *vi* and *ā* and the verbal root *dhā*, meaning "to stand apart," or "be scattered." Vyāsa explains the word as "an imbalance of the 'instruments' [i.e., the sense organs], the secretions, or the humors." Vācaspati explains: "The humors—wind, bile, and phlegm—are [so called] because of their sustaining the body. Secretion is a special modification of food that is eaten or drunk. The 'instruments' are the senses. An imbalance in them is a condition of deficiency or excess." The *Bhoja-Vritti* gives "fever, etc." as an example of a cause for such imbalance, as do the *Candrikā* and the *Yoga-Sudhākara*. Bhāva Ganesha has *kapha* instead of *shleshma*—both meaning "phlegm"—and explains *karana* (instrument) as "skin, eyes, etc." He paraphrases *vaishamya* (imbalance) as "loss of essence" (*svabhāva-pracyava*), that is, forfeiture of the natural balance or health of the body. The *Yoga-Sudhākara* likewise speaks of the three *doshas* (i.e., the humors or *dhātus*).

Shankara Bhagavatpāda has "imbalance is the condition of inequity (*vishama-bhāva*)." He further explains that the imbalance is due to "the excessive employment of one or the other substance, etc." He adds that a *dhātu* may increase of its own accord or by outside factors. Shankara Bhagavatpāda speaks of seven kinds of *rasa*: plasma (also called *rasa*), blood (*lohita*), fat (*medas*), flesh (*māmsa*), bone (*asthi*), marrow (*majjā*), and semen (*shukla*). "Imbalance of the [sensory] instruments," according to him, refers to blindness, deafness, and so forth. Vijnāna Bhikshu, again, states that when Vyāsa has *saha iti* (together with [the mental fluctuations]), then it should be understood that there is no complete simultaneity, but that Vyāsa has ignored the very small fraction of time between the presentation of an obstacle and its disturbing effects on the mind.

APATHY (*Styāna*)

Styāna (from the verbal root *styā* meaning "to grow dense") is mental apathy. The *Yoga-Bhāshya* (1.30) defines it as "inactivity of the mind." Vācaspati has "incapacity for action." Vijnāna Bhikshu explains *akarmanyatā* or inactivity as follows: "Inactivity is an inability to perform Yoga. Even though [there may be] inactivity of the body [due to] constipation, etc., [there is] no obstruction to Yoga relative to the mind. Hence [Vyāsa] stated 'for the mind.'" Shankara Bhagavatpāda simply quotes the *Yoga-Bhāshya* and so does Bhoja, while Bhāva Ganesha and Nāgoji Bhatta follow Vācaspati Mishra's exegesis. The *Mani-Prabhā* has "laziness is an incapacity for action even when there is longing [for it] in the mind." The *Candrikā* has simply "laziness is inactivity," while the *Yoga-Sudhākara* has more specifically "laziness is inactivity of the mind." This could be interpreted as procrastination, a form of mental inertia by which action is postponed.

DOUBT (*Samshaya*)

From earliest times, doubt has been named one of the major obstacles to spiritual realization. We can only come to know Reality, declares the *Brihad-Āranyaka-Upanishad* (4.4.23), when we are free from doubt. The *Bhagavad-Gītā* (4.40) states that doubt afflicts the person who lacks faith (*shraddhā*). Its effect can be devastating and ultimately even self-destructive. The *Matsya-Purāna* (110.10) notes that the doubting individual reaps suffering rather than Yoga.

The *Yoga-Bhāshya* (1.30) explains: "Doubt is knowledge touching on both extremes [of a dilemma] such as 'this might be so, this might not be so.'" Vācaspati Mishra has "Even though there is this by means of staying in the form, doubt and error there being nondifference both extremes touching and nontouching." Shankara Bhagavatpāda states: "Doubt is the notion touching on the two extremes of the dilemma whether there is a post or a man." This is a classic Vedānta example to illustrate the vacillation experienced in the mental state of doubt: We see something at a remote distance and are not sure of its identity. It could be a wooden post or a human being.

Our life is filled with such perceptual uncertainties, but more important are those uncertainties that are not merely perceptual but cognitive: Is there an eternal Self or not? Am I identical with the body or not? And so forth.

HEEDLESSNESS (*Pramāda*)

The yogic path depends on mindfulness and is thwarted by heedlessness, or carelessness. The *Yoga-Bhāshya* (1.30) explains this fault as "not cultivating the means of ecstasy," which can be understood as a lack of self-application. Shankara Bhagavatpāda glosses this with "a lack of persistence."

SLOTH (*Ālasya*)

If *styāna* is mental apathy, *ālasya* is laziness due to physical heaviness (such as from overeating). According to the *Yoga-Bhāshya* (1.30), it is lack of effort owing to heaviness of the body and the mind, which, Vācaspati Mishra informs us, respectively spring from a preponderance of phlegm and the presence of *tamas*, Nature's principle of inertia. This interpretation, however, does not allow us to adequately distinguish *ālasya* from *styāna*. Unfortunately, none of the commentaries is very helpful on this point.

DISSIPATION (*Avirati*)

Virati stems from the verbal root *ram* meaning "to stop" but also "to delight in." It means "cessation," often in the sense of "renunciation," but at the same time it is closely related to *rati*, meaning "sexual pleasure." *Avirati* is here intended as the opposite of "cessation," and many translators have chosen "dissipation" to convey the meaning of this Sanskrit term. James Houghton Woods, however, translated it as "worldliness," on the strength of the *Yoga-Bhāshya* (1.30), which defines the word as "the mind's greed in the form of attachment to things." The mechanism of attachment and greed was articulated long ago in the *Bhagavad-Gītā* (2.62–63):

> When a man contemplates objects, attachment to them is produced. Attachment creates desire, and desire leads to anger.
>
> Anger gives rise to confusion. Confusion results in loss of mindfulness. Loss of mindfulness destroys wisdom. As a result of the destruction of wisdom, he perishes.

The *Bhagavad-Gītā* (2.64) also provides a counter-measure: to roam among the sense objects with the mind and senses under control. In the Vedānta tradition, the term *uparati* (quiescence) is often used to indicate the kind of nonattachment that the sage is asked to cultivate in order to overcome negative emotions and attitudes, not least the penchant for dissipation (*avirati*).

FALSE VISION (*Bhrānti-Darshana*)

Even though doubt is a significant block on the yogic path and brings with it a certain emotional distress (unsettledness), it is potentially a jumping board for a deeper vision and certainty. By contrast, false vision involves a (premature) sense of certainty and therefore does not share doubt's agony; yet it is potentially more seriously damaging. For false vision is basically an error (*viparyaya*). The *Yoga-Bhāshya* (1.30) explains that if a Yoga practitioner were to mistakenly think of a particular stage of yogic attainment as adequate or sufficient, he or she would automatically cease to grow spiritually. Only clear understanding, or what is called "discernment" (*viveka*), can serve as a reliable guide on the razor-edge path to liberation.

NONATTAINMENT OF THE STAGES (*Alabdha-Bhūmikatva*)

Progress on the yogic path varies from person to person and depends on the individual's psychological capacity and, at a deeper level, his or her *karma*. Whatever we represent at the present moment is because of our past volitions (whether or not expressed at the physical level). Our DNA is the product of the sum total of our karmic past, and so, according to Yoga, are our life circumstance and the experiences that we have and that impinge on us. Since much of what we call "mind" depends on brain functions and since our brain is DNA driven, our mental life too is largely determined by our *karma*. Were it not for our essential nature (i.e., the Self or *purusha*), which is transcendental and eternally free, we would be complete robots. By consistently choosing the Self, or pure Consciousness, we can overcome our karmic baggage. Choosing the Self translates as cultivating mindfulness and deactivating negative thoughts, emotions, and attitudes.

This is a gradual process that, according to Yoga philosophy, extends over many lifetimes and involves many instances of apparent failure. Life is a school, and unless we learn from our mistakes we must repeat the same lesson over and over again. Persistence is key to success in Yoga. As the *Yoga-Sūtra* (1.13) states:

> . . . [practice] is firmly grounded [only after it has been] cultivated properly and for a long time uninterruptedly.

Those who have not yet acquired the necessary stamina and determination are unable to reach the next higher stage or level in the unfolding spiritual process. Also a sudden irruption of *karma*—perhaps in the form of sickness or other adversity—can prevent the Yoga practitioner from moving onward.

The *Yoga-Sūtra* (1.30) recognizes the inability to attain the next stage of inner growth as one of the nine obstacles. The *Yoga-Bhāshya* (1.30) tells us that by "stages" (*bhūmi*) are here meant the four stages that Vyāsa describes later in his commentary (3.51): (1) *prathama-kalpika* (initial phase), (2) *madhu-bhūmika*, which the *Yoga-Bhāshya* (1.30) also calls *madhu-matī* (honeyed), (3) *prajñā-jyotis* (wisdom-light), and (4) *atikrānta-bhāvanīya* (in the process of transcending [everything]).

The *prathama-kalpika-yogin* is the practitioner (*abhyāsin*) for whom the inner light is just dawning. The *madhu-bhūmika-yogin* has the truth-bearing wisdom (*ritam-bharā prajñā*) mentioned in the *Yoga-Sūtra* (1.48), which is as sweet or precious as honey. The *prajñā-jyotir-yogin* is in full control of the bodily organs and the elements and is completely capable of realizing the remaining stage. The *atikrānta-bhāvanīya-yogin* transcends everything, and has as his only purpose the resolution (*pratisarga*) of the mind back into the transcendental core of Nature (*prakriti*).

To complicate matters, the *Yoga-Bhāshya* (1.1) also applies, as noted above, the term *bhūmi* to the levels of mental activity, and hence the legitimate question poses itself, which set of stages is intended. Since Patanjali is not specific, nonattainment of a given stage or instability in it may be taken to refer to any stage whatsoever. The author of the *Yoga-Bhāshya* (1.30), however, clearly has the above four levels in mind.

INSTABILITY (*Anavasthitatva*)

If attaining a particular stage of Yoga is difficult, stably remaining in it is an even greater challenge for most practitioners. The higher the stage (*bhūmi*), the more energy (commitment, one-pointedness, etc.) it takes to attain and maintain it. Yogic folklore (especially as found in the *Purānas*) is filled with stories of *yogins* who, after reaching great spiritual heights, took a steep fall out of attachment or pride. There is no real safe stage until liberation is attained. *Anavasthitatva* is the negative of *avasthitatva* (stability), which is formed of the prefix *ava*, the verbal root *sthā* (to stand, abide), and the suffix *tva* ("-ness/-ty"). All of Yoga can be looked upon as an effort to achieve stability in the midst of the unending fluctuations (*vritti*) and transformations (*parināma*) of Nature. Ultimate stability is found only in the transcendental Self, which is considered to possess *aparināmitva* or "immobility" or constancy.

Patanjali is not content with listing the nine obstacles; he makes the following additional statement in his *Yoga-Sūtra* (1.31):

> Pain, depression, tremor of the limbs, [faulty] inhalation and exhalation are accompanying [symptoms] of the distractions.

When, through inattention or the fructification of karma, one or more of the nine obstacles are encountered, these often have unpleasant repercussions. Patanjali names the following four: pain, depression, tremor of the limbs, and faulty breathing.

PAIN (*Duhkha*)

Yoga is designed to help the practitioner overcome suffering (*duhkha*). Yet when he or she falls prey to any of the obstacles, the practitioner exacerbates rather than reduces his or her experience of suffering, or pain. The word *duhkha* is composed of *dur* (bad) and *kha* (space/axle hole) and literally means "having a bad axle-hole," that is, having or being a wheel that is out of balance. The opposite of *duhkha* is *sukha*, which is derived from *su* (good) and *kha*. A contemporary English rendering would be "good space." The dictionary meaning of *sukha* is "joy," "ease," or "pleasure." All nine obstacles are apt to lead to pain or suffering. In fact, they are associated with a mind that is experiencing limitation and thus suffering. In sickness, *duhkha* might be on the physical level but more likely also on the mental level. Or a Yoga practitioner might experience doubt, which brings its own form of suffering. Languor, again, often has painful consequences, as does heedlessness, sloth, and dissipation. It is also easy to see how not attaining a particular stage or losing one's hold on it is attendant with pain.

The *Yoga-Bhāshya* (1.31) describes pain or suffering (*duhkha*) as being threefold: (1) *ādhyātmika* — self-caused, (2) *ādhibhautika* — caused by other beings, and (3) *ādhidaivika* — caused by deities or natural forces (acts of God).

DEPRESSION (*Daurmanasya*)

When obstacles visit a practitioner, it is difficult for him or her to cultivate a positive attitude. Often the *yogin* or *yoginī* becomes discouraged, which leads to emotional collapse, as Arjuna experienced it on the battlefield in the company of his *guru*, Lord Krishna (see the description in the *Bhagavad-Gītā*). Arjuna was overcome with compassion (*kripā*) for his kinsfolk and grieved for them at the prospect of their imminent slaughter. Krisha admonished the prince to shed his grief (*shoka*) and not to succumb to attachment (*rāga*), faint-heartedness (*hridaya-daurbalya*), or the "state of a eunuch" (*klaibya*). In the final analysis, dejection (*vishāda*) or what Patanjali calls depression (*daurmanasya*) is a form of self-indulgence and a failure to practice self-transcendence.

TREMOR OF THE LIMBS (*Angam-Ejayatva*)

The *Bhagavad-Gītā* (1.29) describes Arjuna as trembling in the face of his dilemma. We also tremble out of anger, or really whenever our nervous system is overstimulated. Thus tremor of the limbs is the external manifestation of mental agitation (*kshobha*).

FAULTY INHALATION AND EXHALATION (*Shvāsa-Prashvāsa*)

The traditional commentaries seem to understand the compound *shvāsa-prashvāsa* simply as the involuntary breathing that happens unless we practice deliberate breath control (*prānāyāma*). It would seem, however, that Patanjali had something more in mind: the kind of irregular breathing pattern that comes with mental agitation, which we can characterize as "faulty." This word cannot be found in the *Yoga-Sūtra* but, from the context, seems implied in the compound *shvāsa-prashvāsa*.

The nine obstacles can be directly tackled at the level of the mind. Yet undoubtedly body-based interventions—such as proper diet and exercise—can help as well. But to acknowledge and make use of such physical remedies, we must already have a certain degree of correct view (*samyag-darshana*). All the many practices of Yoga form an integrated whole, but we must begin somewhere. Fortunately, the Yoga tradition offers many options for taking the first step and then steadfastly cultivating our spiritual practice.

❧ 35 ❧
In Praise of Study

KNOWLEDGE IS POWER. But is it? Personally I think this popular maxim is grossly misleading. Nevertheless, knowledge that leads to self-understanding is invaluable, because it is self-understanding that empowers us to live a life that is not dictated by the mechanism of our unconscious. And this is what Yoga and all other spiritual traditions are ultimately about.

Hence in the Yoga tradition *study* is considered an important means of self-knowledge. The Sanskrit word for study is *svādhyāya*, which means literally "one's own (*sva*) going into (*adhyāya*)." It stands for the serious and systematic study of the Yoga tradition and of oneself. Both knowledge of the tradition and self-knowledge go hand in hand. The traditional scriptures contain the distilled wisdom of sages who have climbed to the pinnacle of self-knowledge, and therefore these texts can contribute to our own self-knowledge. Study, in the yogic sense, is always a journey of self-discovery, self-understanding, and self-transcendence. Since ancient times, it has been a regular component of the yogic path. Patanjali, in his *Yoga-Sūtra* (2.32), lists it as one of the constituent practices of self-restraint (*niyama*), the second "limb" of his eightfold path.

Study is an integral part of Yoga's pragmatic orientation. Yoga does not call for blind faith, though it stresses the superlative importance of real, deep faith (*shraddhā*), or trust. Mere belief cannot help us realize that which abides beyond the conditional or egoic personality. Instead, Yoga has always been intensely experimental and experiential, and study is one aspect of this sound approach. In the *Vishnu-Purāna* (6.6.2), an old encyclopedic Sanskrit work, we read:

> From study one should proceed to practice (*yoga*), and from practice to study. The supreme Self is revealed through perfection in study and practice.

Many Western Yoga practitioners, especially those with a dominant right brain, shy away from study. They would much rather learn a new breathing technique or polish their performance of one or the other posture. Yet, it would seem they often miss the mark, because they do not know the proper context in which these techniques must be cultivated. Often they do not even have an accurate knowledge of the techniques themselves. They sometimes seek to compensate for their ignorance by trying to reinvent the wheel and producing their own versions of yogic practices. While innovation is commendable—our whole civilizational adventure is based on it—in the case of Yoga, we would do well to be modest; after all, the Yoga tradition can look back upon at least 5,000 years of intense experimentation.

Just as a predominantly right-brain (action-driven) approach to Yoga has its pitfalls, a purely left-brained (thought-driven) approach is equally precarious, if not altogether futile. "Armchair Yoga" cannot replace actual experience. If our practice is merely nominal, so will be our attainments. In Yoga, both theory and practice form a continuum, like space-time. It requires from us a full engagement, as the Buddhists put it: with body, speech, and mind. Yoga, as the *Bhagavad-Gītā* (2.48) reminds us, is balance (*samatva*). Hence we ought to engage both cerebral hemispheres when applying ourselves to the yogic path. Let us also recall here that one of the meanings of the word *yoga* is "integration."

An ancient scripture, the *Shata-Patha-Brāhmana* (11.5.7.1), declares that, for serious students, study is a source of joy. It focuses the student's mind and lets him or her sleep peacefully. It also yields insight and the capacity to master life. What more could one ask for?

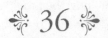

36

Silence Is Golden
The Practice of Mauna

Most of us know the age-old saying, "Speech is silvern, silence is golden." But what does it mean? We seldom reflect on our ancient wisdom anymore, and so we fail to notice many useful things that people were once taught by their elders. On one level, the maxim simply means that silence is better than speech. But, as I will show, there is another, deeper, meaning to it. Let us begin with the obvious, however. Why should silence be better than speech? When we speak, after all, we communicate with others, which is to say, we are in relationship. Silence, on the other hand, can cause awkwardness and misunderstanding. At least, this is how some might view the situation.

But how often do we communicate falsehoods in our speech? Or how frequently do we fail to communicate adequately? That is, how often do we misunderstand each other as a result of the spoken word? The answer is: most of the time. We can easily test this fact by playing a party game, which could be called "rumor": We whisper a message in someone's ear. That person has to pass the message on to the next person in the same way, and so on. By the time the message reaches us again, we will be surprised to find how little is left of our original message. Speech frequently distorts information, because the speaker seldom pays attention to what he or she is saying, and the listener generally is listening with only one ear.

Sacred speech stands in striking contrast to casual speech. In sacred speech, both speaker and listener are attentive to what is being communicated. Hence in the spiritual traditions of humanity, which originally were oral traditions, the sacred teachings have been remarkably well preserved from generation to generation. Memorization was a sacred art and obligation. The invention of books has undermined this art.

We may recall here the primary meaning of the Greek word *mythos*, which stands for the sacred utterance or story told by the tribal elder who had been initiated into the secrets of life. This word stems from the verb *mytheomai*, meaning "to talk, to speak." But, significantly, its root *mu* has yielded another word, *myein*, which means "to close." Thus, myth implies both the closing, or guarding, of the mouth in order to receive the inner, visionary revelation, and the opening of the mouth in order to communicate that revelation. On this point, the Swiss cultural philosopher Jean Gebser offered significant insights in his epochal work *The Ever-Present Origin*.[1]

Silence, to be sure, also is a kind of communication. Therefore it can be either understood correctly or misinterpreted. People are silent for many reasons: to withhold information, to feel superior, to repress their feelings, to stand off from a difficult situation, to underscore what they have just said, to communicate feelings with their eyes or other parts of their bodies, to feel more intensely, to express disapproval, and so on.

But there is another kind of silence, which, in India, is known as *mauna*. This Sanskrit word is generally translated as "silence," but it conveys much more to native speakers of Sanskrit. It stems from the same verbal root as the word *manas*, meaning "mind." The root is *man*, meaning "to ponder" but also "to meditate." *Mauna* is not simply "thinking." On the contrary, it is the absence of thought, while being intensely present in the inner environment. *Mauna* is sacred silence. It is meditation.

The practitioner of *mauna* is called a *muni*. Now, a *muni* is never described as an individual who is merely silent. Rather, he is known as an ecstatic. Thus we may ask: What have sacred silence and ecstasy in common? In sacred silence, we transcend our human condition. We stand (*stasis*) outside (*ex*) our ordinary egoic personality. This self-transcendence fulfills itself in the state of ecstasy, in which our psychic conditioning is temporarily suspended in utter bliss.

The spiritual discipline of silence—and it *is* a discipline or a voluntary self-chastening—is thus not merely the absence of speech or utterance. What appears from the outside to be a negative condition is inwardly experienced as an immense richness, or fullness. For the discipline of silence is practiced not only in regard to the organ of speech, but also in regard to the mind itself. It includes the silencing of the mental chatter that characterizes the ordinary person. This deep inner silence is experienced as peace and, ultimately, as an abundance of bliss. As the British essayist Thomas Carlyle, in his work *Sartor Resartus* (1834), put it, "Silence is the element in which great things fashion themselves together."

Sacred silence, then, is an activity that is really a counteractivity, for it engenders stillness. It is stillness. And that stillness opens up the dimension of spiritual existence—that luminous world that awaits our discovery as soon as we redirect our attention from external things to our own radiant depths. In the *Īsha-Upanishad* (vs. 17), an esoteric Hindu text composed in the centuries before Christ, the anonymous author prays:

> The face of Truth is covered with a golden lid. Remove it,
> O Fosterer, for him who adheres to the Truth.

Sacred silence leads to and beyond the lustrous "golden orb" in the nucleus of our own being. Through silence, we traverse the bright inner dimensions until we penetrate to the blinding Light of the ultimate Reality itself, and become one with It. *So'ham,* "I am He," declared the Upanishadic sages in their rapture.

In many spiritual traditions, this transcendental Reality is symbolized by the Sun. The reason for this is not far to seek: Like the Sun, the transcendental Reality is experienced by the mystics of all ages as life-giving and radiant. It is Life itself. As one Upanishadic sage put it long ago, it is by the power of that Reality that the Sun and all the myriad other stars do their work.

Silence is not merely a discipline; rather, it is primarily a state of being. It is in, through, and as silence that we discover our authentic identity, the Self *(ātman, purusha).* Thus silence partakes of the golden nature of the ultimate Reality. By comparison, speech is like the silver-bodied Moon, which has no light of its own but is illuminated by the radiance of the Sun.

Through silence we can attune ourselves to the supreme stillness of the single Being, which is utter silence that is never disrupted by sound. Jean Klein, a twentieth-century exponent of Advaita Vedānta, comments:

> The Self is silent awareness and cannot be defined in terms of a silence as opposed to noise. How should we react towards silence or its opposite? If you want to rid yourself of agitation so as to attain a state of silence, you reject, you fight, you defend yourself. But if on the contrary you were to accept it, the agitation—which is part of this silence—will disappear within it. Then you will reach the silence of the Self, beyond silence and agitation.[2]

Once that great, sustaining Reality has been discovered, all our actions, thoughts, and utterances become spontaneous signals of that infinite silence, which is sheer bliss. Thus, the words of the enlightened adepts have transformative power, because they address that part in us which instinctively knows of that unsurpassed silence.

Just as in ordinary life, speech and silence are intimately interwoven, so also in spiritual life do they complement one another. This has been recognized particularly in Taoism. In the language of the *I Ching*, speech is *yang*, or the masculine pole of silence; silence is *yin*, or the feminine pole. Together they are responsible for the creativity of human interaction. In spiritual life we cultivate sacred silence to regenerate our inner being so that we can return to our daily activities and to speech from a new perspective.

In his monumental work *A Study of History*, the great British historian Arnold Toynbee has written about the creative withdrawal of the spiritual heroes of the past—the founders and inspirers of religions. They sought out the wilderness in order to find the fountain of truth within their own being. Then they returned, strengthened and ready to uplift humanity by sharing with others their extraordinary discovery. "Silence," said Ovid, "is strength." We need not have the spiritual standing of a Moses, Jesus, Mahāvīra, or Gautama the Buddha to practice sacred silence and benefit from it.

✤ 37 ✤
Die While You Live and Last-Hour Yoga

THERE IS AN OFT-QUOTED verse in the *Bhagavad-Gītā* (8.6) that is widely understood as declaring that a person's last thought on the death-bed determines his or her postmortem destiny. In Juan Mascáro's popular English translation, the stanza in question reads as follows:

> For on whomsoever one thinks at the last moment of life,
> unto him in truth he goes, through sympathy with his nature.

On first hearing, this sounds as if death furnishes us with a magic wand by which we can transmogrify ourselves into absolutely anything that captures our imagination when we draw the last breath, even divinity. And this is in fact how popular Indian tradition has caricatured the God-man Krishna's utterance. In the following I will show that Krishna's teaching is less comical but far more subtle and practically demanding.

To begin with, we must note that if indeed the more facile interpretation were correct, we would have to discard one of the fundamental principles of Krishna's metaphysics, namely the idea that the cosmos is a process guided by an immutable moral law. It would be perfectly feasible to picture, for example, the following extreme case: A mass murderer who, until the penultimate moment of his life, pursues his ugly trade and then, cunning as he is, spends his very last instant of embodiment thinking about the Absolute. In keeping with a simplistic exegesis of Krishna's word, the murderer would most certainly become instantly coessential with the ultimate Reality. His string of heinous crimes would be forgiven and forgotten in an instant, and he would be rewarded with unexcelled bliss. This possibility rightly offends our sense of justice.

Let us frame another extreme case: A saint who, until the penultimate moment of his life, has not once transgressed the moral laws of the universe, dies in a car accident and his very last thought is one of compassion for the unfortunate driver—the mass murderer of our previous example who is also killed. In terms of the popular interpretation, the saint's fate is definitely sealed. He would take a very steep fall from the heights of spiritual attainment to which he had ascended through life-long struggle.

It seems improbable that Krishna should have taught such an outrageous doctrine, which would make nonsense of his whole ethical teaching, the path of Yoga, and the orderliness of creation. So, what did Krishna really say all those many centuries ago? A more literal rendering than Juan Mascáro's widely read paraphrase provides important clues:

> Whatever state of existence he remembers when at last he sheds the body, even that [state of existence] does he attain, O son-of-Kunti, always forced to become that state of existence.

First of all, we find that the enlightened adept Krishna does not speak, as the above-quoted translator would have it, of "someone" upon whom one should fix one's mind, but of a "state of existence" (*bhāva*). Furthermore, there is a world of difference between "thinking" about something and "remembering" it, which is Krishna's well-chosen term.

Now, "state of existence" is not just anything. Rather, the word denotes a whole *category* of existential possibilities within the immeasurable Body Divine. In the most radical sense there are only two major *bhāvas*, or levels of being: the mutable (*kshara*) or impermanent realm and the immutable (*akshara*). From our human perspective, the first level is of course the space-time universe, which is the familiar arena of our conditioned experiencing. But the world as we know it is but the outer shell of a vastly more magnificent structure of hierarchically interlocking levels of existence. At the apex of it all, pervading and upholding the entire creation, is the Immutable, or Divine.

The *Bhagavad-Gītā* distinguishes three more subordinate levels. Closest to the Divine, which is Krishna in his true nature, are the innumerable transcendental Selves called *ātman* (Self) or *akshara-purusha* (immutable Person). This multitude of eternal Selves forms as it were the cells of the Divine Body. These Selves are also referred to as the Divine Person's "higher nature" (*parā-prakriti*). When these eternally free Selves are associated with particular body-minds, they become *kshara-purushas* or "perishable persons," or finite psyches. These are the many individuals in bondage to the material universe. Ourselves.

In Yoga metaphysics, the cosmos is conceived as a composite of three cardinal levels of existence. Over and above the material realm there is a vast suprasensible world that is the level of the mind or subtle body. This extends up to the very matrix (*prakriti-pradhāna*) of the objective universe, the playground of the transcendental Selves. Diagrammatically, this progressive inclusiveness looks as follows:

1. The Whole, Lord Krishna, the Supreme Person (*purushottama*)
2. The countless transcendental Selves (*purusha*)
3. The transcendental ground of the world (*brahman = prakriti-pradhāna*)
4. The various suprasensible realms (*sūkshma-loka*)
5. The material universe, or coarse realm (*sthūla-loka*)

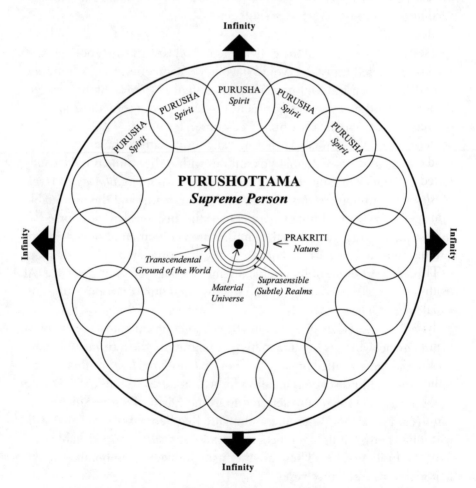

The Ultimate Reality and Its Manifestations According to the Bhagavad-Gītā

Looked at differently, these various levels are possibilities of "bodily" existence. Depending on which "body," or state of existence, we set our heart on, we will obtain that very form of embodiment once we have quit our present physical vehicle. Thus we may resume a human form, become an angelic being *(deva)* inhabiting the subtle realm, sink into the cosmic matrix itself as a *prakriti-laya,* or recover our true identity as the Self in the blissful "company" of the Divine Person, Lord Krishna.

The phrase "to set one's heart on something" is perhaps more expressive of the intended meaning of "remembering" than is "thinking." The latter has too abstract a flavor, while the former is indicative of a deep-level process. This becomes clear when one realizes that one of the synonyms of "meditation" is in fact "remembering."

Meditative remembering means sending taproots down into the hidden recesses of our being, into the depth-mind *(buddhi).* The depth-mind is the storehouse of the essence (i.e., karmic deposits) of our world experience. It has been likened to a net whose knots are the impressions left behind by our volitional activity.

Meditation is a partial enactment of the process of dying. Conversely, death is the meditative process taken to its logical conclusion. At death, the mind disentangles itself from the physical body, and the center of identity is shifted to the subtle vehicle—the so-called astral body or "subtle vehicle" *(sūkshma-sharīra).* The quintessence of the contents of the mind, in the form of the subliminal impressions *(samskāra)* stored away in the depth-mind, is the factor that determines the after-death fate of the deceased according to the iron-law of moral retribution or *karma.*

This event is a kind of "remembering," for it is by the power of the depth-mind, the hidden memory, that justice is done to the virtuous individual and the sinner alike, each according to his or her deeds or, more precisely, volitions. People who have been on the verge of death, or who have been resuscitated after having been clinically dead, often report that they saw their life's journey flash past their inner eye. Everything is stored away in the mind.

We can easily imagine what this remembering on the threshold of death would consist of in the case of an ordinary man. He would be presented with fleeting scenes from his childhood, his adolescence, his love affairs, marriages, career, and leisure activities, his role as a parent, friend, and colleague. He would momentarily relive all the joyous and sad moments of his life and understand their deeper significance. He would recognize an overall pattern that is the essential structure informing his mode of existence in the hereafter and his eventual rebirth.

Self-transcending spiritual practitioners will undoubtedly have many of the above experiences in common with worldly individuals. But they will presumably look back upon fewer missed opportunities for self-improvement and inner growth. In their depth-mind there will be powerful impressions that are incompatible with re-embodiment in the material realm. If the practitioners are advanced, these subliminal activators (*samskāra*) will outweigh all others. Individuals who have always lived typical human lives invite rebirth (*punar-janman*) as typical human beings. But those Yoga practitioners who model their whole existence not on mere human standards but on the ultimate Reality will, if they have succeeded in setting up incisive enough impressions in their depth-memory, merge with that Reality.

And if these practitioners are sufficiently advanced on the spiritual path, they will be able to monitor the process of dying and so ensure that no vestiges remain in their depth-mind, which would force them to assume another physical body. In fact, the conscious departure from this world is one of the sure marks by which one can recognize a genuine *yogin* or *yoginī*. The Self-realized adept regards the body like a vessel that is engulfed by space, both within and without, the space being the omnipresent Reality itself.

Death does not shake an adept in the least. Many moving stories are told by disciples who have witnessed their *guru's* exit from the world—"with a single breath" and a smile. A dying *yogin* in agony or a state of stupor is almost a contradiction in terms. The maxim holds: Show me how you die, and I show you who you are.

But, the reader may ask, what if the Yoga adept drowns unexpectedly or is killed by a stray bullet? Will the element of surprise not outwit him or her? The traditional answer is a most emphatic No. There can be no surprise for the enlightened being—hence the smile. Otherwise we would have to assume that the universe is ruled by chance, which is an assumption that is explicitly rejected by the Yoga masters.

In whichever way the masters of Yoga take leave from this world—and, as the poet knew, death has ten thousand doors—they will have foreknowledge of their death. There are too many well-attested examples for this to be purely fictional icing on the cake of hagiolatry. How such knowledge is obtained remains a mystery that need not concern us here.

The process of conscious exit from the body, however, is not a secret—at least not in principle. The archaic *Chāndogya-Upanishad* (8.6.5–6) discloses the following:

Now, when he thus departs from this body, then he ascends upward with these rays [of the Sun]. Uttering [the sacred syllable] *om*, he dies. As soon as the mind is cast off, he goes to the Sun. This, verily, is the "world door," an entry for the knowers, [but] a blockage for the ignorant.

On this there is the following verse:

There are a hundred and one channels of the heart. One of these runs to [the crown of] the head. Going up by it, one reaches immortality. The others are for departing to various [lower levels of being]; [they] are for departing to various [lower levels].

In conscious dying, attention is focused on the axial current of the body, or what is known as the *sushumnā-nādī*. This is the only pathway of the life energy *(prāna)* that extends from the lowest psychosomatic center (at the base of the spine) to the crown of the head, which is the location of the thousand-petaled lotus, the seat of the mystical Sun. This intense focusing of the mind and the life force within the central channel, and especially on its upper terminal in the head, coincides with the condition of ecstasy *(samādhi)*. Then, as the author of the *Hatha-Yoga-Pradīpikā* (4.17) observes, time stands still. Such knowledge is implied in the words of the God-man Krishna who, in the *Bhagavad-Gītā* (8.5, 9f.), admonishes his would-be devotee thus:

He who goes hence at the "end time," abandoning the body and remembering Me alone—he reaches My state of existence.

He who remembers the Ancient Bard, Governor [of all the world], smaller than the small, Supporter of all, of inconceivable form, Sun-colored [and abiding] beyond darkness—that [*yogin*], at the time of going-forth, with unmoving mind, yoked by love and by the power of Yoga, directing the life force *(prāna)* to [the spot in] the middle of the eyebrows, comes to that supreme divine Being.

The first verse of this passage includes a term that invites closer inspection. This is the Sanskrit word *anta-kāla*, which I have rendered literally as "end time." A more conventional translation would be "last hour," but "end time" has more instructive connotations. For the term *anta-kāla* is also used in regard to the final dissolution of creation during the onset of a cosmic "night," when the Creator is asleep and when all manifestation is resolved into a state of latency. By extension, *anta-kāla* can also be applied to the segments of the flux of events—those spells of creative respite of the world process that cause the pulse of life. Time, we know, is discontinuous. This modern insight has long been anticipated by the Yoga masters of yore who talked of time-quanta (*kshana*), which alone are imbued with reality, whereas time itself is but a mental construct.

What does this have to do with our main theme? If time is merely a series of infinitesimally small "instants," which are perceptible only to the *yogin*, then we must conclude that we die and are reborn in rapid succession. Life and death, in this view, are intimately and inseparably linked. If we now transfer Krishna's ethical imperative that we should remember him at the "end time" to this situation, we arrive at an important insight: We must remember the Divine Person not only when the Reaper knocks on our door, but in every moment of our life.

Students of the *Bhagavad-Gītā* know that this is precisely what Lord Krishna expects from his devotees. The vocation of the practitioner of Yoga is a full-time occupation. Only thus can he or she hope to conquer *kāla*— a Sanskrit word that means both "death" and "time."

Death borders upon our birth, and our cradle stands in the grave.
—JOSEPH HALL, *Epistles*

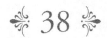

38

Living in the Dark Age (Kali-Yuga)

THE IDEA THAT WE live either at the brink of Armageddon or at the dawn of a new golden age was becoming ever more prominent as we approached the end of the second millennium C.E. Some critics acidly observed that people throughout the ages have always believed they were living in particularly crucial times. There is some truth to this criticism, because human history is indeed continuously decisive, for in humanity's march through time every step determines the future of our species. But only the cynic would sneer at the idea that some steps, some historical periods, are more decisive than others—not only in the shaping of a particular race or nation, but for humanity as a whole. Possibly one such decisive historical threshold was what the German philosopher and psychiatrist Karl Jaspers styled the "axial age"—the period between 800–500 B.C.E. when "thought turned back upon thought": the epoch of Confucius, Lao Tzu, Buddha, Zoroaster, Heraclitus, Plato, and Socrates.[1]

In the West, this development gradually led to what can only be described as the enthronement and autarchy of cold reason and the consequent suppression of nonrational modes of consciousness. As many contemporary thinkers have shown, this inflation of ratio lies at the root of today's moral and spiritual bankruptcy, and its disastrous effects can be witnessed all around us (and in us, if we care to look). What is perhaps most disheartening is that this lopsided orientation to life is now being thrust upon the "underdeveloped" world, which merely magnifies the existing threat to our planet's ecology and to the survival of countless life forms, not least our own human species. When we take stock of the folly of humankind we begin to realize the extent of the global problems induced, in the last analysis, by hypertrophied (egocentric) reason. We may also be impressed with the traditional Hindu explanation of the particular spirit of our era. For, according to the computations of the Hindu pundits, we are well into the "dawn phase" of the *kali-yuga*, or "dark age."

Like so many premodern mythologies, Hinduism views the evolution of humanity as a cyclical process of progressive moral degeneration from an original state of purity and spiritual wholeness. The Sanskrit sources distinguish four stages in this drama: (1) *Krita-yuga*, also called *satya-yuga*, the golden age of harmony and truth (*satya*), (2) *Tretā-yuga*, literally, the "age of the thrice (-lucky)," (3) *Dvāpara-yuga*, literally, the "age of the twice (-lucky)," and (4) *Kali-yuga*, literally, the "unlucky age.

This intriguing doctrine was elaborated in the late pre-Christian centuries, perhaps around the same time that the founding fathers of our Western civilization, the philosophers of Greece, Ionia, and Italy, started to express the new mode of consciousness. The strange-sounding designations for these four epochs (*yuga*) are explained by the fact that they were adopted from the earlier Vedic tradition, where they stood for certain throws of dice — *krita* being the most accomplished, or "luckiest," and *kali* being the unlucky throw. It is not clear how these gambling terms came to acquire their new meaning, but why they did can be gleaned from the respective duration postulated for each world age. This is best conveyed in tabular form:

	DIVINE YEARS	HUMAN YEARS
Krita-yuga-samdhyā (Morning Twilight Phase)	400	144,000
Krita-yuga	4,000	1,440,000
Krita-yuga-samdhyā-amsha (Evening Twilight Phase)	400	144,000
Tretā-yuga-samdhyā (Morning Twilight Phase)	300	108,000
Tretā-yuga	3,000	1,080,000
Tretā-yuga-samdhyā-amsha (Evening Twilight Phase)	300	108,000
Dvāpara-yuga-samdhyā (Morning Twilight Phase)	200	72,000
Dvāpara-yuga	2,000	720,000
Dvāpara-yuga-samdhyā-amsha (Evening Twilight Phase)	200	72,000
Kali-yuga-samdhyā (Morning Twilight Phase)	100	36,000
Kali-yuga	1,000	360,000
Kali-yuga-samdhyā-amsha (Evening Twilight Phase)	100	36,000
	12,000 =	4,320,000

From the above tabulation we can see that while the *krita-yuga* comes in fours, the *tretā-yuga* is based on a computation of threes and the *dvāpara–yuga* of twos. The world ages are thus considered progressively less auspicious. The computation further indicates that we are dealing here with "divine years" which, when translated into human terms, yield immense spans of time.

But Hindu chronology does not stop there. The four world ages are collectively known as a *mahā-yuga* or "great age," and it is thought that two thousand of these supercycles form but a single dawn and night (called *kalpa*) in the life of the Creator (God Brahma). His life-span extends over a "century," that is, a period of 311,040,000,000,000 human years. At the demise of the Creator, the whole manifest universe becomes dissolved. After an immeasurable period, the process is reversed and the whole cycle of space-time existence starts all over again. A truly awesome vision! It leaves no doubt about the utter insignificance of the human race, never mind the individual.

Only liberated beings (*jīvan-mukta*) have cause for humor, for they alone stand well clear of this cosmic *perpetuum mobile*. Their dissolution is not merely a temporary respite from the whirling wheel of existence, but it amounts to a permanent establishment in the transcendental condition of Being-Consciousness-Bliss. This unsurpassable attainment is called "absolute dissolution" (*atyantika-pralaya*) and is distinct from both *pralaya* and *mahā-pralaya*.

Where do we of today stand in this immense time game? As I have mentioned already, we find ourselves in the opening phase of the last of the four world ages. According to the Hindu mythochronologers, the present *kali-yuga* (morning twilight phase) commenced on February 18, 3102 B.C.E. This date is supposed to mark the memorable battle on the *kuru-kshetra*, the great war recorded in the *Mahābhārata* epic. Some traditional authorities, however, place the beginning slightly later to commemorate the ascension of the incarnate God Krishna, thirty-six years after the Bharata war. There are several more views, however, that converge on roughly the same century. But these differences are of marginal significance only.

What is of interest here is the characterization of the *yugas* in general and of the *kali-yuga* in particular. We find that the descriptions are remarkably uniform in the various scriptures dealing with the world ages, such as the *Smritis* (ritual texts), the *Mahābhārata* epic, the *Purānas* (popular encyclopedias), and also works on astronomy. The following is a quotation from the *Mahābhārata* that describes our present era and the immediately preceding *yuga*, revealing a progressive deterioration of humanity's moral fiber.

Again, in the *dvāpara-yuga* the moral order *(dharma)* exists [only] half. [God] Vishnu becomes yellow, and the *Veda* is now fourfold [i.e., the original wisdom is split into the four Vedic hymnodies].

Thence, some [adhere to] four *Vedas*, others to three *Vedas*, or two *Vedas*, or a single *Veda*, while yet others have no hymns [at all].

Thus, owing to the broken traditions, rites become manifold and creatures, fond of austerities and almsgiving, become *rajas*-motivated[2].

Due to ignorance about the single *Veda*, the *Vedas* become multiple and because of the collapse of truth, few adhere to truthfulness.

Many diseases appear for those who have fallen from truth, and there are desires and disasters caused by fate. Afflicted by these, [some] men perform very severe austerities; others, filled with [worldly] desires or desiring heaven, conduct sacrifices.

Thus with the onset of the *dvāpara*, creatures perish through their lawlessness. In the *kali-yuga*, O Kaunteya, the moral order *(dharma)* exists by one quarter only.

With the onset of this *tamas*-motivated[3] age, O Keshava [i.e., God Vishnu] becomes black *(krishna)*. The Vedic ways of life end, and so do the moral order, sacrifice, and rites.

Plagues, disease, sloth, blemishes such as anger, as well as calamities, sickness, and afflictions prevail.

In the course of the *yugas*, the moral order diminishes increasingly. With the diminution of the moral order, the people *(loka)* diminish.

This description of the *kali-yuga* is not as daunting as it is in some other scriptures. But the message is clear enough: Ours is a sinister age. What thinking person would not agree? Can we not, by now, fill a whole library with tales of human foolishness, of humanity's thoughtless interference with the life-world and its almost unbelievable lack of concern for fellow beings, both human and nonhuman?

Is there no hope, then, for humankind? Is historian Oswald Spengler's dark prophecy of the decline of the West (and with it, also of the East) coming true?[4] Or are there, today, forces at work that countermand the *Zeitgeist*, the spirit of the age? This latter appears to be the case. It could not be otherwise. Or else our species would have perished long ago, right at the outset of the *kali-yuga*. The *kali-yuga*, then, does not signal *total* spiritual darkness or inevitable doom. Inverting a popular maxim, one can perhaps say that where there is shadow there is also light. Here and there, the present dark age is pierced by shafts of light. It is not without its benign counterbalancing influences.

According to the Hindu tradition, shortly before the dawn of the *kali-yuga*, on the first morning of one of the fiercest wars fought in antiquity, the Divine critically intervened in human affairs. It revealed itself in the form of the God-man Krishna, who acted as a charioteer on the side of Prince Arjuna's military force. Just before the first battle between the two mighty armies, representing good and evil respectively, Lord Krishna instructed the virtuous prince in spiritual matters. Krishna's message is of particular interest not least because it is a teaching that was framed in response to an imminent "holocaust"—the kind of disastrous human action that is typical of the *kali-yuga*. It requires no special imaginative skills to perceive the parallel between the fateful situation faced by Prince Arjuna and our present-day crisis. At that time—just as today—the evil machinations of a few power-hungry individuals with no regard for the larger good had created an intolerable situation demanding to be redressed. As is so often true, circumstances and human will conspired that this restoration of law and order should be accomplished by an all-out military confrontation.

Prince Arjuna, though born into the warrior estate, was at heart a peace-loving man. When the two colossal armies lined up on opposite sides, he began to have serious doubts about his task. It was not so much personal fear of death that swayed his heart but, rather, acute moral qualms. Has anyone the right, he wondered, to use force in order to promote the larger good? His dilemma was greatly aggravated by the fact that among those whom he was supposed to fight—maim and possibly kill—were kinsmen and revered teachers.

Arjuna's duty as a warrior was clear enough; he had to fight. But the moment he contemplated the larger implications of this action, he was terrified to abide by his decision to reconquer his lost kingdom. Arjuna's attitude is typical of human life itself. We are all the time engaged in decision-making or in decision-avoidance. The more consciously we live, the more we realize that life is really an incessant stream of potential decisions.

Arjuna, as we know, did fight his war and also emerged victorious. But first he had to learn an important spiritual lesson. Lord Krishna, who acted as his charioteer, convinced the prince that his whole confusion was the result of a faulty perspective. The God-man demonstrated to the prince that the problem that caused him such anxiety was a problem conjured up by the ego. It had no existence apart from the ego. The divine teacher made Arjuna understand that we can never transcend our circumstances merely by closing our eyes, by avoiding action, by dropping out. Even avoidance is an action, which will have its inevitable repercussions since avoidance is rooted in the ego.

What Lord Krishna recommended instead was a cognitive shift, a new view of the whole matter: away from the delimiting, anxious ego and toward the boundless Self. All action must be sacrifice, he explained. We must not hold on to any conventional ego-derived scheme. Only when we abandon the delusion that we, as ego-personalities, are the ultimate initiators of actions can we have knowledge of what is truly right and good. That is to say, when we discover the "witness," the transcendental Self, we realize that life unfolds spontaneously and mysteriously, and that the ego is merely one of the countless forms arising within the flux of life.

For the Hindu authorities, the general deterioration of spirituality and the decline of humanity's psychological health in no way precludes the possibility of spiritual aspiration and success. It is nowhere denied that contemporary humanity, feeble as it may be in comparison to its ancestors, can swim against the stream. On the contrary, all spiritual teachings affirm that we must do our utmost to cultivate spiritual values in the midst of the great darkness surrounding us.

In fact, the tradition of Tantrism or Tantra, which emerged in the early post-Christian centuries, purports to be a spiritual discipline specifically for the dark age. It is clearly based on the belief that we can and must improve our spiritual destiny. Whatever the age, we are inherently capable of transcending the particular circumstances of our time. However dense the *kali-yuga* may become, human beings will always be able to conjure up within themselves the characteristics of the golden age, the *satya-yuga*, marked by freedom, joy, and love.

This is so because whatever degree of moral corruption may befall us, in our essence we are neither space-bound nor time-dependent. Therefore, by an act of will, we can always remove ourselves from the values and attitudes of our particular epoch or culture and cultivate those values and attitudes that reflect the purer characteristics of the *dvāpara-*, the *tretā-*, or even the *satya-yuga*. Yet, it appears, exceedingly few people today exercise their radical freedom to choose higher values and forms of life surpassing the conditions of the dark age. As we have learned from the above-quoted passage from the *Mahābhārata*, lethargy is a function of our time, which is ruled by *tamas*, or the principle of inertia.

The general pessimism of the Hindu mythochronologers is not shared by many Western enthusiasts of astrology. They celebrate the passage of the equinoxes through the constellation of Aquarius, in March 1948, as ushering in a new age in which humankind will come to fulfill its earthly destiny. The symbol of this new age is the Water Bearer who, with the Water of Immortality contained in a pitcher, irrigates and thus fertilizes Nature. This new era has been explained as coinciding with the realization of true humanity on earth: the unification of humankind through science and technology on one hand, and through the biological-spiritual ideal of "friendship" on the other. There are high hopes and expectations in new age circles.

This optimism has given rise both to a new mythology that tends toward the baroque and to a number of rather eccentric cults. There are, however, also more serious manifestations of new age thought, and these are slowly gaining influence in the larger society. They coexist side by side with the destructive forces of our age, which extend from rampant consumerism, scientific materialism, and technocratic ideology to religious fundamentalism, racism, and militarism.

One of the more sober efforts to articulate the *Zeitgeist* is found in the monumental study by the Swiss cultural philosopher Jean Gebser (1905–1973).[5] In his work *The Ever-Present Origin*, he presented a large body of evidence that something new is indeed trying to crystallize in our midst. In his penetrating analysis of the history of human consciousness, Gebser arrived at the startling conclusion that the present global crisis is but the outer reverberation of a drastic "mutation" of consciousness, the transformation of the dualistic-rational mode of world perception into what he calls the "integral" structure of consciousness. After a careful scrutiny of the sciences, music, architecture, painting, and—with particular illumination—language itself, Gebser discovered a host of significant signposts pointing out the direction that this emergent consciousness might take if we but nurture it. Whatever else it might bring about, it will first and foremost help us to actualize *ego-transcendence*. Gebser felt that without this realization humanity cannot possibly hope to master the problems that lie ahead.

It is reassuring that Gebser's general thesis, first conceived in 1932, has independently been voiced by at least two other intellectual giants—the

Hindu philosopher-sage Sri Aurobindo and the French priest and paleon-tologist Pierre Teilhard de Chardin.[6] Whereas Sri Aurobindo spoke of the descent of the "Supermind," Teilhard de Chardin invented the concept of the "Omega point," the spiritual evolutionary destiny of humanity. During the past two decades, numerous other thinkers have formulated their own version of what is happening today. I have discussed a cross-section of their work in my book *Structures of Consciousness*.[7] Our era's perils notwithstanding, many feel that we are witnessing a growing concern to create a more benign future for our species, which is an encouraging sign. What is more encouraging still is the fact that these voices are part of a small but increasingly vociferous minority. Should the spiritual wasteland become arable once again? Or are these hopeful signs only so many will-o'-the-wisps? Is the Aquarian Age only a sub-cycle within the larger cycle of the *kali-yuga*, or is the Hindu view simply in error?

Leaving aside for the moment certain occult reinterpretations of the *yugas* (which are drastically shortened to suit astrological purposes), a number of the *Purānas* contain a puzzling but undoubtedly significant statement. According to these Sanskrit scriptures, the whole bold structure of the *yuga* theory applies only to Bhāratavārsha, that is, India! Admittedly, this smacks of a critical afterthought by editors or scribes who have come into contact with non-Indian chronologies and obviously felt the need to justify their own native tradition. But their qualification is nonetheless fascinating.

Whatever the truth about the Hindu model of world ages may be, in determining our individual response to life we can rely neither on the *yuga* theory nor on any of the contending new age explanations of the spirit of our times. Rather, we must realize that, as individuals and to some extent as a group, we determine our own future. We can embody either the dark actualities of our age or its luminous potential. We can help shape gloom and doom or increase the light in the world. The choice is always ours.

39

Yoga and Terrorism

Our contemporary problems of overpopulation, pollution, ozone deple-
tion, dwindling of natural resources, threat of nuclear war, terrorism, and
so forth are global problems and require that we tackle them together.
Many of us—individuals and nations—are still trying to resist this globalization process, but it is inevitable if we are to survive as a species. No one
country or belief system can solve these problems independently. What
happens on the other side of the world can profoundly affect us where we
live. It is increasingly becoming apparent that the only solution to the
present world crisis is to build a global civilization, which requires a clearly
articulated view of one humanity.1

THE ABOVE SENTENCES were published in a 1995 book of mine. Two years
later, in *Lucid Waking,* I wrote about the presence of irrationality in our "rational" human society and particularly referred to the terrorist attack on innocent Japanese commuters by the Japanese Aum Shinrikyo sect. Since that
time, my thoughts have intermittently returned to the problem of terrorism.
The horrible terrorist attacks on September 11, 2001, killing thousands of
people on American soil, have brought the magnitude of the problem to the
attention of the whole world. I think many people are still too much in
shock to think clearly and others prefer denial out of complacency or fear.
It is my belief, however, that the "Ground Zero" event may only be the beginning of a horrifying specter that in the years to come will claim many
more lives and challenge the economic, military, political, and moral resources of numerous countries in the world.

Although terrorism is a unique development that has no parallels in premodern times, humankind is not new to war and its material and moral dev-
astations. The 1.1 million casualties claimed for all the American wars since
the Revolution of 1775–1783 pale into insignificance when we know that, in
the twentieth century alone, an estimated 185 million people have been
killed through political action (war, persecution, etc.).[2]

If I am right—and I hope I am dreadfully wrong—then we must expect to live in something of a combat zone for an indefinite period of time during which we will never know when, where, or how the next attack will occur. Today, thanks to the irresponsibility, machinations, and shortsightedness of governments, terrorists are in possession of a variety of weapons of mass destruction, which some experts fear may include biological, chemical, and nuclear means. Governments will have to find their own solutions to this formidable challenge. But how should we as individuals conduct our lives in the shadow of these developments?

Apart from whatever political and other steps we may choose to take to protect ourselves and our interests and those of the country we live in, we also must face the moral issues involved. I believe that no complete moral consideration is possible without including the question of the spiritual destiny of our species. This is where the wisdom of the East, notably Yoga, becomes immediately relevant.

On the assumption that terrorism is a form of warfare, the philosophy of the *Bhagavad-Gītā* (Lord's Song)—a 2,500-year-old Sanskrit scripture that "Mahatma" Gandhi called his "mother"—is an obvious first choice for our consideration. The *Gītā*, which is to Hinduism what the New Testament is to Christianity, in fact contains teachings that were given by the God-man Krishna on the morrow of one of the fiercest wars fought on Indian soil. They were intended to provide a spiritual framework for dealing with war and violence and are as relevant today as they were then.

The gist of Krishna's teachings is that as long as we are alive, we are forced to act. His message came at a time when large numbers of spiritual seekers were abandoning their householder existence and heading into the forests or remote mountain caves to pursue a contemplative lifestyle. He conceded that there is some legitimacy to such a world-weary quest for inner peace, but questioned both its philosophical foundations and the motivations of many of those who were choosing that particular path. In his view, action is simply superior to inaction. The problem with action, however, is that it leads to karmic consequences, which may be positive (auspicious) or negative (inauspicious). Of course, inaction also has repercussions in the realm of karma (or the law of moral causation). The reason for this is that both action and inaction involve the human mind, which is the seedbed of all karma.

Every thought or intention, depending on its moral quality and emotional charge, leaves a residue in the depth of our mind. This imprint is not passive, but rather, as the Sanskrit word *samskāra* suggests, a potent "activator" that constantly seeks to express or fulfill itself. In other words, by our thoughts and intentions we are actively shaping our destiny. Therefore the sages of India have been eager to discipline the mind by means of Yoga in order to avoid disastrous karmic consequences. In fact, they have always sought to overcome not only negative karmic activity but *all* karmic activity.

Here is Krishna's formulation of the yogic position:

> Not by abstention from actions does a person enjoy action-transcendence (*naishkarmya*), nor by renunciation (*samnyāsa*) alone does he approach perfection (*siddhi*).

> For, not even for a moment can anyone ever remain without performing action. Every [being] is unwittingly made to act by the constituents (*guna*) born of Nature (*prakrti*).

> He who restrains his conative organs (*karma-indriya*), but sits remembering in his mind the objects (*artha*) of the senses, is called a hypocrite, a confused self.

> But more excellent, O Arjuna, is he who, controlling the [cognitive] senses (*indriya*) with the mind, embarks unattached on Karma-Yoga with the conative organs.

> You must do the allotted (*niyata*) action, for action is superior to inaction; not even your body's processes (*yātrā*) can be accomplished by inaction.

> This world is bound by action, save when this action [is intended] as sacrifice (*yajna*). With that purpose [in mind], O Son of Kunti, engage in action devoid of attachment.

> —*Bhagavad-Gītā* (3.4–9)

Action, inaction, wrong action, and action transcendence are four concepts proposed in the *Gītā*, which we must understand clearly. The first three leave a karmic residue, and only the last represents a way out of the maze of karma. Not only does Krishna strongly urge us to be active but also to engage in proper (*niyata*) action, or action that is in accord with our place in life and our inner capacity. In contemporary terms, proper action means action that arises for us when we are "in the flow" of things. Action transcendence is proper action done without egocentric motivation or attachment, as a "sacrifice." It is service of the highest order.

This teaching of Karma-Yoga (the path of self-transcending action) was given to Prince Arjuna, who led the army of the Pāndavas. He and his four brothers had been cheated out of their kingdom and were now reclaiming it. Alas, when Arjuna saw family members, friends, and honored teachers standing with the enemy army, he wavered in his mission. Krishna had to remind him that he was not fighting for any selfish purpose but to restore *dharma*.

This vital concept can be translated as "morality," "virtue," "order," "norm," "duty," "law," etc. The Sanskrit words stems from the verbal root *dhri* meaning "to bear" or "to carry." Thus *dharma* is that which sustains human life, namely the moral order, which is reflected in us in the form of life-enhancing values or virtues. The Kaurava princes, cousins of the Pāndavas, were unjustly and unfairly governing the country and had thrown it into moral and spiritual darkness. Krishna, acting without self-interest and only out of the spontaneity of full enlightenment, had incarnated on Earth to restore the moral order, and the Pāndava princes were merely the instruments for executing his plan. The Hindus look upon Krishna as a theophany (*avatāra*), but we can also see in him simply a prophet, visionary, sage, or spiritual teacher who wishes to promote the spiritual and moral welfare of the people of his time.

Moral lines are not always as clear cut as they are traditionally painted in the case of the Pāndavas and Kauravas. Today the world is far more complex, and the nations of the world are entangled in a long common history of political intrigue, economic competition, ideological division, and not least warfare. In Hindu terms, every nation on Earth is suffering from an overdose of heavy-duty karma. There are no black and white sides, only a lot of gray areas. Thus the September 11 attack on the United States also did not occur in a vacuum. Terrorism, inexcusable as it is, has definite causes, and these need to be understood before terrorism can be overcome; but this is not within the scope of the present discussion.

What is relevant, however, is to appreciate the fact that our society—humankind as a whole—is in exactly the state of moral and spiritual decline that Krishna spoke of. Contrary to New Ageism, which is principally confined to the middle class of the United States and the developed nations of Europe, we are not at the cusp of a great spiritual upliftment. The accomplishments of the "Aquarian Age," which are hailed as harbingers of a better world, are at best minipeaks in a valley of unfortunate developments. Let us just recall that every year some 100 million people are dying of hunger and a similar number are killed in wars, revolutions, and persecutions. These are surely not signs of a current or an imminent golden age. Writing in 1964, C. G. Jung accurately observed:

> Modern man does not understand how much his "rationalism" (which has destroyed his capacity to respond to numinous symbols and ideas) has put him at the mercy of the psychic "underworld." He has freed himself from "superstition" (or so he believes), but in the process he has lost his spiritual values to a positively dangerous degree. His moral and spiritual tradition has disintegrated, and he is now paying the price for this break-up in worldwide disorientation and dissociation.[3]

Once we accept that we do not live in the best of all possible worlds, we can perhaps also see that we are coresponsible for our present situation. As Jung observed, we must see the shadow in our own psyche if we want to perceive reality clearly or, as the Buddhists put it, "see things as they really are." We cannot become whole without this work on our shadow, the swampland consisting of all those aspects of our personality that we prefer to deny and instead project onto others: egotism, fantasy, greed, cowardice, laziness, irrationality, fanaticism, etc.

To put it starkly: In order to become whole, we must discover the potential of terrorism in the complex circuitry of our own psyche. Terrorism is an expression of spiritual deafness, moral blindness, and irrational anger. Only when we can acknowledge the presence of these dark forces within us can we take responsibility for them. This brings me back to the mental discipline of Karma-Yoga by which action is transformed in such a way that it is not rooted in the shadow and therefore is not karmically tainted.

Morally and spiritually sound action must be accompanied by self-observation, self-understanding, self-acceptance, self-transformation, and self-transcendence. Without these disciplines, we are likely to succumb to projection and wrong action (*vikarma*). These, in turn, are not conducive to inner and outer peace. On the contrary, if our behavior fails to be anchored in sound spiritual virtues and practices, it will predictably cause disturbance, disharmony, harm, hurt, and even chaos in the world.

Krishna taught that there are circumstances when it is not only appropriate but essential to take a firm stand against evil. He was not a romantic pacifist who, in the interest of an abstract principle (however noble), allows evil to conquer good. When the moral or spiritual order is at stake, we must actively oppose the forces that seek to undermine it. He even condoned war to accomplish this end, though a war not tinged with hatred and conducted for selfish reasons.

The question that presents itself here is: Which or whose moral or spiritual order justifies war and violence? According to the Muslim terrorists, the Western capitalist system that they wish to destroy is inherently evil. Their own belief system, however, is intrinsically right, lawful, and absolutely deserving of their support, protection, and if necessary violent promulgation. When they speak of *jihād*, they do mean "holy war" against a nation or interest group that, in their eyes, falls short of Muslim morality. This use of the concept, however, is a misuse. The Arab word means literally "striving"—the endeavor to live a just and virtuous life, both individually and collectively.

Even though many Muslims dangerously consider the conquest and conversion of non-Muslim peoples as a religious duty, the *Qur'ān* itself sanctions war only against an aggressor who is threatening the moral order. The verses dealing with *jihād* in the familiar sense of holy war can be understood from the sociopolitical context of the early Muslim community, which was widely opposed by the Arab society of its day. That these *sūras* should now prove the seed for fundamentalism and unreasonable hostility is profoundly regrettable but a fact of life that both Muslims and non-Muslims need to examine carefully in their endeavor to build a prosperous and peaceful future for themselves.

To be sure, the original and moderate concept of *jihād* meshes with the Hindu position, as mapped out by Krishna, who also urged his disciple Prince Arjuna to fight on moral grounds. When we examine the Muslim notions with what constitutes a morally sound and virtuous life, we quickly find that they are not in contradiction to the core values of Christianity, Hinduism, Buddhism, and any of the other great religious-spiritual traditions of the world. In all these traditions, including Islam, hatred has no place but love, kindness, mercy, tolerance, generosity, and forgiveness are recommended to all. There have of course been failures to live up to these great ideals in all traditions, though some of them, more than others, have a history of severe infringements, notably Islam and, yes, Christianity.

When we look at the traditional concept of "moral order," we are looking at moral universals, not culture-specific moral rules or expectations. The morality recommended by Krishna, the Buddha, Jesus of Nazareth, and Mohammad consists of the moral values and attitudes that arise spontaneously in any pure heart, whatever the culture or religious affiliation may be. These values and attitudes are intrinsically life enhancing and promote inner freedom and peace.

When Krishna recommended combative action to Prince Arjuna, he took into account Arjuna's *sva-dharma*, or "inner law." Arjuna was an aristocrat, whose duty was to defend the state and protect its citizens from harm and exploitation. As a member of the warrior estate (*kshatra*), it was his obligation by birth to uphold the moral order (*dharma*). He was trained to lead soldiers into battle.

Krishna would not have given the same advice to a member of the priestly or merchant estate. While today the boundaries between social classes are drawn differently and also are perhaps more fluid than in the days of Krishna, the notion of *sva-dharma* still deserves our attention. It is closely associated with the notion of *sva-bhāva* or "inner being," which is our personal makeup—the quality of our mind, character, or personality. From a traditional perspective, a person who is by dint of his mind, character, or personality more artistic than combative is considered constitutionally unfit for aggressive action such as a war demands. It would be morally questionable—as well as psychologically unsound—to expect such an individual to pick up arms and fight at the frontline. Similarly, it would be outright wrong for a member of the priestly estate (*brāhmana*) to join in aggressive action. His or her appropriate task would be to pray and conduct rituals for the success of a military campaign.

We must come to know our own *sva-bhāva* and the *sva-dharma* connected with it, and then we must act in accordance with our moral and psychological constitution and the attendant moral obligations. As a writer with strong pacifist leanings, I myself would make a bad soldier. In fact, I have not had any military training, for which I am grateful. However, as a writer I have the capacity and obligation to support the high moral and spiritual values that help create or sustain the kind of environment in which humankind can thrive. I wield my pen instead of a sword, just as a farmer employs the plow.

"Mahatma" Gandhi, a lawyer by profession, used the weapon of passive resistance to end the hegemony of the British in India and helped to achieve India's independence in 1947. He found violence abhorrent and held high the ideal of *ahimsā* or nonharming. Yet even Gandhi admitted:

> Whilst all violence is bad and must be condemned in the abstract, it is permissible for, it is even the duty of, a believer in *ahimsa* to distinguish between the aggressor and the defender. Having done so, he will side with the defender in a non-violent manner, i.e., give his life in saving him.[4]

Gandhi realized that we live in an imperfect realm, and so he allowed for the existence of a military and police but regretted that there was a need for them. This dilemma demonstrates that while we must uphold and aspire to the highest moral and spiritual values, we cannot turn away from the realities of the "real world." In our daily life, we are constantly confronted with situations of potential or actual conflict. How we react depends on who we are. Gandhi was an extraordinary individual who, in his homeland and abroad, is remembered as a saint. To his credit, he had a more modest opinion of himself. Few of us have the courage of our convictions. He died for his idealism on January 30, 1948, while on his way to evening prayer. Applying the existing law, the government was unforgiving and promptly executed the assassin Nathuram Godse, a brahmin who fanatically objected to Gandhi's pro-Muslim stance.

We must find our own response to all situations of violence. As Yoga practitioners, we certainly must pay due attention to the superb moral imperative of nonharming. But we can always only act in accordance with our *sva-bhāva* and *sva-dharma* lest we should animate a false sense of self. In this context, the *Gītā* makes the important statement that it is better to fulfill one's own law (*sva-dharma*) imperfectly than another's perfectly. To do so we must know who we are and behave truthfully. If our inner truth, or conscience, leads us to abandon the guiding ideal of nonharming, then we must act accordingly and also courageously accept the consequences of our action. If, however, our inner voice prompts us to adopt nonharming as our foremost principle, then we must choose stillness and boldly accept the repercussions of the pacifist path, even if it costs us our life.

Like Hinduism, Buddhism holds nonharming in the highest regard and recommends it for both monastics and lay followers. The Dalai Lama's nonviolent response to the invasion of his country by the Chinese is a superb example of the Buddhist stance. Yet, according to *World Tibet Network News* (March 30, 2000), the exiled leader of the Tibetans and winner of the Nobel Peace Prize in 1989, too, admitted:

> . . . theoretically, violence can be permitted depending on the motive and if a greater goal is sought. But in practice, it is very difficult. The nature of violence is very unpredictable. In today's world, destruction of your neighbor is destruction of yourself.[5]

We have here the same contrast, already noted in Gandhi's comments, between the theoretical or abstract principle of nonviolence and day-to-day reality. While the Dalai Lama has consistently maintained a nonviolent orientation to the atrocities committed in his homeland and advocated the same principle in all other situations of violence, it is interesting that at least theoretically he allows violence "if a greater goal is sought." As a Buddhist monk, he is absolutely committed to nonharming. As the leader of an exiled nation, he steers the same course but not without concern and perhaps a certain unease that his pacifism has caused a schism among Tibetans and not done anything to stop or even slow down the raping of his country.

Those of us who are nonmonastics, living in the world with families to worry about, must find our own answer to the present crisis—any crisis involving violence. Krishna tried to show a middle path long ago, which emphasized not only skillful action in the world but also skillful inner action—through mental discipline. When we are free from anger and feelings of revenge, we may—with a centered and peaceful mind—take appropriate action to defend what would be considered good and life enhancing by any person of sound and clear mind.

If terrorism is here to challenge us in the years to come, we must not let it poison our heart but, on the contrary, strengthen our resolve to spread peace and happiness to all our fellow humans. We must cultivate this higher orientation even if, in specific situations, we feel the need to defend ourselves and others.

There has been much talk of a new world order. Often this concept is promoted by ruthless industrialists and politicians, who are motivated by greed and power rather than the betterment of the material and spiritual welfare of all peoples on Earth. In their hands, this is indeed a dangerous concept. At the same time, commerce has brought disparate nations closer together, and slowly everyone is realizing that humanity is one and that all of us are interdependent. Globalization is happening. The challenge before us is to give it the right direction. We can contribute to this commission by cultivating, in our own relationships, the sublime values that are upheld by all the religious-spiritual traditions of the world. World peace starts with inner peace and mental clarity, or wisdom. When we have no ax to grind but possess serenity, we also enjoy tolerance, compassion, and love. These are the great, universal virtues that are recommended on the path of Yoga. Who could reasonably argue against them?

PART THREE

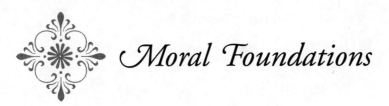 *Moral Foundations*

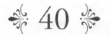

40

Yoga Begins and Ends with Virtuous Action

VIRTUE IS FOR MOST Westerners an old-fashioned word and an equally antiquated and impractical concept. In the spiritual traditions, however, virtue is considered a foremost principle of action. While, in Yoga, the ultimate Reality is thought to lie beyond good and evil, there is a recognized need for the cultivation of virtuous deeds, words, and thoughts. Virtue is traditionally connected with the idea of merit. Thus thoughts or actions are deemed meritorious or demeritorious depending on whether they spring from virtue or vice. Merit (*punya*) is really the fruit of good *karma*, that is, the positive momentum generated in the mind as a result of positive physical, verbal, or mental behavior. Positive behavior is associated with kindness, compassion, love, nonharming, generosity, patience, contentment, correct understanding, etc. It leaves imprints of a positive nature in the depth of the mind. Negative behavior is connected with self-delusion, anger, greed, harming, miserliness, inconsiderateness, impatience, etc. It too creates karmic deposits in the deep levels of the mind. These imprints or deposits serve as seeds that will sprout in the future, bringing good or bad consequences. As Je Tsongkhapa, the founder of the Gelugpa Order, notes in his magnificent *Lam-Rim Chen-Mo* (chapter 13):

> All happiness in the sense of feelings of ease—whether of ordinary or noble beings, including even the slightest pleasures such as the rising of a cool breeze for a being born in a hell—arises from previously accumulated virtuous karma. It is impossible for happiness to arise from nonvirtuous karma.
>
> All sufferings in the sense of painful feelings—including even the slightest suffering occurring in an arhat's mind-stream—arise from previously accumulated nonvirtuous karma. It is impossible for suffering to arise from virtuous karma.[1]

The question is how can virtuous behavior lead to the ultimate transcendence of good and evil, as aspired to in all yogic traditions? Should we not expect that virtuous behavior simply leads to greater goodness? Does the belief in an ultimate Reality that is inherently transmoral not make nonsense out of all ethical behavior? The masters of Yoga do not think so. Nonvirtuous behavior, according to them, results in future suffering, whereas virtuous behavior brings joyous experiences. Put in theological terms, one culminates in Hell, the other in Heaven.

Significantly, however, the Yoga adepts have as little interest in heaven as they have in hell. They endeavor to go beyond all conditional states of existence and attain liberation or *nirvāna*. The only reason they are eager to cultivate virtuous behavior is that it reduces the mental factors causing suffering (*duhkha*). But even joyous experiences are inherently limiting, because they presuppose an ego-personality who has experiences of enjoyment and very likely becomes attached to them, thus keeping the vicious cycle of conditional existence (*samsāra*) perpetually in motion.

Only liberation is total freedom from suffering, that is, from the law of cause and effect. Liberation, or enlightenment, alone guarantees that we end the beginningless chain of karmic conditioning leading to lifetime after painful lifetime in various limited realms.

After carefully pondering the question of the relationship between ethics and liberation, Je Tsongkhapa offered the following answer, as disclosed to him by Buddha Manjushrī himself:

> Suppose you fail to devote some part of your practice to thinking over the various problems of cyclic life, and the different benefits of freedom from it. You don't sit down and meditate, keeping your mind on trying to open your eyes to the ugliness of life, or holding it on the wonders of freedom. You don't reach the point where you never give a thought to the present life. You never master the art of renunciation.
>
> And let's say you go out then and try to develop a skill in some great virtuous practice — the perfection of giving, or that of morality, or forbearance, effort, or staying in concentration. It doesn't matter what. None of it can ever lead you on to the state of freedom. People who really long for freedom then should forget at first about all those other supposedly so deep advices. They should use the "mental review" meditation to develop renunciation.
>
> People who are trying to practice the greater way should set aside some regular periods of time for considering how harmful it is to concentrate on your own welfare, and how much good can come from concentrating on the welfare of others. Eventually these thoughts can become habitual; nothing that you ever do without them will ever turn to a path that leads you anywhere.[2]

Thus there are three necessities—called the "three principal paths"—for a successful spiritual life: the cultivation of correct view, renunciation, and the wish to attain enlightenment for the benefit of others. Correct view consists in recognizing that there is no independent self in us or anything; everything is, in the language of Mahāyāna, "empty" (*shūnya*). Yet, everything is arising in interdependence by the force of karma. Renunciation is simply letting go of attachment, especially our attachment to the notion of being an independent entity, or self. The phrase "concentrating on the welfare of others" captures the practice of *bodhicitta*, or the intention or firm resolution to attain enlightenment *for the sake of all beings*—the essence of the Mahāyāna Buddhist ideal of the *bodhisattva*. Following these three "paths," the practitioner accumulates merit (*punya*) and wisdom (*prajnā*).

For virtuous behavior to have not merely moral/religious but *spiritual* relevance, it must unfold in the context of the above three "paths," or their equivalents. Virtue is an integral part of authentic spiritual practice. In Classical Yoga, morally sound behavior is the first limb of the eightfold path leading to liberation. The same is true of other forms of Yoga as well. We cannot be rogues and hope to grow spiritually. Rather, as practitioners, we are expected to harmonize our interpersonal relationships through the time-honored virtues of nonharming, nonstealing, truthfulness, greedlessness, and chastity. These and others are recognized as universally valid principles of behavior in all religious and spiritual traditions of the world. They should be bountifully present in those claiming to be enlightened or close to enlightenment. Even in the case of initiates employing the unconventional tactics of a "holy fool" or "crazy adept," we should see clear evidence of their having mastered their "lower" impulses and stably realized the great virtues.[3] The path to freedom goes through rather than around morality—not the bourgeois morality of anxious individuals but the heartfelt morality of those who profoundly care for the welfare and freedom of others.

❧ 41 ❧

Is Nonharming (Ahimsā)
an Old-Fashioned Value?

Homo homini lupus, "Man is a wolf among men." Sigmund Freud, who quoted this Latin saying, remarked gloomily: "Who has the courage to dispute it in the face of all the evidence?" An array of psychologists, sociologists, and philosophers have reiterated the same view, arguing that aggression is innate in human beings, that we are programmed to attack, maim, and kill.

But if aggression is an innate impulse, so is gentleness and the ability to go beyond our murderous instincts. Only an utter pessimist would deny that it is impossible for us to live in peace and harmony with our fellow beings and Nature at large. We do not *need* to murder 100 million people by warfare and torture, as we did in the twentieth century alone. We are free to follow a different course of action. We can cultivate nonviolence, or nonharming (*ahimsā*), as a viable lifestyle.

Nor is this a mere utopian ideal. Here and there in past eras, and even in our own time, men and women have succeeded in living together cooperatively, without war and strife. Some monastic communities have achieved this great ideal at least during part of their history. A few village communities in sheltered environs, which are too remote for curious tourists, are still achieving it today. It is done not for any high metaphysical reasons, but simply because everyone's survival depends on the spirit of cooperation — an important insight that seems to become lost as societies grow more complex.

However, at a particular level in a person's spiritual development, nonviolence becomes something more than an economic or social exigency. It becomes an expression of the inner feeling of unity with everything.

Nonaggressiveness, or nonharming, has been hailed as a cardinal virtue in all major religio-spiritual traditions of the world. Thus, it has for centuries been central to Yoga. In Patanjali's *Yoga-Sūtra*, nonharming is introduced as one of the five practices constituting the "great vow" of the moral disciplines (*yama*).

What does the virtue of nonharming mean to the contemporary Western Yoga student? Is *ahimsā* merely a romantic ideal? Or is it, as Patanjali insists, universally and unconditionally valid? Is this still plausible in our far more complex world? In the twentieth century it was "Mahatma" Gandhi, a master of Karma-Yoga (the path of self-transcending action), who upheld the ancient ideal of *ahimsā*. He also demonstrated its political effectiveness through his policy of passive resistance. Gandhi inspired the modern philosophy and practice of nonviolent social action through demonstrations, sit-ins, teach-ins, petitioning, fasting, and so on. Nonviolent campaigns of social reform have been surprisingly successful, bearing witness to the transformative power of nonharming.

The answer to the question posed above must be: *Ahimsā* is as relevant today as it was at the time of Patanjali and of Gautama the Buddha, another stalwart spokesman for nonviolence. What we need to examine is *how* we can translate the ideal of nonharming into daily practice—for ourselves, our local community, and our global society.

The Buddha's older contemporary Mahāvīra, the founder of historical Jainism, furnished extensive rules about nonharming. More than any other religio-spiritual culture in the world, Jainism abhors violence in all its numerous forms. Even today members of some Jaina sects in India still wear a mask to filter the air, lest they should unwittingly inhale and take the life of small creatures. This is a religious custom that few of us would want to follow. Nevertheless, upon closer inspection this extreme practice contains a useful lesson: our life is built on the sacrificial death of others. We are involuntarily murdering creatures with every breath—a massacre that not even a mask can prevent. For, we constantly annihilate billions of invisible microbes so that we may live. We ourselves are a link in the great food chain of life, destined to die and be food for microbic creatures.

We need not stop breathing or feeding ourselves, or constantly "turn the other cheek," but we must appreciate how we owe our life to other beings and how they owe their lives to us. When we truly see this vast interconnectedness, it becomes easy for us to cultivate an attitude of reverence for life, which is essentially an attitude of nonharming and of ego-transcending love.

We must train our sensitivity to the fact that we are not alone in the universe but are interdependent cells of a cosmic body. Spiritual life is largely a matter of taking responsibility for the things we have understood about ourselves and the world we live in. This includes assuming responsibility for our destructive aggression, as it reveals itself to us in ever subtler forms.

As Patanjali states, nonharming must be practiced under *all* conditions—in thought, word, and deed. Our self-inspection can begin with our active life. For instance, we may ask ourselves whether our livelihood involves harming others in ways that are not morally justifiable. As a writer I have become progressively aware of the fact that I am co-responsible for the destruction of forests, which are the habitat of countless species, not least human tribal groups. I have begun to take remedial actions, though I have an uneasy feeling that I should do much more.

Another important area of self-inspection concerns our social relationships—our family life, friendships, and business relationships. How are we destructively aggressive in them? Where could we begin to practice *ahimsā* more seriously? How do we typically express our unlove and lack of compassion or empathy? One way of going about this is to ask our relatives and friends to give us their undoubtedly painful feedback. We may find that we tend to come across as overly aggressive, cold, or unapproachable. We may be told that we do not let others express themselves, or that we are poor listeners. There are numerous ways in which we can practice unlove, just as there are countless ways in which we can be loving and compassionate.

We can cause harm not only by our physical actions but also by our speech. Words spoken in anger or out of inconsiderateness may hurt others as much as or more than a slap in the face. Another area of psychological harming is our competitiveness when it becomes callous. We try to outstrip each other and in the process strip ourselves and others of all dignity.

Then there is the whole matter of how we maintain our body's energies and health. Unless we are strict vegetarians, we consume meat, fish, eggs, and dairy products. Quite apart from any religious considerations, we must be concerned about the fact that our dietary habits are locked into a vast industry that is not known for its moral scruples. The meals we eat tend to come from factory-farmed animals that are widely treated with unbelievable cruelty ("because animals don't feel pain as we do"). Cows are kept artificially pregnant to yield milk, while their calves are deprived of motherly affection, forced to eat a monotonous milk-replacing diet to ensure that their flesh will be as white as the market demands; chickens are debeaked and cooped up in torturously small cages; pigs are taildocked and kept in miniscule pens in the dark, forced to eat from sheer boredom, doing nothing but waiting to be slaughtered in an often brutal way. The most horrendous practice of animal husbandry is that of feeding cows the pulverized meat of their own species (cannibalism), which is the cause of mad cow disease. Bovines are by nature vegetarians and feeding them meat violates their own biology and recently led to the slaughter of hundreds of thousands of cows in Europe.

Thus our food habits endorse an industry, running to some 50 billion dollars a year, that blatantly violates the ideal of nonharming. It also contributes in a major way to the massive degradation of the environment. Our medical needs and choices have a similarly tragic effect, for they support the often gruesome exploitation of animals in laboratories. Similarly, our hunger for entertainment leads to animal abuse in a variety of ways—from hunting to rodeos and races to seemingly innocuous zoos and circuses. Much could also be said about how our conspicuous consumption directly or indirectly disadvantages other nations, causing hunger and plight to millions of fellow-humans.

All our actions have moral repercussions. For instance, doing our duty as an upright citizen involves paying taxes every year. But our taxes help support a vast military industry that revolves around violence, and which in effect leads to countless deaths and untold pain around the world. It would be foolish to withhold taxes, but we can work for a long-overdue tax reform and, more importantly, protest against the ways in which our tax money is spent.

Finally, the ideal of nonharming is not confined to physical or verbal expression. Our very thoughts are powerful. They determine the subtle ways in which we relate to life, especially how we interact with others. If we are down, we tend to drag our environment down. If we are emotionally buoyant, our happiness uplifts those around us. Even if we do not mean to harm another person, our coldness or indifference is a form of harming. Whenever we are not present as love, we inevitably reduce our own life and the life in others. Hence we are responsible for how we are present in the world, even when we are on our own, because our field is interconnected with the fields of everyone and everything else.

Ahimsā, as a manifestation of self-transcending love, is a building block of spiritual practice. Genuine Yoga is impossible without it. Nonharming is certainly not an old-fashioned value.

❧ 42 ❧
Nonharming According to Jaina Yoga

THE THREE MAJOR cultural traditions of India—Hinduism, Buddhism, and Jainism—all promote the supreme moral value of nonharming, or ahimsā. In the *Yoga-Sūtra* (2.30) of Patanjali, representing Hindu Yoga, nonharming is listed among the five observances or disciplines (*yama*), which are said to be universally applicable. Patanjali's position has its precise parallels in Buddhism and Jainism. Of these three great traditions, Jainism offers the most comprehensive treatment of nonharming.

Historical Jainism was founded in the sixth century B.C.E. by Vardhamāna Mahāvīra, an older contemporary of Gautama the Buddha, but tradition knows of twenty-three earlier teachers, who are known as "ford-makers" (*tīrthankara*). The sacred canonical literature of the Jainas (or Jains), which comprises some sixty scriptures, has three main divisions: the fourteen *Pūrvas* (which have all been lost), the twelve *Angas* (spoken by Mahāvīra), and the thirty-four *Angabāhyas*, consisting of *Upāngas* and *Sūtras* (composed by various elders)—all written in the archaic Magadhan language.

Like Hinduism and Buddhism, Jainism offers a spiritual path leading to liberation and originally was a strictly monastic community that later also acquired lay followers. Jainism is marked by vigorous asceticism (*tapas*) and has produced a long line of great world-renouncing adepts. The degree of asceticism can be seen in the early dispute over whether Jaina monastics should wear clothes or go about naked. Around 300 B.C.E., the community split into those wearing clothes (i.e., the Shvetāmbaras) and those clad only with space (i.e., the Digambaras). The lifestyle of Jaina monks and nuns has exerted a strong influence on the laity, and so we find that even ordinary householders are keenly practicing the ideal of nonharming.

The oldest and in many ways most important extant scripture is the *Ācārānga-Sūtra* spoken by Mahāvīra. This text outlines the proper conduct for monks and nuns and includes a lengthy consideration about nonharming. For Jainas, "nonharming is the supreme virtue" (*ahimsā paramo dharmah*).

According to Hemacandra's *Yoga-Shāstra* (2.31), spiritual practice is worthless if it is not based on the abandonment of all harmful activity. The *Dashā-Vaikālika-Sūtra* (1.1–4) of the Shvetāmbara branch, which was possibly composed in the fifth century B.C.E., opens with the following verses:

Dharma is the greatest blessing: Nonharming, restraint, and asceticism. Even the deities honor a mind always set on *dharma*.

As a bee is satisfied with drinking the nectar of tree blossoms, without damaging the blossoms, so also do here on Earth the liberated ascetics, who, seeking food among the blossoms as it were, delight in devoted offerings.

Like bees from flowers we subsist on whatever has been prepared, without burdening anyone.

Thus even in such a vital aspect of life as nutrition, the Jaina monastics walk lightly on this planet, wishing to avoid harming or even inconveniencing others. Nonharming is the great vow (*mahā-vrāta*). As the *Dashā-Vaikālika-Sūtra* (1.11) puts it:

Sir, the first great vow is abstention from harming living beings. Sir, I will abstain from harming any living beings, be they small or large, mobile or immobile. I myself will not harm any living being. I will not harm any living being through another. I will not condone the harming of any living being. For as long as I live, I will not cause, instigate, or condone [harming others] through the threefold means of body, speech, and mind.

The Jaina moral code forbids monastics to dig in the soil with a piece of wood or with their fingers, to mold lumps of clay, or to deliberately dry out lakes or even puddles. Everything must be left as undisturbed as possible, for life is to be found everywhere. They are not even to make or put out a fire because fire too has its own life forms that must be neither molested nor destroyed.

When walking, the Jaina monastics must gaze at the ground to avoid stepping on living beings, including vegetation. They must gently remove any insect that happens to have landed on their body, being careful not to place it where it would cause inconvenience to other life forms. Some monastics — the Sthānakavāsins — wear a strip of cloth called *muhpatti* over their mouth to avoid accidentally swallowing insects, and so forth. For the same reason, the Jaina monastics abstain from fanning themselves and swimming or even wading in water.

All harmful acts cause karma, which then binds the person to the finite world (*samsāra*) characterized by suffering. According to the *Tattva-Artha-Sūtra* (7.13) by Umāsvāmin, harming (*himsā*) is cutting off another's life out of carelessness. Harming can be intentional (*samkalpa-ja*) or accidental (*ārambha-ja*) in the performance of one's allotted work.

Needless to say, the Jainas abhor hunting, vivisection, capital punishment, animal sacrifice, personal revenge, and war. The rules for the laity are far less strict than those for the monastics, as lay people are permitted, within reason, to defend their own life.

The key to nonharming is constant vigilance or attentiveness (*apramāda*). As the above scripture explains (7.4), this is to be cultivated by means of the following five practices:

1. *vāg-gupti*, guarding one's speech
2. *mano-gupti*, guarding one's thoughts
3. *īrya-samiti*, care in walking
4. *ādāna-nikshepana-samiti*, care in lifting and laying down things
5. *ālokita-pāna-bhojana*, careful inspection of one's food and drink

The *Tattva-Artha-Sūtra* (7.11) also recommends the following four practices:

1. *maitrī*, benevolence toward all beings
2. *pramoda*, delight in all beings
3. *kārunya*, compassion for all beings
4. *madhyastha*, forbearance toward all those who are misguided in their behavior

We become inattentive and negligent through negative mental states, notably pride, passion, anger, greed, and delusion. These cloud reason and cause carelessness, which may lead to the injuring or even killing of other beings.

Clearly, the Jaina moral code demands acute awareness. This is even more impressive when one knows that the vow of nonharming belongs only to the second of eleven stages of spiritual development in the life of a lay practitioner and fourteen stages in the case of a monastic.

A balanced moral life serves to free attention for the meditative process and the cultivation of those higher virtues that lead to liberation. Non-Jaina Yoga practitioners can learn a great deal from the exemplary nonviolent lifestyle of the adherents of Jainism.

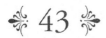

43

Yoga and Vegetarianism

THE FACT THAT MOST Tibetan practitioners of Vajrayāna Buddhism (a Tantric Yoga) eat meat tells us that Yoga does not inevitably subscribe to a vegetarian diet. Most forms of Yoga, however, do recommend or even insist on vegetarianism. The Tibetans are a special case, because their sparse mountainous land does not easily lend itself to crop cultivation that would make for an adequate diet in the cold Himalayan climate. Without meat they would likely suffer the ill effects of malnutrition. Not so excusable is the continued consumption of meat among the expatriate Tibetan community living in India or Western countries. It is simply a habit, and one that at least some of the Tibetan leaders have wrestled with. The Dalai Lama, for instance, made these unequivocal comments:

> I do not see any reason why animals should be slaughtered to serve as human diet when there are so many substitutes. After all, man can live without meat. It is only some carnivorous animals that have to subsist on flesh. Killing animals for sport, for pleasure, for adventures, and for hides and furs is a phenomenon which is at once disgusting and distressing. There is no justification in indulging in such acts of brutality.
>
> In our approach to life, be it pragmatic or otherwise, the ultimate truth that confronts us squarely and unmistakably is the desire for peace, security and happiness. Different forms of life in different aspects of existence make up the teeming denizens of this earth of ours. And, no matter whether they belong to the higher group as human beings or to the lower group, the animals, all beings primarily seek peace, comfort and security. Life is as dear to a mute creature as it is to a man. Just as one wants happiness and fears pain, just as one wants to live and not to die, so do other creatures.[1]

A Buddhist practitioner who has studied with the Dalai Lama added the following encouraging sidelight to the above statement:

I have had the privilege of being a Buddhist student of His Holiness and he stated that on doctor's orders he does eat meat every other day. He does not eat much as it is against the precepts but has been working on being vegan.[2]

More recently, in an interview with World Tibet Network on December 26, 2000, the Dalai Lama stated:

I am not a vegetarian. From 1965 to 1967, for almost two years ago I tried to become a strict vegetarian. But because of some liver problem, hepatitis, I had to resume the meat diet. However, during my childhood in Tibet, I tried to transform many Tibetan government festivals into vegetarian festivals. So, although I am not a vegetarian, but I always try to promote vegetarianism.[3]

The Dalai Lama is clearly moving toward the original Buddhist practice of vegetarianism and might by now be a vegetarian if he had access to up-to-date medical and dietary information.

Sometimes an argument is made that Gautama the Buddha was not a strict vegetarian but consumed meat. There is a highly controversial statement in the Mahāparinibbāna-Sutta, a canonical Pali text, that has been interpreted as a count against the Buddha's vegetarianism. According to this Sutta (4.20), which is included in the Dīgha-Nikāya, the Buddha ate on at least one occasion sūkara-maddava—a Pali word meaning something like "pig's delight"—in the mango grove of Cunda, the smith. Early Buddhist authorities understood this term to refer to pig's flesh; others interpret it to mean a plant desired by pigs (i.e., truffles), yet others as a kind of mushroom. Whatever sūkara-maddava may have been, it was the physical trigger of the Buddha's death. Curiously, before being served the meal, the Buddha is recorded to have asked Cunda to serve him sūkara-maddava alone while offering the other members of his community other foods. After the meal, the Buddha asked Cunda to bury the remainder of the sūkara-maddava as no one but a tathāgata (i.e., the Buddha himself) could possibly digest it. So, from the outset, the Buddha considered this substance problematical. Indeed, he promptly fell ill and suffered violent pains and vomited blood, suggesting dysentery. However, because of his extraordinary mental control over the body, he was able to move on to Kusinara where he gave some more instructions, including the complete exoneration of Cunda, and then he shed his body the next morning.

The highest moral injunction in the Buddha's teaching is not to harm other sentient beings, including killing them. At the same time, he instructed his monastics to accept whatever food was placed into their begging bowls, so that no attachment could arise. It is true, however, that the Buddha forbade his monastic community to eat meat when the animal had been killed specifically for the purpose of feeding the monks and nuns. Apparently, the Buddha refused to formulate an injunction that would exclude meat altogether.

Vegetarianism is definitely the rule within Hindu Yoga, and it is unquestionably an imperative within Jaina Yoga. Behind this dietary preference lies the strong moral conviction that in order to reach enlightenment, we must avoid harming others. Meat eating clearly involves harming, especially today with the egregious practices of the so-called meat industry. Already the term "meat industry" drives home the point that animals are being treated as objects that can be processed for consumption without regard to their inner life (i.e., sensations of pain and feelings of fear). Yet, there were and still are groups of Hindus who feel it necessary to slaughter animals for ritual purposes—a practice the Buddha definitely opposed.

For the Yoga practitioner, animals are first and foremost sentient beings, and as such they deserve our full considerateness. Few meat consumers ever stop to consider the process by which a living being is reduced to neatly packaged meat in the supermarket. They do not know—or do not want to know—that to suit their palate billions of animals every year are treated with a callousness and cruelty that, if applied to fellow humans, would be considered psychopathic.

Apart from moral considerations, Yoga practitioners tend to avoid meat also for health reasons. Research has shown over and over again the great disadvantages of meat consumption and the undeniable benefits of a vegetarian diet.

Furthermore, according to tradition, Yoga practitioners have long promoted vegetarianism for reasons of purity. Meat is considered impure, because it is composed primarily of *tamas* and *rajas*, the principles of inertia and dynamism, whereas the *yogin* and *yoginī* seek to increase *sattva*, the principle of lucidity in Nature. *Tamas* and *rajas* are said to produce sluggishness and aggressiveness respectively, which must be fully mastered on the yogic path. They can be mastered through the systematic cultivation of *sattva*, which lies at the heart of all authentic forms of Yoga.

❧ 44 ❧
The Practice of Eco-Yoga

ALL LIFE IS INTERCONNECTED and ultimately interdependent. This is the subject matter of ecology. Very simply, ecology is the study of the vital relationships between plants and animals (or humans) and the environment in which they live. Often the word is used to refer to the living being/environment nexus itself, though more accurately, ecology is the study of that nexus.

Our planet has been likened to a gigantic spaceship whose resources are limited. While it is true that the Earth's resources are by no means inexhaustible, a far more important fact is that our home planet is vastly more complex than any technological device could ever be. It is, as biologist James Gordon Lovelock reminded our generation, a living organism, which he called "Gaia."[1] As a living organism, the Earth is a finely balanced system of forces.

Over the past several decades, this equilibrium has been seriously disturbed by unecological patterns of life characteristic mainly of the "civilized" countries of the world, leading to what is called the "ecological crisis." Many factors are involved in this very serious crisis, notably overpopulation, disadvantageous population distribution (e.g., huge metropolitan areas), overconsumption, wasteful patterns of consumption, inappropriate use of technology, and, not least, egocentric, shortsighted ways of thought.

What does all this have to do with Yoga? *Everything.* Yoga is intrinsically ecological. All Yoga is what has been called "Eco-Yoga."[2] As the *Bhagavad-Gītā* (11.48) puts it, Yoga is balance (*samatva*). We need not understand this in purely psychological terms. When we are inwardly balanced, we are also balanced in relationship to our environment. This is borne out by the comprehensive and rigorous ethical code of Yoga, which covers the whole range of the Yoga practitioner's relationship to the environment and other living beings.

This code is expressed in the five moral disciplines (*yama*): nonharming, truthfulness, nonstealing, chastity, greedlessness. Thus, nonharming (*ahimsā*) consists in reverence for all forms of life. This implies, for instance, that we should choose a lifestyle that will not rob other creatures of their ecological niches. Also, if we take this rule seriously, we must adopt a vegetarian diet. Failing this, we should ensure that our consumption of animal products (meat, eggs, and dairy products) at least does not in any way support the cruel practice of factory-farming of animals.

The yogic rule of nonstealing (*asteya*) implies, for example, that we should not take more than we need for the upkeep of our body-mind. Few of us are willing to live in the Spartan fashion to which *yogins* are accustomed. However, there are many things we can do to adapt to this moral obligation. Thus, we can avoid what has been called "conspicuous consumption," including the needless wasting of food. Instead, we could learn to use our surplus (which is often simply destined to become garbage) to improve the living conditions of our less fortunate fellow humans.

Similarly, the moral rule of greedlessness (*aparigraha*) is understood as a comprehensive demand to relate to life in a balanced, nongrasping manner, which respects the right of others to share the resources of our planet. Conscious living is a balance between giving and taking. So, for instance, when we have to cut down a tree on our property, we should plant at least one new tree. Eco-yogic thinking demands that we help replenish our planet's resources.

The yogic call for purity (*shauca*), which is a part of the rules of self-restraint (*niyama*), can also be understood in a wider ecological sense. We should do our utmost to eliminate pollution in our own life and to support those efforts that seek to clean up our environment at large.

"Eco-Yoga" is a way of describing the now necessary convergence between traditional yogic spirituality and social activism focusing on ecological concerns. At the beginning of the third millennium, we are facing an increasing environmental crisis affecting all our lives deeply. We cannot afford any longer to exclusively pursue quietistic goals. We must also take responsibility for the environment in which we live, and that means recover our sense of the sacredness of this planet and to actively participate in its ecological recovery.

Metaphysically speaking, the challenge confronting us is to learn to respect both transcendence and immanence. To put it concretely, we cannot hope to find ourselves, never mind the Divine, so long as we obstruct our view by piling up mountains of garbage or by opaqueing the air with toxic pollutants. Instead, we must learn to cooperate with Nature, which is the very basis for any spiritual effort we wish to make. We must be willing to be loyal not only to our chosen spiritual path but also to our habitat.

The yogic tradition of Tantra has hailed the body as a most valuable instrument for realizing the Divine, or Reality. We must similarly recognize the immense value of our planet. The Earth is our body, and it is the only one we have. If we destroy it, we commit suicide. Here are some guidelines for cultivating the eco-yogic process:

Making a serious attempt at understanding our present age and the historical forces shaping it. Since we live in a complex pluralistic civilization, our lives are inevitably subject to all kinds of sociocultural currents, which we need to understand in order to cultivate our own authenticity. Recommended reading (in alphabetical order): Morris Berman, *The Re-enchantment of the World* (1981); Marilyn Ferguson, *The Aquarian Conspiracy* (1980); Jean Gebser, *The Ever-Present Origin* (1985); Carl Gustav Jung, *Modern Man in Search of a Soul* (1963); Gordon Rattray Taylor, *Rethink* (1972); Theodore Roszak, *Person/Planet* (1978); Alvin Toffler, *Future Shock* (1970) and *The Third Wave* (1980); Ken Wilber, *Up from Eden* (1981) and *Sex, Consciousness, Spirituality* (1995).

Becoming fully aware of and informed about the problem. Recommended reading: Thomas Berry, *The Dream of the Earth* (1988); Lester Brown, *State of the World* reports; Paul and Anne Ehrlich, *The Population Bomb* (1968) and *The Population Explosion* (1990); Duane Elgin, *Voluntary Simplicity* (1981); Francesca Lyman, et al., eds., *The Greenhouse Trap* (1990); Mihajlo Mesarovic and Eduard Pestel, *Mankind at the Turning Point* (1974); John G. Mitchell and Constance L. Stallings, eds., *Ecotactics* (1970); Jonathan Porritt, *Seeing Green* (1984); Barbara Ward, *The Home of Man* (1976). All these publications, and many other good books, contain a wealth of valuable information that has immediate relevance. But there are a few books that can be particularly recommended as practical manuals: *The Global Ecology Handbook: What You Can Do about the Environmental Crisis* (1990), edited by Walter H. Corson; *50 Simple Things You Can Do to Save the Earth* (1989), *50 Simple Things Kids Can Do to Save the Earth* (1990), and *The Recycler's Handbook* (1990) by the EarthWorks Group in Berkeley, California; *The Simple Act of Planting a Tree* (1990) by Treepeople with Andy and Katie Lipkis, published by J. P. Tarcher. We do not have to become experts, but we ought to know what is happening around us that affects us and the life of our children and grandchildren.

Living a simpler, ecologically sensitive life. We should take stock of our consumption patterns and decide how we can help reduce energy consumption and pollution in our own immediate environment. For instance, we might ask ourselves: Do I need to have so many lights on? Do I really need to run the air conditioner or heater, or could I insulate my house better and thus cut down energy wastage? Do I need to use the car quite so often, or could I plan my trips more wisely and perhaps use car pools? Do I need to flush the toilet with every use, or have fifteen-minute showers every day? Why couldn't I recycle cans and bottles? Can I really not afford to buy healthier organic food? Am I simply too lethargic to use vegetable waste to make a compost heap in the garden? And so on. Big change begins by doing the "little" things—now.

Joining forces with a local ecology group and becoming politically active. Yoga is not merely inwardness. Nor are Yoga and political commitment incompatible. All too often Yoga practitioners are concerned exclusively with their own salvation, ignoring the larger context in which they live. In the final analysis, this is not only selfish and contrary to the spirit of Yoga but also counterproductive. For the environment impinges on us. How can we, for example, hope to cultivate breath control in a polluted neighborhood? Or how can we maintain a healthy body-mind when the soil on which our food grows is poisoned by chemicals? Or how can we hope to achieve the necessary inner stillness for meditation and prayer to transform our psyche when our eardrums vibrate from the constant cacophony on the streets and in the sky? At the very least, we should support activist groups like Greenpeace, Friends of the Earth, Sierra Club, National Wildlife Federation, or the Elmwood Institute.

Cultivating self-understanding by scrutinizing the motives behind our spiritual odyssey, and being willing to recognize and work with neurotic tendencies masquerading as spiritual ideals. We should not necessarily trust our own self-image, but consult benevolent others who may serve us as more accurate mirrors of our character. Inadequate self-understanding frequently leads to wrong action.

Studying the spiritual traditions of the world to deepen our understanding of our preferred path. This will help us appreciate the complementarity of the Earth's religious and spiritual traditions. It will also reduce the tendency toward parochialism, cultism, spiritual elitism, and other forms of exclusivism. Such study can help us cultivate the admirable and indeed essential virtues of compassion and tolerance, which facilitate cooperation and ecological living.

Staying in touch with our natural environment. Living in cities seduces people into having a merely abstract relationship to the Earth. It is important to touch the soil, tend flowers or trees, taste clean spring water, see the exuberance of wildlife, and so forth. Inwardness without such grounding is often little more than neurotic escape. Wholeness requires the transformative touch of the Earth as well as blessing from the "heaven within."

Daily reminding ourselves that life is a precious gift, which must not be squandered, neglected, or abused. If our heart is open, gratitude and praise will flow easily from our lips. Our Western upbringing, generally speaking, does not make us predisposed to express our gratitude (or our other emotions), and it teaches us to be critical rather than full of praise. There is, of course, no need to withhold criticism where it is due, but it is often received more readily when it is tempered with compassion and praise (which can be viewed as an active form of compassion).

Living in our postmodern world has wounded us all in one way or another, and there is much need for healing. Praise and the expression of gratitude are excellent means of soothing our pain *(duhkha)* and restoring hope. When we experience life as a spiritual opportunity for which we are grateful, the world ceases to be our enemy. We will still share in the harvest of our collective karma and feel sorrow at the exploitation of the Earth, but we will also begin to feel a deeper affinity for everyone and everything— which is healing in itself. We become true citizens of the ecosystem, consciously casting our vote for its future by the way we live in each moment.

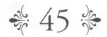

Overcoming Greed

Hɪɴᴅᴜ Yᴏɢᴀ ᴘᴏɪɴᴛs ᴛᴏ three motivating factors in ordinary life, often called the "three poisons" or "three flaws:" ignorance (*moha*), anger/hostility (*krodha*), and greed (*lobha*). The same triad can also be found in the Buddhist literature. Some Buddhist texts, however, speak of the following three mental poisons: attachment (*rāga*), hostility (*krodha*), and ignorance (*moha*). Here attachment takes the place of greed in the Hindu Yoga version. In the well-known image of the Wheel of Life, the innermost of four concentric circles contains the images of a dove (or cock), a snake, and a pig, each biting the tail of the one in front. The dove (or cock) stands for lust, the snake for hostility (*dvesha*), and the pig for ignorance.

Jaina Yoga, too, considers greed as a major obstacle. Thus the *Tattva-Artha-Sūtra* (8.10) mentions four passions (*kashāya*): anger (*krodha*), pride (*māna*), deceitfulness (*māyā*), and greed (*lobha*). The Jainas acknowledge that greed is present in the psyche of the practitioner for a long time, and they speak of "flickering greed" even at the tenth of fourteen stages of inner development.

All these factors derive from spiritual ignorance (*avidyā*), which is the root cause of all our ills. It keeps us in the dark about our true nature, which is infinite Consciousness. Out of ignorance we presume ourselves to be an independent individual identifying with a limited body-mind and the many limited experiences this yields. As apparently limited subjects, we consider ourselves separate from everything else, and thus we experience a need to extend ourselves into the apparent objective world. We reach out to appropriate more and more of the world from which we have artificially separated ourselves. This reaching out or grasping is what the Yoga tradition refers to as "greed" or "attachment." All it takes is to follow the lead of our senses. The *Bhagavad-Gītā* (2.62–63) portrays this situation very well:

> When a person thinks of things, contact with them is made. From contact springs desire; from desire arises anger.

Anger leads to bewilderment (*sammoha*); bewilderment [brings] confusion of the memory; confusion of the memory [leads to] obliteration of wisdom (*buddhi*). Upon the obliteration of wisdom, one is lost.

Human consciousness is characterized by a strong extravert tendency that reaches for objects via the senses. Hence the Yoga masters call for the control of both the mind and the senses, *citta-nigraha* and *indriya-nigraha*.

Buddhist Yoga speaks of three types of "thirsting" (*trishna*), or grasping: (1) thirsting for things of the world, (2) thirsting for rebirth, and (3) thirsting for liberation. While thirsting for liberation is preferable over the other two, it still represents a limitation. Therefore it, too, must be overcome. *Nirvāna* (nonblowing) was originally defined as the nonblowing of the wind of desire—for anything, including the impulse toward liberation. *Nirvāna* is realized only when every form of grasping is transcended.

According to an old Buddhist model, human life unfolds as a play of twelve factors of dependent origination (*pratītya-samutpāda*):

1. Ignorance (*avidyā*), which gives rise to
2. Volitional activity (*samskāra*), which can be bodily, vocal, or merely mental and which represents either meritorious or demeritorious karma; this leads to
3. Consciousness (*vijnāna*), which causes
4. "Name and form" (*nāma-rūpa*), which stands for what today is called the body-mind as a whole and which gives rise to
5. The "six bases" (*shad-āyatana*) consisting of the five senses and that part of the mind which processes sensory input; this leads to
6. Contact (*sparsha*) with sense objects, which gives rise to
7. Feeling (*samveda*), comprising pleasant, unpleasant, or neutral sensations; this evokes
8. Craving (*trishna*), or the desire to unite with pleasant or separate from unpleasant experiences, which leads to
9. Grasping (*upadāna*), which consists in one's holding onto specific experiences, views, behaviors, or the sense of self as such; this causes
10. "Becoming" (*bhava*), or a particular state of existence that corresponds to a person's inner constitution, which leads to
11. Birth (*jāti*), or the actual incarnation as a specific individual, which brings
12. Ageing and death (*jarā-marana*).

This causal nexus seeks to explain cyclic existence (*samsāra*) in terms of an individual's journey from birth to death to rebirth, ad infinitum. This model makes it clear that cyclic existence is not due to any outside agency but the human mind itself. In other words, we are creating our destiny in every moment. Yoga further tells us that *samsāra* is not inevitable but that we can stop the vicious cycle by modifying our volitional activity and behavior. This good news is fundamental to all forms of Yoga.

Greed is a phenomenon of the unregenerate psyche, which is under the spell of the conditioned nexus and has not taken control of its own destiny. Freedom from greed comes with nongrasping (*aparigraha*), which is based on the recognition that we are inherently complete and need nothing for our perfection.

❧ 46 ❧
Authenticity, Integrity, Unity

AUTHENTICITY, INTEGRITY, and unity can serve as solid guiding ideals for all Yoga practitioners and organizations and could also be adopted with benefit by anyone outside the field of Yoga.

"Authenticity" is meant to remind us that only authentic, genuine Yoga practice can bear positive fruit. That is to say, our practice must be informed by the highest standards of the Yoga tradition. This entails acknowledging the fact that Yoga is a *spiritual* way of life, not merely a system of physical or mental exercises for improving one's bodily health or psychic well-being. From the beginning, Yoga has had the purpose of assisting men and women in their impulse to go beyond the self or egoic personality and to connect with or realize the ultimate Reality whatever it may be called—Spirit, transcendental Self, Divine, or God/Goddess. This impulse is acknowledged as an essential prerequisite in all schools of Yoga and is called desire for liberation (*mumukshutva*).

In the absence of a deep connection with the ultimate Reality, we basically live inauthentic lives—revolving around self-centered expectations, assumptions, and projections. Yoga seeks to systematically undermine this falsity and restore us to our true identity as Spirit (*purusha, ātman, brahman*, etc.).

"Integrity" is intended to remind us that we should approach Yoga and life in general as whole beings, with wholeheartedness. We cannot hope to succeed in Yoga if we compartmentalize our yogic practice and our life. For instance, if we are keen meditators but ignore the moral rules of Yoga, we do violence to the wholeness of the yogic teachings and to our own wholeness. Or, if we are fond of the postures but ignore the spiritual context in which they occur, we likewise fall short of the ideals of Yoga. The yogic term for "integrity" is *ārjava*, which means literally "rectitude."

"Unity" is a reminder that we are not alone and also that we cannot succeed in isolation. Westerners, including Yoga practitioners, tend to be individualistic, which is fine. But we must always remember that our personal efforts could be greatly enriched by others, and that we could enrich the life and practice of others in turn. This is particularly true when we try to live a sane way of life in our contemporary society, which is scarcely supportive of personal growth and the spiritual quest. But even in earlier ages, the masters of Yoga emphasized the advantage of seeking out "good company" (*sat-sanga*).

It is essential that we cooperate with each other as much as possible — both on the individual and the organizational level. Strife between individuals and between one teacher or school and another simply has no place in the world of Yoga. One of the meanings of the Sanskrit word *yoga* is, after all, "union."

If we allow the three ideals of authenticity, integrity, and unity to invigorate our Yoga practice and our life in general, we will not only empower our personal growth but also the growth of other practitioners and the Yoga movement as a whole. The Yoga movement could become a powerful agent of social change in our confused world. Then it would benefit many more people than is the case at present.

✦ 47 ✦

The Power of Truth

ASSUMING EVERYONE WERE to lie about everything all the time, could we as individuals and as a society survive? The answer is a resounding No. For even if we were to convert in our heads every lie into its opposite, we would still not arrive at the truth in each and every case. Most of the time we would be guessing at the truth, and clearly this would complicate our lives infinitely. More than that, one can think of any number of instances where telling lies would have fatal consequences for the other person, possibly even for ourselves.

Truthfulness, on the contrary, is inherently life enhancing. Not only does it simplify our interactions with one another, it also is ennobling and dignifying. For in sharing the truth with another person, we affirm that person's intrinsic worthiness. Above all, through truthfulness we participate in Truth itself. It will become clear what I mean by this.

We can readily observe the chaotic effect of untruthfulness in daily life, especially among our leaders. Politics has become almost synonymous with lying and cheating. Big business is another area where lying is considered expedient, lest the truth should require sounder ecological and other standards and hence lead to a reduction in profits.

But lying may go even deeper than that. Two and a half millennia ago, the Greek philosopher Plato wondered in his *Republic* whether one could contrive a "noble lie" that would carry enough conviction for a whole community? In fact, such a core lie—though it may not be all that noble—is very much operative in our Western society. That lie is the belief, spawned by scientific materialism, that life is one-dimensional and that all talk about a higher Reality is mere fantasy or wishful thinking.

From this central lie springs an entire outlook on life that deprives us of our participation in the higher dimensions of existence and thus of our full human potential and dignity. For as long as we think and reinforce in each other the belief that we are mere meat bodies destined to vanish into oblivion at the hour of death, we are living a lie that diminishes us.

Little wonder that truthfulness has traditionally been celebrated as the highest moral virtue, and the foundation of all other virtues. Thus in the *Mahānirvāna-Tantra* (4.75–77), composed several centuries ago, we find the following declaration:

> There is no virtue greater than truth; there is no sin greater than falsehood. Therefore a mortal being should take refuge in truth with his entire self.

> Worship without truth is futile. Recitation (*japa*) without truth is useless. Asceticism (*tapas*) without truth is as unfruitful as seed on barren soil.

> The nature of truth is the supreme Absolute. Truth is the most asceticism. All actions should be rooted in truth. Nothing is superior to truth.

The above excerpt expresses a sentiment that once was global but that today is generally little more than a pretty saying. However, the spiritual traditions of the world, notably Yoga, contain many poignant considerations of the nature of truth and truthfulness, which have lost none of their relevance.

For the traditional *yogin*, truthfulness is a manifestation of the absolute Truth, which is the ultimate spiritual Reality itself. That is to say, when we are truthful we participate in some way in that ultimate Truth. To be true means to respect, adhere to, and even commune with that Reality. Therein lies the power of truth.

By being truthful we are true to our higher, divine or spiritual nature. The Sanskrit word for truthfulness is *satya*, which is both etymologically and semantically related to *sat*, denoting that which is real or truly existent. We transmute a part of the cosmos—our immediate circumstance and life—into a piece of heaven. This is the central task of all spiritual work: to transform nature, our own as well as nature in general, and to make it conform to that which is ultimately real. Truthfulness is the moral foundation upon which the Yoga practitioner can build his or her temple of spiritual discipline and conscious living. This is as true today as it was thousands of years ago.

Truthfulness has many aspects. One above all is sincerity, which is absolutely essential on the spiritual path. As the great Hindu scriptures remind us, so long as we are prone to deception, self-deception, dishonesty, pretense, hypocrisy, and posturing, our spiritual seeds will fall on barren soil. Lies are like quicksand, sucking even our best endeavors into darkness.

These thoughts seem almost outlandish to our modern mind, which is so used to a wide variety of deceptions. We are surrounded by pretense and lies—from advertising to politics to relationships. For many of us, truth is what is expedient in the moment. We have little white lies and large gray areas where neither truth nor falsehood reigns supreme. While there is something appropriate about our having jettisoned the intolerant black-and-white outlook of an earlier era, since life is a web of many colors, we tend to apply this newly found wisdom rather indiscriminately, usually in the hope of gaining personal advantage.

There are occasions when it would be brutal to tell the truth, as when a young child eagerly anticipating Santa Claus is told that Santa Claus does not exist. (It would presumably be better not to indoctrinate children with this myth from the sixth century C.E., which has been highly commercialized.) But there are many more occasions when telling the truth may hurt in the moment but bring about wholeness in the long run, as when we confess a transgression. But truthfulness takes courage and trust, two qualities that call for what was once called the heroic disposition.

Sincere Yoga practitioners are constantly challenged to bear the ultimate Truth in mind (and in their hearts). Yet their highest aspiration is sustained by those countless little truths that demand to be respected throughout the day. Yoga expects us to be heroes and heroines—not of the swashbuckling kind but of the sort that go about their daily routines with integrity and in the knowledge that truthfulness is a great power and integral to self-actualization and self-transcendence.

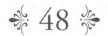

48

Compassion

ONE OF THE MOST sublime ideals of Yoga is that of the *bodhisattva*, the person dedicated to enlightenment for the benefit of all beings, which was the great contribution of the masters of Mahāyāna Buddhism. Moved by profound compassion (*karunā*), the *bodhisattva* engages the spiritual struggle toward perfection not merely for his or her own sake, but for the sake of sentient beings everywhere. To this the masters of Vajrayāna (Tantric) Buddhism added the sense of urgency. Since all unenlightened beings are inevitably suffering, the *bodhisattva* must waste no time on the spiritual path, so that their suffering can be ended as soon as possible. Of course, the Mahāyāna and Vajrayāna adepts were not ignorant of the fact that since there are infinite numbers of beings in the world of change (*samsāra*), the challenge to liberate them is practically impossible. Yet, this must not deter the *bodhisattva* from making absolutely every effort to attain enlightenment, or liberation, on behalf of everyone.

The Mahāyāna and Vajrayāna masters also were and are well aware of the following apparent contradiction in their teachings. They believe that every being and thing's innermost core is the Buddha Nature or *dharmakāya* and that we are merely ignorant of this unshakable fact. Therefore, from a higher perspective, everyone is already liberated and free from suffering and no one needs to make any effort to attain liberation either for himself or anybody else. Another way Buddhist philosophers have put this is to say that at the heart of everything is emptiness (*shūnyatā*) and therefore any possible thought, feeling, or action—including the impulse to free others from suffering—must be empty too. Thankfully they have not been stupefied by this apparent doctrinal contradiction but have always sought to integrate the ideal of compassion with that of wisdom (*prajnā*), realizing that "form is emptiness and emptiness is form."

It is sometimes thought that the *bodhisattva* ideal was radically innovative and that there is nothing like it in earlier Buddhism or other yogic teachings. This is not the case. While it can be said that the Mahāyāna masters developed the *bodhisattva* ideal into a full-fledged doctrine, concern for the welfare of others—especially their spiritual well-being—is present in Hīnayāna Buddhism as much as branches of Hindu and Jaina Yoga.

When we examine the spiritual paths and moral values of Hīnayāna, Mahāyāna, and Vajrayāna, we quickly find that all three "vehicles" (*yāna*) praise and recommend compassion in its various forms. The *bodhisattva* ideal can be viewed as an elaboration of earlier teachings on friendliness (*maitrī*) and compassion (*karunā*) toward all beings. In his book *Buddhist Images of Human Perfection*, Nathan Katz has clearly shown that goal and path in each of the three vehicles of Buddhism are, contrary to much popular and scholarly opinion, equivalent.[1]

When we turn to Hindu Yoga, we find a similar emphasis where a compassionate concern for others is considered an integral part of moral practice. Thus Patanjali, in his *Yoga-Sūtra* (1.33), names the same four disciplines that, in Buddhism, make up the *brahma-vihāras* or "brahmic abidings": friendliness (*maitrī*), compassion (*karunā*), joy (*muditā*), and equanimity (*upekshā*). These are to be contemplated, cultivated, and projected toward all beings. As the Sanskrit name *brahma-vihāra* suggests, this was in all probability originally a Hindu teaching, which was so significant and widespread that the Buddha readily adopted it (see *Majjhīma-Nikāya* 1.38).

We find the same four disciplines mentioned also in the Haribhadra Sūri's *Yoga-Bindu* (402), a Jaina work dating from the eighth century C.E. Jainism, in general, lays great store by reverence for all beings and the virtue of kindness (*dayā*).

Many other instances could be cited for all these traditions which would show the pervasiveness of such moral virtues as compassion or kindness in Hindu, Buddhist, and Jaina Yoga. How could it be otherwise? The path to freedom unfolds through the purification of our own mind—a process that, in the language of Hinduism, can be characterized as the progressive *sattvification* of one's being. *Sattva*, according to Hindu Yoga, is the highest aspect of the conditional universe. As one of three fundamental forces of Nature (*prakriti*), it is present to varying degrees in everything, but is present to a superlative degree in all those states of mind that we would consider noble and highly desirable. By cultivating virtues like compassion, the *yogin* automatically increases the *sattva* content of the mind, thus bringing him closer to inner freedom. Ultimately, *sattva* has to be transcended in favor of a state that is beyond all qualities and forms. Apart from its spiritual value, compassion clearly also has merit from a more conventional point of view. As the Dalai Lama put it:

> Compassion, loving kindness, altruism, and a sense of brotherhood and sisterhood are the keys to human development, not only in the future but in the present as well . . . Thus, we find that kindness and a good heart form the underlying foundation for our success in this life, our progress on the spiritual path, and our fullfilment of our ultimate aspiration, the attainment of full enlightenment. Hence, kindness and a good heart are not only important at the beginning but also in the middle and at the end. Their necessity and value are not limited to any specific time, place, society, or culture.[2]

49

Ethical Guidelines for Yoga Teachers

Yoga is an integrated way of life, which includes moral standards—traditionally called "virtues"—that any reasonable human being will find in principle acceptable. Some of these standards are encoded in the first limb (*anga*) of Patanjali's eightfold path (*ashtānga-yoga*), called *yama* (discipline or restraint). According to Patanjali's *Yoga-Sūtra* (2.30), this practice category is composed of the following five virtues: nonharming (*ahimsā*), truthfulness (*satya*), nonstealing (*asteya*), chastity (*brahmacarya*), and greedlessness (*aparigraha*). These have been explained by traditional authorities and also by modern interpreters. In other key scriptures of Yoga further moral principles are mentioned, including kindness, compassion, generosity, patience, helpfulness, forgiveness, purity, and so on. All these are virtues that we connect with a "good" person and that are demonstrated to a superlative degree in the lives of the great masters of Yoga.

In light of this, it seems appropriate for contemporary Yoga teachers to endeavor to conduct their lives in consonance with the moral principles put forward in Yoga. As teachers, they have a great responsibility toward their students, and they can be expected to clearly demonstrate the qualities one would associate with a good teacher. As practitioners and representatives of Yoga, their behavior can be expected to reflect the high moral standards espoused in Yoga. At the same time, we must take into account the present-day sociocultural context, which differs in some ways from the conditions of pre-modern India.

The following guidelines were formulated for the Yoga Research and Education Center as part of its effort to help preserve the traditional legacy of Yoga and improve the quality of Yoga teaching and practice in the modern world.

- Yoga teachers understand and appreciate that teaching Yoga is a noble and ennobling endeavor, which aligns them with a long line of honorable teachers.

- Yoga teachers are committed to practicing Yoga as a way of life.
- Yoga teachers are committed to maintaining impeccable standards of professional competence and integrity.
- Yoga teachers dedicate themselves to a thorough and continuing study and practice of Yoga, in particular the theoretical and practical aspects of the branch or type of Yoga that they teach others.
- Yoga teachers are committed to avoiding substance abuse and, if for some reason, they succumb to chemical dependency will stop teaching until they are free again from drug and alcohol abuse. In that case, they will do everything in their power to stay free, including full accountability to a support group.
- Yoga teachers will accurately represent their education, training, and experience relevant to their teaching of Yoga.
- Yoga teachers are committed to promoting the physical, mental, and spiritual well-being of their students.
- Yoga teachers, especially those teaching Hatha-Yoga, will abstain from giving medical advice, or advice that could be interpreted as such, unless they have the necessary medical qualifications.
- Yoga teachers particularly embrace the ideal of truthfulness in dealing with students and others.
- Yoga teachers are open to instructing all students irrespective of race, nationality, gender, sexual orientation, and social or financial status.
- Yoga teachers are willing to accept students with physical disabilities, providing they have the skill to teach those students properly.
- Yoga teachers will treat their students with respect.
- Yoga teachers will never force their own opinions on students but appreciate the fact that every individual is entitled to his or her worldview, ideas, and beliefs. At the same time, however, Yoga teachers must communicate to their students that Yoga seeks to achieve a deep-level transformation of the human personality, including attitudes and ideas. If a student is not open to change or if a student's opinions seriously impede the process of communicating yogic teachings to him or her, then the Yoga teacher is free to refuse to work with that individual and, if possible, find an amicable way of dissolving the teaching relationship.
- Yoga teachers will avoid any form of sexual harassment of students.
- Yoga teachers wishing to enter a consensual sexual relationship with a present or former student should seek the immediate counsel of their peers before taking any action.
- Yoga teachers will make every effort to avoid exploiting the trust and

potential dependency of students and instead encourage them to find greater inner freedom.

- Yoga teachers acknowledge the importance of the proper context for teaching and agree to avoid teaching in a casual manner, which includes observing proper decorum inside and outside of class.
- Yoga teachers strive to practice tolerance toward other Yoga teachers, schools, and traditions. When criticism has to be brought, this should be done in fairness and with appropriate regard for the facts.

These ethical guidelines are not exhaustive, and the fact that a given conduct is not specifically covered by these guidelines does not say anything about the ethical or unethical nature of that conduct. Yoga teachers always endeavor to respect and, to the best of their abilities, adhere to the traditional yogic code of conduct as well as to the law current in their country or state.

PART FOUR

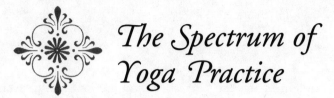 *The Spectrum of Yoga Practice*

❧ 50 ❧
Āsanas for the Body and the Mind

A Brief History of Āsana

The *Vedas*, India's oldest scriptures, do not mention the Sanskrit word *āsana* anywhere, though they make use of the verbal root *ās* meaning "to sit," which is closely connected with the root *as* meaning "to be." Both verbal roots suggest the sense of "abiding." The cognate term *āsandī* occurs already in the *Atharva-Veda* (15.3.2), which in its final version must have existed by 2500 B.C.E. or so. This refers to a "seat" or "stool." Thus the *vrātya*, a type of ascetic in Vedic times, is said to have sat on an *āsandī* while contemplating the mysteries of life. This term was also used in the *Brāhmanas* and *Āranyakas*, but it was not until the *Brihad-Āranyaka-Upanishad* (6.2.4), possibly the earliest text of the Upanishadic genre (c. 1500–1000 B.C.E.), that the synonym *āsana* came into vogue.

Originally, like its cognate *āsandī*, *āsana* simply referred to a seat upon which the sage would settle for meditation or sacrificial rituals. This is exactly the usage in the *Brihad-Āranyaka-Upanishad* and the archaic *Taittirīya-Upanishad* (1.11.3). The old *Kaushītaki-Upanishad* (1.3 and 1.5), however, still uses *āsandī* instead of *āsana*. This might be due to local usage or suggest an earlier date for this *Upanishad* than is normally assumed. Even in the *Bhagavad-Gītā* (6.11–12; 11.42), which can be dated to c. 500 B.C.E., *āsana* is still understood in the sense of a sitting platform. The *Maitrāyanīya-Upanishad*, which can be dated to c. 300 B.C.E., taught a six-limbed yogic path (*shad-anga-yoga*), which excluded *yama* (moral discipline), *niyama* (self-restraint), and *āsana* (posture) as separate categories. Patanjali recognized *āsana* as the third limb of his eightfold path (*ashta-anga-yoga*) and in his *Yoga-Sūtra* (2.46) tells us that posture should be easeful (*sukha*) and stable (*sthīra*). Vyāsa, in his fifth-century *Yoga-Bhāshya* commentary on Patanjali's work, lists by name eleven postures, all of which appear to have been used for meditation: (1) *padma-āsana* (lotus posture), (2) *vīra-āsana* (hero's posture), (3) *bhadra-āsana* (auspicious posture), (4) *svastika* (hail [posture]), (5) *danda-āsana* (staff posture), (6) *sopāshraya* ([posture] with a support),

(7) *paryanka* (bedstead), (8) *kraunca-nishpadana* (curlew seat), (9) *hasti-nishadana* (elephant seat), (10) *ushtra-nishadana* (camel seat), and (11) *sama-samsthāna* (even arrangement).

Once *āsana* had acquired the sense of "posture," it first clearly referred only to meditation postures, such as the all-time favorite lotus posture (*padma-āsana*) and adept's or accomplished posture (*siddha-āsana*). With the emergence of Tantra, which primarily regarded the human body as a temple of the Divine, the way was open to the development of posture as an instrument for intensifying the life energy (*prāna*), maintaining or restoring health and prolonging life. This aspect of *āsana* was particularly developed in the schools of Hatha-Yoga, a branch of Tantra that emerged c. 1000 C.E. Hatha-Yoga is traditionally considered to be the invention of Goraksha Nātha, who is still remembered as one of the immortal Tantric adepts. One posture even bears his name.

According to the *Goraksha-Paddhati* (1.9), Shiva long ago taught 8,400,000 kinds of *āsana* of which only 84 are particularly useful to Yoga practitioners. The *Hatha-Yoga-Pradīpikā*, a widely used traditional manual dating back to the mid-fourteenth century, describes sixteen postures. The *Gheranda-Samhitā*, a seventeenth-century manual, furnishes practical details on thirty-two postures. Some modern handbooks on Hatha-Yoga contain descriptions of 200 and more postures, and one work published in Brazil shows illustrations of over 2,000 postures, including variations.

TOWARD A PHILOSOPHY OF ĀSANA

Many contemporary Yoga practitioners, especially those in Western countries, look upon *āsana* as a tool for achieving physical fitness and flexibility. The yogic postures have certainly demonstrated their physiological benefits in millions of cases. They improve musculoskeletal flexibility, strength, resilience, endurance, cardiovascular and respiratory efficiency, endocrine and gastrointestinal functioning, immunity, sleep, eye-hand coordination, balance. Experiments also have shown various psychological benefits, including improvement of somatic awareness, attention, memory, learning, and mood. The regular practice of postures also decreases anxiety, depression, and aggression.[1]

All these effects are clearly beneficial and highly desirable. Yet, the traditional purpose of *āsana* is something far more radical, namely to assist the Hatha-Yoga practitioner in the creation of an "adamantine body" (*vajra-deha*) or "divine body" (*divya-deha*). This is a transubstantiated body that is immortal and completely under the control of the adept's will (which is merged with the Divine Will). It is an energy body that, depending on the adept's wish, is either visible or invisible to the human eye. In this body, the liberated master can carry out benevolent activities with the least possible obstruction.

ĀSANA AS A TOOL OF NONDUAL EXPERIENCE[2]

The transubstantiated body of the truly accomplished Hatha-Yoga master is, realistically speaking, out of reach for most of us—not because we are not in principle capable of realizing it but because only very few have the determination and stamina to even pursue this yogic ideal. Does this mean we have to settle for the more pedestrian benefits of posture practice? I believe there is another side to *āsana*, which, while not representing the ultimate possibility of our human potential, is yet a significant and necessary accomplishment on the yogic path. That is to cultivate and experience *āsana* as an instrument for tasting nonduality (*advaita*). Almost all Yoga authorities subscribe to a nondualistic metaphysics according to which Reality is singular and the world of multiplicity is either altogether false (*mithyā*) or merely a lower expression of that ultimate Singularity.

Typically, Yoga practitioners assume that the experience of nonduality is bound to the state of ecstasy (*samādhi*) and that this state is hard to come by and is likely to escape them at least in this lifetime. But this belief is ill founded. In fact, it is counterproductive and should be regarded as an obstacle (*vighna*) on the path to enlightenment. While we might not have an experience of ecstasy, we *can* have an experience of nonduality. The ecstatic state is simply a special version of the nondual experience. As Karl Baier, a German professor of psychology and practitioner of Iyengar Yoga, has shown, posture practice can be an efficient means of nondual experience in which we overcome the most obvious and painful duality of body and mind. In his own words:

> There is no duality between body and mind insofar as we are personally living the body; only when we are looking at the body as an external, corporeal thing—a point of view that is not in accordance with its essence—then the problem of body and mind relationship may arise. But if you look closer at what is happening, you may find that it is never a mind without a body that objectifies the body; it is always the living body that objectifies parts of itself.[3]

Through the medium of attention, or present-mindedness, we can in fact integrate body and mind in any given moment. This is the process underlying meditation. It also is fundamental to the performance of yogic postures. This is why B. K. S. Iyengar was able to write that in the practice of *āsana*, the five "sheaths" (*kosha*) "come together in each and every one of our trillions of cells."[4] The five "sheaths" or "casings" are: (1) the sheath composed of food (*anna-maya-kosha*), or physical body, (2) the sheath composed of vital energy (*prāna-maya-kosha*), (3) the sheath composed of the lower mind (*mano-maya-kosha*), (4) the sheath composed of understanding (*vijnāna-maya-kosha*), and (5) the sheath composed of bliss (*ānanda-maya-kosha*). When these five levels of our being are integrated through the medium of attention or mindfulness, *āsana* becomes what Iyengar calls a "contemplative pose." Thus *āsana*, correctly performed, is meditation.

Iyengar also observed that the typical body is dull, or defined by a preponderance of *tamas* (the principle of inertia).[5] *Āsanas* introduce *rajas* (the principle of dynamism) into the system and cause the body to become more vibrant. The next step, as he explained, is to increase *sattva* (the principle of luminosity) in the body, so that it can more and more reflect the Light of the transcendental Self (*ātman*).

✣ 51 ✣
Shava-Āsana, or Corpse Posture

ALL YOGIC POSTURES are an effort to unify or simplify our somatic existence. They are as it were one-pointedness (ekāgratā)[1] at the level of the body. Ordinarily we are as distracted on the physical level as we are on the mental level. Our bodily behavior is a direct manifestation of our mental state. This can best be seen when we are waiting for something or someone. We fidget, rock ourselves, drum with our fingers, chew gum, whistle, hum, or talk to ourselves. We cannot sit still or keep quiet, and in fact some people are afraid of silence and inactivity. In other words, our body and mind are in a scattered state.

The yogin behaves in the exact opposite way. He sits for hours without moving and even barely blinks. He is fond of silence and solitude and is content, without need for stimulation from the senses. He is able to do all this because of his deep inner renunciation (samnyāsa), which makes him impartial to all the many things that preoccupy the ordinary individual. There are some yogins who show their impartiality to worldly things by walking about naked wearing only ashes from the cremation ground. This is also how God Shiva, the archetypal yogin, is typically portrayed in Hindu art. The ashes indicate that the yogin has burnt all desires and therefore the seeds of future karma.

The ash-besmeared ascetics are inwardly dead to the world. From a worldly perspective, they are walking dead—though, to be sure, they are full of life on the inside. This combination of outer death and inner life are beautifully exemplified in depictions of Shiva and the Goddess Kālī, who stands fiercely on her reclining divine spouse. Shiva wears only ashes but his sexual organ is stiff with life force, suggesting that he is not at all dead.

The yogic posture of shava-āsana (spoken: shavāsana), meaning the "corpse posture," is outwardly immobile but inwardly very much alive. It combines inner stillness with high energy, thus perfectly symbolizing the essence of Yoga. This goes to show that relaxation, which is the purpose of shava-āsana, is not mere inertia. Relaxation contains a preponderance of *sattva*, the principle of lucidity and easefulness, which demarcates it from sleep, which is defined by the overwhelming presence of *tamas*, the principle of inertia.

Also called *mrita-āsana* (dead posture) or *preta-āsana* (ghost posture), this pose is the yogic name for relaxation exercise, which consists in lying still like a corpse. It is mentioned already in the *Hatha-Yoga-Pradīpikā* (1.32), a fourteenth-century manual, where it is said to ward off fatigue and bring mental repose. *Shava-āsana* is typically performed by lying flat on one's back, with legs slightly (c. 30 degrees) apart and arms somewhat extended to allow one's palms to be comfortably turned up. Some Yoga teachers recommend that the hands should rest on their edges, with the thumbs facing up.

A variation of this posture is mentioned in the *Hatha-Sanketa-Candrikā*, which recommends that it should be executed by resting the hands on the chest (*hrid*, "heart"). No explanation is given for this departure from earlier authorities. Presumably this variant hand position creates a psychoenergetic circuit that revitalizes the heart center. During the execution of *shava-āsana*, the eyes should be closed and the mouth relaxed. Breathing is done through the nose, with the mind observing the movement of the breath or, in modern terms, visualization of oneself floating in the warm waters of a tropical lagoon. According to the *Yoga-Shāstra* (line 46), one should absorb the mind in the left or right big toe. Even five minutes of *shava-āsana* will be found helpful, though it is best to practice it a minimum of twenty minutes. Surprisingly, *shava-āsana* — despite its technical simplicity — is not easy to master.

The benefits of *shava-āsana* have been investigated by various researchers. K. N. Udupa, at Benares Hindu University, published an article on "Disorders of Stress and Their Management by Yoga" in 1978 in which he states that *shava-āsana* significantly reduced plasma catecholamines and nervous system activity in his test subjects.[2] (Plasma catecholamines are chemicals that have hormonal functions.) In the late 1960s, K. K. Datey and his team at the King Edward Memorial Hospital in Bombay demonstrated that *shava-āsana* can be a very effective tool for combating hypertension.[3] The patients were instructed to breathe slowly, rhythmically, and with the diaphragm. They also were asked to pay attention to the flow of the breath, particularly the sensations at the nostrils. It took patients approximately three weeks to adequately learn *shava-āsana*. Those who were taking drugs were able to lower the dosage, and those who were not on medication for their hypertension were able to significantly lower their blood pressure.

C. H. Patel in England reported a similar success with *shava-āsana* in the management of hypertension in various studies in the early to mid-1970s.[4]

In his commentary on the *Hatha-Yoga-Pradīpikā*, Swami Muktabodhananda Saraswati (under the guidance of Swami Satyananda Saraswati of the Bihar School of Yoga) enthusiastically (and with good reason) wrote about the corpse posture as follows:

It is very useful in yogic management of high blood pressure, peptic ulcers, anxiety, hysteria, cancer and all psychosomatic diseases and neuroses. In fact, shavasana is beneficial no matter what the condition is, even in perfect health, because it brings up the latent impressions buried within the subconscious mind. The mind which operates during waking consciousness relaxes and subsides. It is therefore necessary to practice shavasana for developing dharana [concentration] and dhyana [meditation]. Even though it is a static pose it revitalizes the entire system.[5]

❧ 52 ❧
The Breath of Life

WEDGED BETWEEN THE visible material realm and the transcendental Reality is *prāna* (life) or *prāna-shakti* (life energy). This is an all-pervasive power that sustains every material thing. In its cosmic or universal aspect, it is known as *mukhya-prāna*; in its microcosmic or individual aspect, it is simply *prāna*, and the breath is its material correlate. The term is composed of the prefix *pra-* and the verbal root *ān* (to breathe). The word *prāna* is widely used already in the archaic *Rig-Veda*. By the time of the *Atharva-Veda* (Chapter 15), some 4,500 years ago, we encounter the familiar division of the life energy/breath into five aspects as follows:

1. *prāna* (in-breath)—the life energy residing in the chest and which is connected with inhalation
2. *apāna* (out-breath)—the life energy present in the lower abdomen and which is associated with exhalation
3. *udāna* (up-breath)—the life energy present in the area of the throat and head and which is associated with speech and, in particular, the yogic processes of meditation and conscious dying
4. *samāna* (mid-breath)—the life energy residing in the upper abdomen and navel area and which is responsible, among other things, for the digestive process
5. *vyāna* (through-breath)—the life energy circulating throughout the body

In addition to the above principal types of life force, some scriptures also know of five secondary types (*upaprāna*), namely *nāga* (lit. "serpent"), *kūrma* (tortoise), *kri-kara* (*kri*-maker), *deva-datta* (God-given), and *dhanam-jaya* (conquest of wealth), which are respectively associated with vomiting (or eructation), blinking, hunger (or sneezing), sleep (or yawning), and decomposition of the corpse.

All these "breaths" animate the otherwise inert body. Especially *prāna* and *apāna* play an important role in Yoga. As the *Goraksha-Paddhati* (1.38–40), a twelfth/thirteenth-century work on Hatha-Yoga, states:

As a ball hit with a crook flies up, so the psyche (*jīva*), propelled by *prāna* and *apāna*, does not stand still

Under the impact of *prāna* and *apāna*, the psyche rushes up and down through the left and right pathways and on account of this fickleness cannot be perceived.

As a hawk tied to a rope can be brought back again when it has flown away, so the psyche bound to the qualities (*guna*) [of the cosmos, or *prakriti*] is pulled along by *prāna* and *apāna*.

The above stanzas spell out one of the great discoveries of Yoga, namely that mind and breath (or life energy) are closely connected. Influencing the one means influencing the other. When we are upset, we breathe faster. When we are calm, our breathing slows down. *Yogins* understood this early on and invented a battery of techniques for controlling the breath in order to control the mind. These techniques are called *prānāyāma*, which is widely translated as "breath control." The literal meaning of this Sanskrit term is "lengthening of the life energy." This is accomplished through breathing rhythmically and slowly and through the special yogic practice of prolonged retention of the breath, either before or after inhalation.

In Patanjali's eightfold path, breath control constitutes the fourth limb. He did not describe or prescribe any specific technique, and elaboration was left to the adepts of Hatha-Yoga many centuries later. They, like most other Tantric adepts, were eager to explore the *prāna-maya-kosha*, or the "etheric body," and its subtle energetic environment. By contrast, most contemporary schools of Hatha-Yoga ignore *prāna* and *prānāyāma*, just as they ignore the mental disciplines and spiritual goals, and instead promote a plethora of physical postures (*āsana*). This emphasis is problematical, as it has led to an unfortunate reductionism and distortion of the traditional yogic heritage.

The gradual re-inclusion of *prānāyāma* into contemporary Hatha-Yoga, however, is very promising, because this practice sooner or later leads to an experiential encounter with *prāna*, which is distinct from mere oxygen.

According to Yoga, we are meant to live a full 120 years. Since we take 21,600 breaths every day, the total number of breath in our lifetime will be 946,080,000 breaths. This may seem like a lot, but we also know that life goes by very quickly. Therefore it makes sense to want our every breath count, and Yoga makes this possible.

❧ 53 ❧
Cultivating Wisdom

WISDOM ARISES IN US whenever the quality of *sattva* grows stronger in the mind. *Sattva*, which literally means "being-ness," is one of three primary qualities (*guna*) of creation. The other two qualities are *rajas* (the dynamic principle) and *tamas* (the principle of inertia). These primary qualities underlie absolutely everything that is other than the superconscious Spirit, which is pure Awareness. According to Yoga and Sāmkhya, they are the behavioral modes of *prakriti*, often translated as "Nature" but standing for the universe in all its dimensions. Together, in various mixtures, they shape all forms at whatever level of existence, material and mental. Only at the transcendental level of *prakriti*—which is called *prakriti-pradhāna* or "creatrix foundation"—do the three qualities exist in perfect balance. As soon as this primordial balance is disturbed, the process of creation sets in, beginning with the most subtle (mental) manifestations and terminating with the material realm.

Sattva represents the principle of lucidity or transparency, as it manifests in and through wisdom. Just as the moon, which has no atmosphere, oceans, or vegetation, reflects the light of the sun, so *sattva* reflects the superconscious Spirit more faithfully than the other two qualities of creation. By comparison, *rajas* and *tamas* are obscuring factors, which distort our vision of the superconscious Spirit.

Like everything within creation, the human mind is not pure *sattva* but a composite of the three primary qualities. And, significantly, the composition varies from individual to individual. Thus there are as many shades of mental lucidity as there are human beings (or living creatures in general). Even in a single day, our individual mind cycles through a series of qualitative changes that correspond to the relative preponderance of one primary quality over another. For instance, the waking state contains overall more *sattva* than the dream state, which has a predominance of *rajas*, while deep sleep shows a preeminence of the principle of inertia. Or, to give another example, when we are peaceful and calm, our mind is governed primarily by *sattva;* when we are agitated, our mind is ruled by *rajas,* and when we feel bored and dull, *tamas* predominates.

The Sanskrit language knows many words for "wisdom:" *jnāna, vidyā, prajñā, medhā, buddhi,* and so on. I will single out the term *buddhi* here, because it is significant in the Yoga and Sāmkhya traditions. It can stand for both wisdom and the organ of wisdom, that is, the higher mind. The lower mind (*manas*) is bound to the physical senses, which supply it with an incessant stream of information that it then processes to produce knowledge. Thus it is characterized by a preponderance of *rajas,* the principle of dynamism. The higher mind, in which *sattva* is preeminent, does not depend in the same way on the senses and the brain. Traditionally, it is compared to a polished mirror that reflects the light of Consciousness (*cit*) more faithfully than the lower mind. When the light of Consciousness or transcendental Awareness falls into the higher mind, wisdom is produced.

This is a particular kind of knowing, which relates not so much to the finite world of physical or psychological realities but to the Spirit. At the level of the intellect, wisdom can be said to augment Awareness in us. At the level of feelings, wisdom generates such elevated states as universal love, compassion, kindness, patience, tolerance, and other similar virtues. At the level of values, wisdom is responsible for our concern with the ideal of goodness, beauty, and harmony. Not least, the presence of wisdom creates in us the urge toward self-understanding, self-discipline, self-transcendence, and, ultimately, Self-realization. In other words, the impulse toward freedom and liberation, or enlightenment, becomes manifest in us when wisdom harmonizes the otherwise turbulent mind. More than that, wisdom is the means by which liberation or enlightenment is made possible.

Whatever yogic path we may follow, all paths unfold through wisdom. Even Bhakti-Yoga, the spiritual discipline of self-surrender to the Divine Being, relies on the liberating power of wisdom. For before we can practice self-surrender, we must first determine—through applied wisdom—the proper object of our devotion. Otherwise we could end up worshiping "false gods" or confuse the self (ego) with the transcendental Identity or Self. Our emotions are notoriously unreliable if left to their own devices; they require the light of intelligence in the form of wisdom.

Or, how could we practice Karma-Yoga, the yogic path of self-transcending day-to-day action, without having wisdom tell us what course of action is appropriate in any given case? The God-man Krishna addressed this vital point in the *Bhagavad-Gītā* to end Prince Arjuna's mental confusion.

The cultivation of wisdom is clearly a priority on the spiritual path. Since wisdom is a function of the presence of *sattva*, we can invite wisdom to manifest in us through any and all activities that enhance *sattva* in our body and mind: Eating pure and wholesome food, keeping the body healthy through appropriate exercise and other habits, entertaining pure and wholesome thoughts, engaging in virtuous actions, remaining attentive in all situations, speaking kind and helpful words and otherwise practicing silence (*mauna*), cultivating self-observation, self-understanding, and self-discipline, focusing on that which matters rather than scattering our energy and attention, developing concentration and meditation, cultivating a joyful mood, conquering doubt through faith (*shraddhā*) in ourselves, as well as in the process of self-transformation, the ideal of liberation, and the great teachings and teachers.

The more we foster the *sattva* quality in ourselves, the more wisdom will guide us in making the right choices in all areas of life. Whereas the self-divided mind lacking in wisdom is typically problem oriented, the wisdom mind always offers "natural," plausible solutions. Wisdom puts us in the flow of things. By contrast, the unwise mind experiences itself as immersed in a hostile environment that must be fought and conquered. Wisdom shows us that there is nothing to conquer. The universe is not our enemy; only our false sense of being a limited ego-personality encased by a limited body gives us this illusion, which is the source of all our pain and suffering (*duhkha*).

Wisdom is not about yet another piece of information that has to be judged and either accepted or rejected; rather it gives us a view of the whole situation and thus shows us a way out of all dilemma or conflict. Wisdom is marked by wholeness and happiness.

Therefore let us cultivate *sattva* in everything we do, say, and think so that wisdom may illuminate the path before us.

❧ 54 ❧
Buddhi-Yoga

WE FIRST HEAR ABOUT Buddhi-Yoga in the *Katha-Upanishad*, which we may assign to the earlier half of the second millennium B.C.E., and the *Bhagavad-Gītā* (Lord's Song), which in its present form was composed several centuries later. In both these works, the word *buddhi* is used in the context of teachings that are typical of the tradition of Sāmkhya, or rather Sāmkhya-Yoga. The Sanskrit term *buddhi* has a wide range of meanings: "mind," "idea," "intention," "thought," "intelligence," "understanding," "reason," "opinion," "conviction," "belief," etc. It derives from the verbal root *budh* "to be awake/aware" and is closely associated with *buddha* (awakened) and *bodha* (awareness or enlightenment). Understandably, the word *buddhi* is widely employed in the Yoga literature and often in the sense of "wisdom" or "organ of wisdom."

When we examine the ancient *Katha-Upanishad* (1.3.3–4), we find that the term *buddhi* is not to be met with until the third section of chapter 1, where it appears in connection with the well-known chariot metaphor:

> Know the Self (*ātman*) as the chariot-lord and the body as the chariot. Know the *buddhi* as the charioteer and the mind (*manas*) as the reins.

> The senses, they say, are the horses; the sense objects (*artha*) are their pastures. The sages declare the enjoyer [i.e., the Self] to be associated with oneself (*ātman*) [i.e., one's body], the senses, and the mind.[1]

In this passage a clear distinction is made between *buddhi* and *manas* — a distinction that is fundamental in the metaphysics of Hindu Yoga and Sāmkhya. From the stanzas that follow, it is evident that the *buddhi's* allocated function is that of understanding (*vijnāna*). The person who lacks understanding, whose mind is unchecked and whose senses are rampant is assured of continued entanglement in the world of change (*samsāra*). By contrast, the person of understanding, who has understanding for his charioteer, will win the estate of Vishnu, that is, attain liberation.

The above-cited stanzas imply the kind of ontological hierarchy that marks the philosophy of almost all Sāmkhya and Hindu Yoga schools. The following seven main categories are distinguished:

1. Self (*purusha*)
2. Unmanifest (*avyakta*)
3. Great self (*mahān ātman*)
4. Organ of wisdom (*buddhi*)
5. Mind (*manas*)
6. Sense objects (*artha*)
7. Senses (*indriya*)

The *purusha*, equated in stanza 12 with the *ātman*, is our true Identity and the supreme goal of human existence. It can be "seen," or known, only by means of a focused (*agra*) and subtle (*sūkshma*) intelligence (*buddhi*). How this is to be achieved is explained in the next verse, which states that one should constrain one's speech in the mind, the mind in the "knowledge self" (*jnāna-ātman*), the "knowledge (self)" in the "great self" (*mahān ātman*), and that in the "tranquil Self" (*shānta-ātman*). In this sequence, speech stands for all sensory functions, which are to be gathered into the lower mind (*manas*)—a process that is the essence of the yogic practice of sensory inhibition (*pratyāhāra*), which came to constitute the fifth limb of Patanjali's eightfold path. By "knowledge self" is undoubtedly meant the *buddhi*, which corresponds to the "sheath made of knowledge" (*vijnāna-maya-kosha*) mentioned in the *Taittirīya-Upanishad*. When the senses have been brought under control, then the lower mind itself must be focused within the higher mind, which, according to Patanjali (c. 150 C.E.), is accomplished through the integrated process of concentration (*dhāranā*), meditation (*dhyāna*), and ecstasy (*samādhi*). The "tranquil Self" can be none other than the supreme Self (*purusha*).

Thus we find that of the seven categories mentioned above, the process of meditative involution involves only five categories. The remaining two, that is, the sense objects and the Unmanifest (i.e., the core of Nature), refer to the objective aspect of reality. The Unmanifest is the "signless" (*alinga*) objective counterpart to the "signless" transcendental Subject, or Self. Of special interest is the term "great self," which R. E. Hume wrongly assumed to be identical with the *buddhi*. Rather, this is the matrix of cosmic existence, analogous to the concept of the creator (*īshvara*) of later schools and also corresponding to the *mahat* of Classical Yoga. We could speak of it as

the collectivity of all *buddhis* or, in Jungian terms, the collective unconscious or, from a more yogic perspective, as cosmic consciousness. Although
the *buddhi* is attributed with intelligence and understanding, it actually is
a product of insentient Nature and as such does not have consciousness of
its own. This typical Sāmkhya-Yoga doctrine is reiterated in the *Katha-
Upanishad* (2.3.7–8) as follows:

> Greater than the senses is the mind. Superior to the mind is *sattva.*
> Higher than *sattva* is the "great self." Superior to the "great [self]" is the
> Unmanifest.

> But greater than the Unmanifest is the all-pervading and signless *pu-
> rusha,* knowing which a person is liberated and attains immortality.

Here the synonym *sattva* is introduced for the term *buddhi,* which is not
uncommon. R. E. Hume, in his translation of the passage, repeated his mistake of identifying the "great self" with the *buddhi.* In stanza 10 of the same
chapter, it is said that the supreme condition is actualized when the five
"knowledges" (*jnāna*), that is, the cognitive senses, together with the mind,
remain motionless and when even the *buddhi* is not active. The mind is
thought to be closer to the senses than the *buddhi,* which itself is in proximity to the supra-individual "great self."

Buddhi and *manas* are not unlike the German polar concepts of *Vernunft* and *Verstand* respectively. The former is the receptive, intuitive side
of mentation, the latter is the faculty of reasoning, logic and postulation.

Looked at from the viewpoint of the triad of forces, the *gunas,* which in
collaboration unfurl the psychophysical universe, the *buddhi* shows a predominance of the lucidity factor; hence its designation *sattva.* This expression is used in a very similar way in the *Yoga-Sūtra* (see 2.41; 3.35, 49, 55).
Metaphorically speaking, the *buddhi* or *sattva* is that level of the human
personality that is so rarefied as to be capable of receiving the "light" of the
self-luminous *purusha.* In contrast, the mind or *manas* shows a preponderance of the forces of *rajas* and *tamas,* which make it relatively unreceptive
to the *purusha's* brilliance.

Although the *buddhi* is naturally closer to our true Identity than is the
sense-bound mind, it must still be prepared to act as a fit reflector. The
anonymous author of the *Katha-Upanishad,* therefore, speaks of making it
"pointed" or focused, and "subtle" or turned inward or upward rather than
outward and downward. But, as is apparent from verse 2.3.11, the essence of

Yoga is the control of the senses (*indriya-dhārana*), which are inherently unstable. The control of the mind depends on the control of the senses.

We encounter similar teachings in the *Bhagavad-Gītā*, which, like the *Katha-Upanishad*, is a document of the Sāmkhya-Yoga tradition preceding Patanjali's Classical Yoga. At first, before commencement of the great battle, the God-man Krishna instructs his disciple Prince Arjuna in the wisdom of Sāmkhya, consisting in tenets like the following:

• Our true nature is eternal and unmodifiable (and hence indestructible).

• We inhabit body after body so long as we do not know our true nature.

• Since our bodily existence is of no ultimate consequence, we also do not need to be too concerned about it but focus on realizing our immortal Self, or Spirit. This entails not worrying about taking military action when the larger good is at stake.

These basic insights, Krishna explains, make up the wisdom of Sāmkhya (2.39). To them we may profitably add the wisdom of Yoga, specifically Karma-Yoga, which tells us how to act in the world without incurring sin (or karma). Such Yoga is anchored in the grand ideal of action transcendence (*naishkarmya-karman*) grounded in equanimity (*samatva*). When we are inwardly unattached and balanced, our actions cannot defile us, including military actions. As the *Bhagavad-Gītā* (2.47–50) puts it:

> In action alone is your rightful interest (*adhikāra*), never to its fruit. Let not the fruit of action be your motive; neither let yourself be attached to inaction.

> Abiding in Yoga, do [your allotted] work, O Dhanamjaya [i.e., Arjuna], abandoning attachment and remaining the same in success or failure. Equanimity is called Yoga.

> Indeed far inferior, O Dhanamjaya, is [mere] action to Buddhi-Yoga. Seek refuge in the *buddhi*. Those seeking for the fruit [of their actions] are pitiful.

> He who is *buddhi*-yoked casts off both good deeds (*su-krita*) and evil deeds (*dush-krita*). Therefore apply yourself to Yoga. Yoga is skill in action.

Krishna makes it clear to his disciple that so long as one suffers from lack of discipline (*ayukta*), one also has no wisdom (*buddhi*) and is incapable of contemplation (*bhāvanā*), peace (*shānti*), and joy (*sukha*). In the third chapter of the *Bhagavad-Gītā* (3.3), Krishna explains that this Yoga is in fact Karma-Yoga, and that the earlier delineated path of the Sāmkhya tradition corresponds to Jnāna-Yoga. He also reveals that he has taught these two approaches since time immemorial.

Buddhi is the seat or organ of wisdom. It is an integral structure of human nature, but it may be so occluded that it cannot manifest wisdom in us. Then we continue to be enmeshed in the activities of the world and their consequences. Actions, we are told, all happen automatically out of Nature's (*prakriti*) endless creativity. We only superimpose the sense of being the agent onto these activities, whether it be bodily actions or mental-emotional states. When we think "I am doing this or that" or "I am feeling this or that," we are simply projecting an assumed subject into these automatic activities.

Buddhi-Yoga consists in remaining present as pure awareness, or the witnessing consciousness. This is in fact the crux of all Yoga practice. As Krishna puts it in the *Gītā* (5.8–9):

> The knower of Reality (*tattva-vid*) who is yoked (*yukta*) thinks "I do nothing whatsoever," because while seeing, hearing, touching, smelling, tasting, walking, dreaming, breathing,
>
> speaking, emitting, grasping, opening and closing [the eyes], he maintains that only the senses (*indriya*) are busy with the sense objects.

Identification with our true nature allows us to appreciate what is really going on: Nature is reproducing itself, whereas the transcendental Self, or Spirit, is completely still. Thus the Self-realized sage can be perfectly peaceful in the midst of the most hectic activity.

Jñāna-Yoga: The Path of Wisdom

It is a well-established fact that subject and object are opposed to each other like light and darkness. Hence the tendency to superimpose attributes of the object onto the subject is a grave error. It is just as wrong to superimpose attributes of the subject onto the object. Yet, it is precisely from this kind of confusion between subject and object that we obtain such common statements as "I am this or that" and "this is mine." Now, in the final analysis, the subject is none other than the transcendental Self (*ātman*), which can be "known" only through immediate apprehension. The object is also termed the "nonself" (*anātman*). This designation refers to the body, the senses, the mind, and the countless forms of the world. The superimposition is the same as ignorance (*avidyā*). By contrast, the ascertainment of reality as it is, apart from the attributes superimposed on it, is known as gnosis (*jñāna*).

THE ABOVE PASSAGE is a paraphrase of the opening statement of Shankara's celebrated commentary on the *Brahma-Sūtra* (Aphorisms about the Absolute), which is one of the literary mainstays of Vedānta metaphysics. Shankara, medieval India's best known philosopher-sage, wrote his explanatory treatise twelve hundred years ago. His explanations of the process by which we know Reality are fundamental to Jnāna-Yoga, the path of wisdom. This yogic approach consists in the careful discrimination between the Real (*sat*) and the "unreal" (*asat*). The Real is the transcendental Subject, or singular Self, and the unreal is everything that is experienced as "other": people, animals, trees, institutions, beliefs, abstract ideas. These make up what Shankara calls the "object" (*vishaya*), as opposed to the "subject" (*vishayin*).

Contrary to popular opinion, Shankara does not say that the things of the manifold world do not exist, merely that they are not finally real. They are different from what they appear to be inasmuch as, upon enlightenment, they are all found to be the same Reality. Shankara insisted that there are things to be experienced in the unenlightened state. But he also insisted that what we believe to be objective things are in truth the singular *brahman*, or Absolute. We who perceive the world as consisting of multiple independent objects are therefore committing a cardinal error. We need to look more closely. At a distance a scarecrow looks like a man. When we get closer we can see we were fooled. Shankara uses the example of the rope that is wrongly identified as a snake.

Ordinary knowledge and experience are based on a chronic separation of subject and object, as well as a certain confusion between them. That confusion is known in Vedānta as "superimposition" (*adhyāsa* or *adhyāropa*), by which the true nature of the subject, the Self, is obscured. We wrongly equate the Self with the ego-personality, the empirical "I," which is merely a function of the body-mind. Because of this primal error, we are able to constantly make statements like "I am happy," "I am sad," "I am lean," "I am in pain," "I know," "I grow," "I die," as well as "these are my children," "this belongs to me," "I have a body," and so on. The same error is also responsible for our experiencing perceived objects as other than what they are, namely the ultimate Reality. We think objects are external to us and that we must influence or control them in order to fulfill our deep-seated need for happiness. Thus the process of knowledge is inextricably linked with our emotional life as well as our spiritual destiny. Jnāna-Yoga is an all-out effort to overcome the subject-object division by realizing the subject in its true form—as the transcendental Self, which is permanent, indivisible, and inherently blissful. *Jnāna*, or gnosis, is both the goal and the medium of Jnāna-Yoga.

The West knows its own form of knowledge-based Yoga, which was first strikingly formulated by Descartes in his famous essay *Discours de la Méthode* (Discourse on Method), published in 1637. Descartes mused that "the ground of our opinions is far more custom and example than any certain knowledge."[1] But he was bent on acquiring unshakeable intellectual knowledge. His Yoga consisted in suspending prejudice and in analyzing matters so exhaustively that there is no doubt left. This strictly rational procedure is now the basis for the entire Western scientific enterprise, at least in theory.

Intellectually, Shankara and Descartes are on a par; their approaches, however, could not be more divergent. Descartes, who represents the Western way of science, wanted absolute certainty of knowledge so that he could live a morally sound life. He saw humanity's salvation in the acquisition of more and more accurate and expansive knowledge until reality stands revealed in its nakedness. According to Descartes, such knowledge can only be acquired through the discipline of reason. He placed little faith in the evidence of the senses or the faculty of imagination, but he implicitly trusted reason. It was in this way that he arrived at the famous Cartesian dictum: *cogito ergo sum*, "I think therefore I am." For Descartes, thought was the only means of certainty, from which one could even deduce one's own existence and the existence of everything else. Shankara, representing the East, would have been baffled by Descartes' logic and his apparent satisfaction with a merely rational certainty. According to him, being (*sat*) is a self-evident fact, as obvious as sunlight, requiring no intervention of reason, whereas thought is a derivative of Being, even a falsification of it.

More than that, Shankara believed that conventional knowledge is ultimately circular, or what in philosophical jargon is called "tautological." Knowledge which is based on the split between subject and object is a matter of the mind and mental categories and not a matter of Reality. Unlike Descartes, Shankara did not think that reason furnishes us with absolute certainties. On the contrary, he held that for the most part the mind is an obstruction to the truth. Reiterating the wisdom of the ancient Hindu sages, he described the mind as the organ of doubt (*samshaya*). But doubt, for him, was not only not a desirable state but a clear indication that Being or Truth had not yet been realized.

Shankara's position has been reaffirmed in our own century by Sri Aurobindo, a Self-realized *yogin* who also happened to be one of modern India's greatest philosophers and poets. He observed:

> The intellect, it is said, is man's highest instrument and he must think and act according to its ideas. But this is not true; the intellect needs an inner light to guide, check and control it quite as much as the vital. There is something above the intellect which one has to discover and the intellect should be only an intermediary for the action of that source of true Knowledge.[2]

Thus, Aurobindo did not dismiss the intellect altogether. He merely sought to delimit its authority. Similarly, Shankara admitted that, at its best, knowledge (as wisdom) can point beyond itself. In this sense, reason is not entirely illusory or futile as an instrument of knowledge. Shankara was by no means an irrationalist. Yet he understood the limits of reason very clearly. The same can be said of Paul Brunton, a contemporary *jnāna-yogin*, who wrote:

> The mistake of the mystics is to negate reasoning prematurely. Only

after reasoning has completed its own task to the uttermost will it be psychologically right and philosophically fruitful to still it in the mystic silence.[3]

Brunton understood Jnāna-Yoga as the path of "philosophic insight"—an understanding that transforms and grasps our whole being by widening our horizon beyond the ken of the ego. Philosophic insight, *jñāna*, gives us a glimpse of Reality, which all at once or progressively shatters our preconceptions and connects us to our true identity, the Self. It is this connection, or communion, which gives us certainty beyond the canons of logic, dogma, and mere belief. The absolute certainty to which Shankara aspired, and apparently had realized at a young age, visits us only when all conventional knowledge is transcended together with the knower and the known. This realization, which is synonymous with spiritual enlightenment, is the quintessence of Jnāna-Yoga. It is also the core of Vedānta metaphysics, for which Jnāna-Yoga is the path of realization.

Jnāna-Yoga is the path of insight or wisdom. Such insight, however, is not knowledge as commonly understood, but a higher or metaphysical type of illuminative knowledge, which has been called "gnosis" by some scholars. The scriptures of Vedānta distinguish between a higher knowledge (*jñāna*) and a lower knowledge (*vijnāna*). The former pertains to the organ of wisdom (*buddhi*).[4] The latter is largely a product of the brain-dependent "mind," which functions as a processing plant for the input from the senses. This "lower" mind is known in the Sanskrit language as *manas*, the instrument of thought.[5] The *buddhi* is that aspect of our being which is natively like a limpid pool and capable of reflecting the light of the Self, the esoteric "Sun." The *ātman* is described as being self-luminous, whereas all finite objects, including the *buddhi*, depend for their visibility on the transcendental "Light."

To employ a modern metaphor: The *ātman's* radiance is comparable to the bright light emitted by the high-powered lamp of a lighthouse. That light is reflected in the Fresnel lens surrounding the source of light; the lens corresponds to the *buddhi*. The area beyond the lighthouse is progressively darker—an image that depicts very well the dimness into which the material body and the physical world as a whole are plunged. In more literal terms, the cosmos is a fabric woven of light and darkness. Some cosmic structures (black holes) even trap light by curving space-time itself. And yet, as some astrophysicists conjecture, on the other side of black holes are white holes emitting intense light.

The yogic work consists in spotting the beacon, drawing closer and closer to it, until we realize that the source of light beyond the *buddhi's* Fresnel lens is our essential nature. In the moment of that realization, we *become* the source of light only to find that we are also the world beyond the light tower. We are the source of light, Fresnel lens, lighthouse, the cliff upon which the lighthouse stands, the vast ocean beyond it, and indeed all the visible and invisible realms of the unimaginably vast universe. Such is the glory of spiritual enlightenment. It surpasses the so-called enlightenment of rationalists like Descartes by astronomical magnitudes.

Guided by his trusted reason, Descartes arrived at a concept of God and the world that few today take seriously. For him, God was the great mechanic who fashioned the universe like a clock, wound it up, and now, satisfied with his handiwork, watches the world's progress through the ages. This kind of deism makes no allowance for the mystical impulse in us. There is no spiritual poetry in Descartes' philosophy by which we could rise to the recognition of the Divine as our home. God is forever apart from his creatures.

By contrast, the key message of Vedānta is that there is no gulf between the Divine and the world; that to assume such a separation is a distortion of the truth, and is the root cause of our individual and collective experience of suffering *(duhkha)*. On the contrary, the Vedānta philosophers and sages proclaim that our happiness lies in the discovery that there is no unbridgeable chasm between the Divine, or ultimate Reality, and us: The Divine is our true identity beyond all the many personae that we play out in daily life.

Jnāna-Yoga is the path of Vedānta schools. This implies that, unlike Patanjali's dualistic Yoga, Jnāna-Yoga is based on the metaphysics of nondualism. According to most schools of this Hindu tradition, our perception of a universe rich in distinct forms and beings is a distortion of the truth. In reality, those multiple forms and beings are all appearances or forms of one and the same Being, called *brahman* or *ātman*. The term *jnāna-yoga* is first mentioned in the *Bhagavad-Gītā* (3.3), a pre-Christian work. Here the God-man Krishna declares that he has since time immemorial taught two ways of life — Jnāna-Yoga for the *sāmkhyas* and Karma-Yoga (Yoga of action) for the *yogins*. In this context, a *sāmkhya* is not so much an adherent of the classical Sāmkhya school of thought as a practitioner of wisdom, a traveler on the path of illumination, a *jnānin*.

Krishna equates *jnāna-yoga* with *buddhi-yoga*. As we have seen, the *buddhi* is the faculty of wisdom, the higher mind in which the primary quality of *sattva* predominates. *Sattva* means literally "being-ness" or "real-ness." It is the principle of lucidity, which is present to one degree or another in all things and beings. But it predominates in the *buddhi,* which is both a level of existence and an elevated mental function. Every conceivable phenomenon, whether on the physical level or in other dimensions of cosmic existence, is the product of the interplay of the three primary forces of Nature (*prakriti*): *sattva, rajas,* and *tamas.* The *buddhi is* deemed the very first and purest product of the process of evolution by which forms and beings are manifested on various levels of existence.

All this is ancient wisdom. In a certain sense, the *Bhagavad-Gītā* merely articulates what had long been taught in esoteric circles by word of mouth. In essence, Jnāna-Yoga is present already in archaic *Brihad-Āranyaka-Upanishad.* In this scripture, we hear the utterances of great sages like Yājnavalkya and King Janaka, who possess the secret wisdom of the Absolute (*brahman*). They challenged the clever theologians and would-be mystics of their time in dialogues that cost the loser his head, at least figuratively. In this scripture, we also encounter for the first time the teaching of the two types of *brahman,* the lower and the higher. The lower *brahman* is the world of form, and the higher *brahman* is the formless Reality, which alone is immortal and blissful.

In the *Brihad-Āranyaka-Upanishad,* moreover, we find the teaching of *neti neti* (not this, not that), which is the bedrock of Jnāna-Yoga. In fact, Jnāna-Yoga can be characterized as a path of negation, because it does not create new knowledge but merely removes the obstruction to the Truth that is always the same. The procedure of *neti neti* was first communicated by the wise Yājnavalkya when he instructed the brahmin Shakalya thus:

> That Self is not this, not that. It is intangible, for it cannot be grasped. It is incorruptible, for it cannot be corrupted. It is unattached, for it does not attach itself [to anything]. It is unbounded. It is not agitated. It is not injured.[6]

Yājnavalkya further described the nature of the transcendental Self in a conversation with his spiritually inclined wife Maitreyī. He remarked that after death there is no consciousness (*samjnā*), which confused Maitreyā, whereupon Yājnavalkya elucidated his curious comment in the following classic passage:

> [There is no consciousness after death] because [only] where there is apparent duality (*dvaita*), there one sees one another; there one smells one another; there one hears one another; there one speaks to one another; there one thinks of one another; there one understands one another. [But]

where, verily, everything has become only the Self, then whereby and whom would one smell? Then whereby and whom would one see? Then whereby and whom would one hear? Then whereby and to whom would one speak? Then whereby and of whom would one think? Then whereby and whom would one know? Whereby would one know him by whom one knows all this? Indeed, whereby would one know the Knower (*vijnātri*)?[7]

The Self is not conscious in the ordinary sense of the word. However, it is also not unconscious. It is, rather, pure Awareness or Superconsciousness (*cit*). All other attributes are simply superimpositions, projections of the mind. For the Self to reveal itself in its native splendor, all these projections must be withdrawn, or pierced through. This is achieved by means of the *via negativa* of the *neti neti* method. This approach of negation is succinctly illustrated in the *Nirvāna-Shatka* (Six [Stanzas] on Extinction), which is one of the many didactic poems attributed to Shankara. The full text reads as follows:

I am not the mind or the wisdom faculty (*buddhi*), the I-sense, or thought; neither hearing nor the tongue; neither the nose nor the eyes; nor am I ether, earth, fire, or air. I am Shiva in the form of Awareness (*cit*) and Bliss (*ānanda*). I am Shiva.

I am not what is called the life force (*prāna*), nor am I the five airs [circulating in the body]; nor the seven [bodily] constituents; nor the five [bodily] sheaths. I am also not mouth, hands, feet, genitals, and anus. I am Shiva in the form of Awareness and Bliss. I am Shiva. I am Shiva.

I have neither hatred nor passion, neither greed nor delusion; neither exhilaration nor the mood of envy. I am without virtue or prosperity, without lust or liberation. I am Shiva in the form of Awareness and Bliss. I am Shiva.

[In me there is] neither good nor evil, neither happiness nor suffering, neither *mantra* nor pilgrimage, neither the *Vedas* nor sacrifices. I am not food, the eater, or eating. I am Shiva in the form of Awareness and Bliss. I am Shiva.

I am not [subject to] death, fear, or category of birth. I have no father or mother; [in fact, I have] no birth. I have no relatives or friends, no teacher or pupils. I am Shiva in the form of Awareness and Bliss. I am Shiva.

I am undifferentiated, of formless form. Due to [my] omnipresence I am everywhere [present for the benefit of all the senses. I am neither in bondage nor in liberation. [I am] immeasurable. I am Shiva in the form of Awareness and Bliss. I am Shiva.

Here Shiva is not a specific deity of the Hindu pantheon but a symbol for the Absolute itself. The deities (*deva*) are all part of the relative dimension of existence. They belong to the "lower" *brahman*, also called *shabda-brahman* or the "voiced Absolute," that is, Reality as it can be articulated in thought and speech. The Greeks called this the *logos*, a term corresponding to the Sanskrit *shabda*, which also means "word." Ultimately, only the higher *brahman* is real. And it is this real *brahman* with which the sage wants to identify. To do so, he must learn to discriminate between what is Real and unreal. This intuitive act of discrimination, or discernment, is known as *viveka*.

But there is another important ingredient of Jnāna-Yoga, which is suggested in the story of Yājnavalkya. His instruction of Maitreyī coincided with an important turning-point in his life. For he announced to Maitreyī and Kātyāyanī, his second wife, that he had decided to abandon his householder existence in favor of full renunciation (*samnyāsa*). He was about to adopt the lifestyle of a *parama-hamsa* or "supreme swan"—a bird symbolizing self-sufficiency. Discrimination is one wing and renunciation is the other. Both are necessary for the "supreme swan's" flight to the Absolute.

In the fifteenth century, the path of Jnāna-Yoga was systematized by Sadānanda in his *Vedānta-Sāra* (15–25). We see from Sadānanda's outline of the "limbs" of this Yoga of wisdom that discrimination and renunciation are its foundation:

1. *viveka* or discrimination
2. *virāga* or dispassion
3. *shat-sampatti* (six attainments), namely,
   a) *shama* or tranquillity
   b) *dama* or sense-restraint
   c) *uparati* or abstention from actions that are not relevant to the maintenance of bodily existence or the pursuit of enlightenment
   d) *titikshā* or endurance
   e) *samādhāna* or mental collectedness
   f) *shraddhā* or faith, which is not mere belief
4. *mumukshutva* or impulse toward liberation

Shankara, in his commentary on the *Brahma-Sūtra* (1.1.4), mentions the above limbs with the exception of mental collectedness. He adds *shrāvana* or "listening" to the sacred lore, *manana* or "pondering," and *nididhyāsana* or "meditation." These are also defined in the *Vedānta-Sāra* (182; 191–192). The same manual (200–208) even defines the eight "limbs" of Classical Yoga, presumably as an alternative to the above path. In essence, however, they are the same.

Just as important as discrimination and renunciation is the impulse toward liberation (*mumukshutva*), without which there can be no Self–realization. Although Sadānanda and other authorities of Vedānta explain *mumukshutva* as the "desire (*icchā*) for liberation," it is really not so much a desire as a reorientation of one's whole being toward the ultimate Reality. It is the will to receive the revelation of gnosis (*jnāna*), in which the narrow ego-sense is absent and in which the world and our body-mind glow as the all-comprising singular Reality.

❧ 56 ❧

"That Art Thou"

The Essence of Nondualist Yoga

Gārgī Vācaknavī approached the venerable Sage Yājnavalkya, asking him
to instruct her.

"Ask [your questions], Gārgī," he said.

"Across what is that which is above the sky and beneath the Earth
woven?" she asked.

"It is woven across space," replied Yājnavalkya.

"Across what, then, is space woven?" asked Gārgī.

"That the initiates call the Imperishable. It is neither coarse nor fine,
neither long nor short. Indeed, it is without measure. It casts no shadow,
and there is no darkness in it. It is beyond space and energy. It is odorless,
tasteless, and voiceless, as well as fearless, unaging, undying, and immortal. That Imperishable is the unseen Seer, the unheard Hearer, the un-
thought Thinker, the ununderstood Understander. Other than That there
is nothing that sees, hears, thinks, or understands," replied Yājnavalkya.

THIS STRIKING PASSAGE—here only paraphrased in abbreviated fashion—is found in the ancient *Brihad-Āranyaka-Upanishad* (3.6), which is
considered to be the oldest scripture of the Upanishadic genre. The *Upanishads* are Sanskrit works containing esoteric teachings about the "secret" of
the transcendental Self, which were transmitted by word of mouth for
countless generations until they were committed to writing in modern
times. Sage Yājnavalkya was an enlightened adept who taught the sublime
wisdom of nonduality (*advaita*). We know very little about this illustrious
personage, but the scant information we have about him suggests that he
was one of ancient India's most remarkable spiritual teachers.

The esoteric teaching of nondualism—Vedāntic Yoga or Jnāna-Yoga—
can be summarized as follows. The manifold universe is, in truth, a single
Reality. There is only that one Great Being, which the sages call *brahman*,
in which all the countless forms of existence reside. That Great Being is

utter Consciousness, and it is the very essence, or Self (*ātman*), of all beings. *Tat tvam asi*, "That art thou," is one of the great dicta of the *Upanishads*. It expresses the quintessence of their esotericism. It is no accident that in this Sanskrit utterance the word *tat* (that) precedes *tvam* (thou). Stylistic elegance is by no means the only explanation. As hinted at by Paul Brunton, there is a deeper significance as well.[1] And that significance is that *tat* ontologically precedes *tvam*. In other words, our individual life arises against the backdrop of the universal Reality and is in fact entirely dependent on it. Since the One Being is our essential core, we can realize it, and it is realizable through proper discernment (*viveka*) and renunciation (*vairāgya*). By means of the former, we can hold apart that which is real from that which is unreal or illusory (that is, anything that is experienced as manifold rather than Single). By means of the latter, we can inwardly cleave to that which is Single (*eka*) and thereby recover our identity with it.

This, in a nutshell, is the position of Advaita Vedānta, which has for millennia been the most influential of all schools of Hinduism. In the West, its philosophical elegance and mystical cogency have attracted many distinguished thinkers—Arthur Schopenhauer, who regarded the study of the *Upanishads* as the solace of his life, Ralph Waldo Emerson, Walt Whitman, Gerald Heard, Aldous Huxley, and Julius Robert Oppenheimer. *Advaita Vedānta* means "nondual Vedānta." *Vedānta* is literally "the end of the *Vedas*." This can be understood in at least two senses. First, historically speaking, Vedānta is the tail-end of the ancient revelation as embodied in the hymns of the four *Vedas*. Second, it is the final fulfillment of the Vedic revelation.

The *Vedas* are to Hinduism what the Old Testament is to Christianity. The Sanskrit word *veda* stands for knowledge, more precisely the sacred knowledge that is concerned with the archaic sacrificial ritual and the complex symbolism and mythology surrounding it. With the *Upanishads*, just as with the New Testament in the Middle East, a new spirit emerged in India. The knowledge that the sages of the *Upanishads* were communicating was gnostic or mystical in nature. They taught that the real sacrifice occurs on the level of the human psyche, or the human heart. And so they spoke of ways in which our everyday consciousness could be transformed and transcended, so that we would reawaken to our true identity—as the Self or *ātman*. The *Upanishads*, like the *Vedas* and later *Brāhmanas* and *Āranyakas*, are considered "revelation" (*shruti*). They are treasured as the words of inspired and enlightened adepts. Nondualism is the philosophy that is expressed in the *Upanishads*, the "Himalayas of the soul." There are now more than two hundred of these texts, and they continue to be composed by Hindu mystics to this day.

Many of the early *Upanishads* are in dialogue form, which gives us a sense of participating in the disclosure of the Upanishadic secrets. We encounter such charismatic wisdom teachers as Yājnavalkya, King Ajātashatru, and Uddālaka, who were once surely inaccessible to all but the most serious seekers after wisdom. It is quite amazing that today we can obtain inexpensive paperbacks that reveal what was once the most concealed esoteric teaching and the price of which was certainly much higher than a few dollars: it called for obedience and submission to a teacher, often for many long, trying years, before anything at all was disclosed to the student. Perhaps because we think we can come by this wisdom so easily and cheaply, we generally do not really value it. For instance, how many of us have actually changed our lives significantly after delving into these esoteric scriptures?

The transmission of the Upanishadic teachings was not merely a matter of passing on theories. Rather it involved the transmission of the spiritual force or presence of the teacher, who had at least glimpsed the Self, if not fully realized it. Hence the qualified aspirant was expected to be like an empty vessel into which the *guru's* grace and wisdom could be poured. The Upanishadic sages showed little concern about justifying any of their teachings philosophically, precisely because their verity could be demonstrated to the initiate through direct transmission. Only as other metaphysical traditions—both Hindu and non-Hindu—started to rival Advaita Vedānta, did the Vedānta teachers have to become more sophisticated philosophers and defenders of their faith. At this point, Vedānta became one of the six "systems" or *darshanas* (literally, "viewpoints") of Hinduism. The six orthodox Hindu viewpoints are Sāmkhya, Yoga, Vaisheshika, Nyāya, Mīmāmsā, and Vedānta.

Sāmkhya (the name means "number") is often considered the oldest of the Hindu traditions. It consists essentially in an effort to describe the major patterns of existence. The Sāmkhya teachers developed an evolutionary theory and introduced the distinction between the principle of Consciousness or Spirit (*purusha*) and the principle of insentient Nature (*prakriti*), arguing that whereas the former is immutable, the latter is constantly changing. Yoga, which largely adopted the Sāmkhya view of the world, was primarily a practical path of discovering, or recovering, transcendental Consciousness by means of moral, bodily, and mental disciplines. Vedānta taught, as we have seen, the essential Oneness of everything. The three viewpoints—Sāmkhya, Yoga, and Vedānta—were originally closely allied and became separate traditions only in the course of many centuries. The Vaisheshika school of thought was a kind of naturalist philosophy that, like Sāmkhya, tried to make sense of the phenomenal world. The Nyāya viewpoint was essentially a system of logic, closely associated with the Vaisheshika. Finally, the Mīmāmsā school of thought was a form of ritualist philosophy that sought to justify the Vedic sacrificial cult. It is also known as the "Earlier Vedānta" or Pūrva-Vedānta, whereas the teachings of the Upanishadic sages came to be known as "Later Vedānta" or Uttara-Vedānta. These six "systems," which have their own schools and subschools, make up the orthodox fold of Hindu philosophy. Then there are also unorthodox schools of Hinduism, like materialism, that are so classified because they deny the Vedic revelation outright.

Facing these different branches of Hinduism are such ramifying traditions as Buddhism and Jainism. Gautama, the founder of Buddhism, appears to have studied under Sāmkhya and Yoga teachers. He rejected idealistic metaphysics of the Vedānta type and instead promulgated a spiritually based pragmatic realism. Yet, later Buddhist teachers, especially Asanga and Vasubandhu, elaborated idealistic schools of thought that closely resemble Advaita Vedānta. At any rate, all these different teachings cross-fertilized one another. For instance, Gaudapāda—Shankara's teacher's teacher—has often been called a hidden (Mahāyāna-) Buddhist, as has Shankara himself.

The earliest extant (though not the earliest known) systematic treatment of Vedānta is Bādarāyana's *Vedānta-Sūtra*, which is also known as *Brahma-Sūtra*. This compilation, dating back to around 200 C.E., was an attempt to reconcile the various Vedānta traditions. Primarily its teachings are based on the principal *Upanishads* and the *Bhagavad-Gītā*, which, as few people realize, is traditionally considered an *Upanishad*. The *Upanishads*, the *Gītā*, and the *Vedānta-Sūtra* are the scriptural foundation of all later Vedānta schools. Any teacher wishing to establish his own school would write commentaries on all of them. This is exactly what Shankara (788–820 C.E. or a century earlier), the greatest proponent of Advaita Vedānta, did. His school is known as Kevala Advaita or Absolute Nondualism, because of its extreme position relative to the illusory nature of the perceived world. Today when Vedānta is mentioned in Western circles, generally Shankara's school is intended. This is not altogether fair, since other schools, particularly Rāmānuja's Vishishta Advaita or Qualified Nondualism, have a much larger following. But Shankara's philosophical edifice has been found so attractive because it is deemed the most self-consistent.

Although Shankara was clearly a remarkable man, his genius lay perhaps not so much in the field of philosophy as in the areas of theology and practical spirituality. Much of what tends to be attributed to him was actually established by his teachers, though he brought to it an astounding breadth and depth of learning. But, if tradition is correct, Shankara was an accomplished *yogin* and Self-realizer, who commanded the respect and veneration of his monastic and lay followers, as well as the intelligentsia of his day. Whereas his Sanskrit commentaries on the *Upanishads*, the *Brahma-Sūtra*, and the *Bhagavad-Gītā* tend to be as dry as many Christian scholastic treatises, his more popular works reflect his great wisdom and practical experience as a meditator and an ecstatic. His *Upadesha-Sāhasrī* (Thousand Instructions) and *Viveka-Cūdāmani* (Crest Jewel of Discernment) can be especially recommended.[2]

It is Shankara's Absolute Nondualism that, in our century, had its most charismatic representative in the person of the South Indian sage Ramana Maharshi (1879–1950). He was introduced to Western seekers mainly through the works of Paul Brunton and Arthur Osborne.[3] Sri Ramana spontaneously awakened at the age of sixteen and for the rest of his life remained stably in *sahaja-samādhi*, or natural ecstasy.

In recent years, the Marathi sage Nisargadatta Maharaj (1897–1981) has demonstrated to us that Advaita Vedānta is not merely hearsay or an antiquated philosophy, but a living tradition of God-realization.[4] Unlike Ramana Maharshi, who was a life-long ascetic, Sri Nisargadatta lived as a householder, quietly going about his daily business, all the while attracting a growing number of seekers. Like Sri Ramana, Nisargadatta asked his students to deeply enquire of themselves: "Who am I?" In Socratic fashion, he guided them to the point where, if they were at all open, they could intuit—however briefly and incompletely—the great Mystery that there is only "I" and no "me" or "other." That "I" is, of course, not the ego-sense but the transcendental "I-am-ness," the I AM, the Self-Identity, which Ramana Maharshi also called "I-ness" or *ahamtā*. The similarity between their teachings is not accidental either. For if there is indeed only the One Reality that we, in our unenlightenment, habitually fragment into subject and object, then we can talk about it rationally only in a limited number of ways. But, perhaps, by talking about it, as we are fond of doing, we only distract ourselves from the real business at hand: to realize that single Identity in every moment and with every breath. Therefore both teachers agree that, in the end, silence is the best policy. It obliges us to simply be present as That.

❦ 57 ❦
Discernment and Self-Transcendence

WE ALL SEEK TO maximize happiness and minimize pain and suffering. Beneath this fundamental theme is the urge to find our true identity. Few of us are aware of this process or the reason for much of what we do and how we relate to life. Yoga brings awareness to this ongoing project of largely unconscious self-expression and quest for identity. Ken Wilber has called this primal urge the Atman Project,[1] which is the *ātman* or transcendental Self gazing at itself in the mirror of conditioned existence (*samsāra*). Most of human life consists in the Self mistaking its various reflections for its real nature, which in actuality transcends all that is conditional and finite. Yoga is the Atman Project at its finest: the conscious process of recovering our ultimate identity beyond all assumed roles and secondary identities.

Self-realization—the recovery of our true identity as the *ātman*—depends on applying discernment to everything that is presenting itself to our conscious awareness, realizing that whatever is an object of consciousness is necessarily not the Self, which is the ultimate or transcendental Subject. The classic process of this *via negativa* is epitomized in the insight "I am not this" (*idam na aham*), "I am not that" (*tan na aham*).[2] The formulaic expression of this method is *neti-neti* (not thus, not thus),[3] which was first taught in the early *Upanishads*, the esoteric or gnostic scriptures concluding the Vedic revelatory literature. To this classic process the modern Indian sage Ramana Maharshi provided a complementary approach in the contemplative question "Who am I?" Whereas the former process focuses on the object of consciousness and its unreal (not necessarily illusory) quality, the latter approach has the transcendental Subject as its direct target. For when we inquire "Who am I?" we are inevitably led to a series of perceptions about ourselves, which we recognize to be limited and therefore not indicative of our true identity.

Thus "Who am I?" might give rise to the notion that we are our body, but upon closer inspection we realize that this is not the case, that consciousness is not inevitably bound up with our physical existence. Or we might think that we are the mind, but then, again upon closer inspection, we recognize that the mind too is merely a superimposition upon the transcendental Self, which is pure Being-Consciousness quite free from thought or emotion. Deep self-inquiry in the form that Ramana Maharshi taught gradually reveals to us our various layers of habitual misidentification: "I am of a certain gender, race, age, nationality with such and such a social and educational background" etc. If we persist in the exercise of radical self-inquiry ("Who am I?"), the sage of South India assured us, we will discover our true identity.

During this process of meditative self-inspection — called *ātma-vicāra* in Sanskrit — we automatically, if step by step, transcend ourselves. The fact that self-transcendence is even possible indicates that Consciousness exceeds our biological and mental-psychological conditioning. If self-transcendence is so natural to our being, why does it appear to be so difficult? The simple answer is that our conditioning to identify not with our true Self but any number of substitute identities is extraordinarily strong and requires a powerful sustained effort on our part to be overcome. We must dismantle our misidentifications as we become progressively aware of them, not merely once but over and over again until this new habit of discernment (*viveka*) is firmly established. Then, regardless of the circumstance, we can remain in a witnessing disposition instead of losing ourselves in our habit patterns.

The discovery of the Self as the witness (*sākshin*) of all mental contents — whatever the level or state of consciousness — is a most important event in our life as spiritual practitioners. This witnessing is not merely an intellectual activity, for the intellect is transcended in the process of witnessing. Rather it is a tentative or, when the process has fulfilled itself, the actual and permanent recovery of our Self-Identity. The Yoga of witnessing is *buddhi-yoga*, the yogic path of wisdom through which we perceive our habitual and therefore binding (karmic) patterns of thought and behavior. The term *buddhi* stems from the same verbal root (*budh*) as *bodha* meaning "enlightenment/awakening" and *buddha* (awakened). Thus when wisdom dawns in us, our sense of identity shifts from the body and mind and the external world to the witnessing Self. To the degree that this shift has occurred within us we are free. This inner freedom from our karmic conditioning coincides with our realization of undiluted happiness or bliss (*ānanda*), which, like Being and Consciousness is a hallmark of the transcendental Self.

Self-realization is the end of all suffering (*duhkha*). This is the highest human objective. We are not born to suffer. Suffering is merely a function of our spiritual ignorance (*avidyā*), which occludes our innermost identity, the *ātman*.

When we have realized the *ātman*, the body, the mind, and the world at large cease to be objects for us. We recognize them as our very Self. Then our Self-vision (*ātma-darshana*) encircles everything. We realize ourselves as the ultimate essence and foundation of all beings and things. Yet we no longer fix on particular beings and things—i.e., on a particular body, mind, or world—as demarcating us.

We see through all eyes, we hear through all ears, breathe through every breathing being in the universe, illuminate every single mind, shine in every star, and also are spread out infinitely in the interstices between galaxies and even between the infinite universes that constitute the cells of our space-transcending, time-transcending Being-Consciousness (*sac-cid*).

Tat tvam asi![4] That art thou!

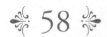

58

Karma-Yoga
The Way of Self-Transcending Action

Of all the philosophical or spiritual questions that we could possibly ask ourselves, there are two big questions to which we must sooner or later find our own answers. The first question is "Why am I here?" This also comes in the form of "Who am I?" or "What does it all mean?" The second and closely related question, which is the focus of the present essay, is "What am I supposed to do with my life?" or "How should I live?"

Our secular Western culture provides us with a great variety of answers to these questions, which is one reason for the moral confusion we are witnessing. The other reason is the inadequacy of those answers, which portray human life as primarily a biological and social adventure, with nothing beyond that: The death of the cellular machine of the human body-mind is supposed to be the end of the story. And, from this point of view, it follows that it does not matter too much what we do with our lives and our planet.

The sacred traditions of the world offer us a different picture—a picture that is not only more compelling but also far more exciting. Thus, according to the Yoga tradition, we are essentially Consciousness-Energy (*cit-shakti*), and the physical body is merely an outer wrapping, a limited appearance of that Consciousness-Energy. There is so much more that is happening besides the familiar material processes. This picture opens up possibilities of experience for us that go far beyond the daily round of eating, drinking, sexing, working, playing, and socializing. The *yogin* discovers dimensions of experience that we barely suspect exist. Above all, however, the practitioner of Yoga assumes a different relationship to the ordinary activities of daily life; in fact, he or she transforms them. He or she makes the activities of daily life extraordinary occasions.

Not everyone is able to meditate profoundly, regularly, and consistently. Everyone is, however, able to practice what in India is known as *karma-yoga*, meaning literally "action Yoga." This Yoga consists in the sacred work of transforming one's everyday activities. It was first taught by the God-man

Krishna, the enlightened teacher of prince Arjuna, on the eve of one of the greatest battles fought on ancient Indian soil. Krishna's teaching has been preserved in the *Bhagavad-Gītā* (Lord's Song), the most famous Yoga scripture. In the third chapter of this "Song of the Lord," Krishna instructs Arjuna—and us—in what is called "skillful action."

Krishna argues that activity is an inseparable attribute of finite existence. Nothing that exists in the realm of Nature is, in the last analysis, inactive. The cosmos (*prakriti*), which is composed of three types of primary qualities (*guna*), is a perpetual motion machine. If it ceased to move even for a moment, the cosmos would collapse. This view coincides with the findings of modern physics, which has revealed to us a universe that is continually vibrating. Therefore, concludes Krishna, it does not make much sense to want to abstain from action. Mere inactivity is not the answer to our existential problems. It is fine to renounce the world and dedicate one's life to contemplating the Divine, providing one can really do it. But few people have the necessary stamina for the rigors of such a solitary lifestyle. Besides, argues Krishna, there is a better way to Self-realization (or God-realization) than renunciation. And that is to continue to be active *but* to act free from egoic attachment. In this way, the continuation of human life is ensured, while at the same time it is being transformed by one's self-transcending disposition.

Krishna's activist gospel, then, does not ask us to carry on as usual. True, the *karma-yogin* continues to get up in the morning, use the bathroom, eat breakfast, go to work, interact with people during the day, return home, eat dinner, spend time with the family, read, listen to music, make love, and sleep. *But* he endeavors, by degrees, to do all this with a subtle yet significant difference: All of these actions are engaged in the spirit of self-surrender. In other words, they are all opportunities to go beyond mere egoic preferences and fixations and to cultivate instead quiet awareness and communion with the Divine.

An important aspect of the practice of Karma-Yoga is the nonneurotic disinterest in what Krishna calls the "fruit" (*phala*) of one's actions. Ordinarily, our actions are governed by so-called ulterior motives—those mostly hidden expectations that would see us rewarded for our deeds. For instance, by putting in an extra hour at work, we secretly, or otherwise, hope to impress the boss. By taking our children to sporting events on Saturdays, we hope for them to share our own excitement, or by sending them to medical school, we seek to live out our own dreams through their lives. By helping an elderly or blind person cross the street, we expect, below the threshold of our conscious mind, to be thanked and thus receive an emotional boost. Or, more subtly, we may do things out of a sense of duty, but without heart. In that case, our actions remain as self-involved as ever. Grim determination is no substitute for the spirit of self-transcendence.

Evidently Karma-Yoga requires a healthy dose of self-knowledge, because in order to engage activities on the basis of self-transcendence rather than self-interest or even self-indulgence, we must first know how that self presents itself in our own case. We must know the patterns of our own egoic personality. Fortunately, we do not have to postpone our practice of Karma-Yoga until we have thoroughly understood ourselves. We can start paying attention—right now—to the hidden motives in our activities, and self-knowledge will grow step by step, as will our capacity to transcend those egoic motives.

Krishna adds another important point to this whole consideration. He argues that we must not only act without egoic attachment, but we must also choose to do the *right* kind of action. For Krishna, who lived well over two thousand years ago, this meant essentially to act in accordance with the social and spiritual wisdom of his day. It would be foolhardy to try to transplant that wisdom to our far more complex contemporary situation, though we can of course learn from it. We must find out for ourselves what is right and what is wrong in each case. For instance, while it is completely appropriate for a practitioner of Karma-Yoga to earn a living, it may not be appropriate for him or her to work in an ammunitions factory or a slaughterhouse, or in a stressful environment. This is where one must exercise discrimination.

At any rate, for the practitioner of Karma-Yoga, work is not merely a means of economic survival or psychic gratification; it is primarily service (*sevā*). And this, in a way, is true of all his or her actions, whether in the workplace or at home. What the *karma-yogin* is serving is the physical, mental, and spiritual welfare of others, including nonhuman beings. The *Bhagavad-Gītā* speaks of this as the ideal of *loka-samgraha*, which literally means "world gathering," or the bringing together of the world, that is, the protection and nurturing of all beings on this planet and anywhere else. "Mahatma" Gandhi embodied this ideal to perfection, and it is not surprising that we learn from his autobiography that early in his life he had imbibed the spirit of the *Gītā*, which he tried to memorize. In his own words:

> . . . to me the Gita became an infallible guide of conduct. It became my dictionary of daily reference. Just as I turned to the English dictionary for the meanings of English words that I did not understand, I turned

to this dictionary of conduct for a ready solution of all my troubles and trials. Words like *aparigraha* (nonpossession) and *samabhava* (equability) gripped me. . . . I understood the Gita teaching of nonpossession to mean that those who desired salvation should act like the trustee who, though having control over great possessions, regards not an iota of them as his own. [1]

Upon closer examination it will be found that skillful action—that is, right action performed without egoic attachment—is inherently loving. When we dethrone the ego, which thinks of itself as the "owner" of objects, beings, ideas, and experiences, we also cease to exert our will over them. Instead, we are more likely to treat others, including apparently inanimate things, with reverence and kindness. We see the greater Life manifesting in everything. This "vision of sameness" (*sama-darshana*) is the foundation for the crucially important attitude of nonharming (*ahimsā*), which Gandhi exemplified in his personal and political life. As he put it:

To see the universal and all-pervading Spirit of Truth face to face one must be able to love the meanest of creation as oneself. And a man who aspires after that cannot afford to keep out of any field of life. That is why my devotion to Truth has drawn me into the field of politics; and I can say without the slightest hesitation, and yet in all humility, that those who say that religion has nothing to do with politics do not know what religion means.[2]

Gandhi continued:

Identification with everything that lives is impossible without self-purification; without self-purification the observance of the law of Ahimsa must remain an empty dream; God can never be realized by one who is not pure of heart.[3]

Self-transcending action thus presupposes both love (*bhakti*) and discernment (*jnāna*) between what is real and unreal. This makes Karma-Yoga ultimately as demanding a way to Self-realization as any other spiritual orientation. However, it seems particularly suited to the active Western disposition, and therefore of all the Yogas, it is the most accessible starting-point for anyone seriously interested in applying the ancient Yoga wisdom in daily life.

If we apply ourselves to the principles of Karma-Yoga, we may well find, as Sri Aurobindo noted, that our actions remain outwardly the same. The real work we are challenged to undertake concerns our inner life.[4] Yet, our new inner disposition will inevitably shine through our actions as well. We may still perform the same steps in washing dishes, for instance, but our movements and comportment will be calm and balanced.

In fact, we should fully expect a subtle but significant difference in any-one who has genuinely been inwardly reborn. That difference is a matter of the Spirit's or Self's luster irradiating, to whatever degree, our body-mind and actions. When this is the case, life is lived in simplicity and with a quiet strength. We become transparent to ourselves and to others, and our inner radiance spontaneously kindles the spiritual flame in others.

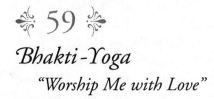

59

Bhakti-Yoga
"Worship Me with Love"

"All you need is love . . ." The Beatles and the flower children of the 1960s knew it: Love is what this world is all about. Not the world of competitiveness, apartheid, social problems, espionage, sabotage, economic progress, and war, but the world *in essence*. We have to step out of our daily skins to appreciate this fact, as did, to some extent, the dropouts of twenty or thirty years ago.

Of course, they were incurable romantics, reacting to the buttoned-down mentality of the older generation. But it is regrettable that their troubadour days are over, because our era is in need of the message of love. I do not mean sophomoric crushes, gushy emotionalism, syrupy neighborliness, or even the New Age kind of idealistic love between so-called soul mates. Rather, what we need is love as an expression of the greater Reality in which we all inhere without distinction.

When we relax our habitual image of ourselves as egos wrapped in flesh, when we cut through our primal fear (*bhaya*), we get in touch with the power of love. Yoga tells us that our essential nature is bliss (*ānanda*) or happiness, which is another word for love. But love suggests a more active involvement than does bliss or happiness. Perhaps it would not be altogether wrong to say that love is the *practice* of happiness.

In the Hindu tradition of Bhakti-Yoga, such love is variously called *bhakti* or *preman*. This love comes not from the mouth or the head. It is a matter of the heart, which epitomizes the entire bodily being. Love wells up from the *anāhata-cakra*, the heart center, where the *yogin* perceives the "unstruck" (*anāhata*) sound, the boom of eternity, the immortal resonance *om*.[1]

Love, or bliss, is a radiant force that bubbles up in us and, in its characteristic superabundance, flows out from us. When we are in love with a person, our love spills over to everybody and everything; it is not confined to our beloved. We embrace all, and our loving embrace is infectious. Love is ecstatic, and it engenders love. There is a great lesson in this, but a lesson that we seldom really learn, because as soon as we fall out of love with our beloved, we fall out of love with everyone and everything, including ourselves. Life looks drab again, or at least no longer quite as extraordinary, whereas our love or abundant happiness infused it with a vibrant vitality that made it enormously attractive.

Few people in our society know such love. It requires a great depth of feeling, and feeling is largely outlawed in our heady, patriarchal world. Feeling is different from emotionality. Feeling is almost an extended form of the sense of touch. In contrast, emotions are mere local disturbances of the bodily field-anger, sorrow, fear, grief, excitement, envy, jealousy, or lust, even such apparently positive emotions as pleasure, self-satisfaction, or warm regard. Feeling transcends them all, just as it transcends our self-sense and our bodily image. In feeling, we reach out beyond the apparent walls of our body-mind.

Feeling—free feeling—is the carrier for the power of love. Bhakti-Yoga is thus the discipline of self-transcending feeling—participation in the world at large. Significantly, the Sanskrit word *bhakti* comes from the verbal root *bhaj,* meaning "to participate in." Through and in love, we participate in the larger Life, in what the teachers of Bhakti-Yoga call the Divine Person. That transcendental Person, or *purusha-uttama,* is the universal soil from which springs all life.

Perhaps the flower children intuited something of this. But their "Yoga" was an unconscious one. It lacked self-knowledge, discipline, and the renunciation of what clear insight has revealed to be unreal or false about oneself. There can be no Yoga, no spiritual life, without self-understanding, disciplined self-application, and renunciation. So, Bhakti-Yoga contains elements of Jnāna-Yoga (the path of discriminative wisdom), Karma-Yoga (the path of self-transcending action), and Samnyāsa-Yoga (the path of renunciation).

At the beginning of his *Bhakti-Sūtra* (Aphorisms on Love), the legendary Sage Nārada notes that *bhakti* is not a form of lust because it entails the spirit of renunciation (*nirodha*).[2] He explained renunciation as the consecration of all one's activities, whether religious or secular, to the Divine Person. Through this act of offering up one's works, a state of unification with the Divine is achieved.

This single-minded self-dedication is best epitomized in the spiritual passion of the cowherd girls for the God-man Krishna. According to legend, the cowherd girls (*gopī*), some of whom were married, were filled with a great longing whenever Krishna would play his flute.[3] Like the Pied Piper he beguiled and distracted them from their daily chores, irresistibly drawing them to him. When they had completely fallen in love with him, their hearts would be with the God-man even in his absence. The story of Rādhā, Krishna's favorite shepherdess, relates how she pined for him like a love-sick girl. He would fuel her passion by prolonged periods of absence. The story is a wonderful allegory of the play between the psyche and the higher Reality, which reveals itself in all its glory now and again, leaving us with a growing desire for divine union. The love mystics of medieval Christendom, notably Saint Bernard of Clairvaux, Saint Theresa of Avila, and Saint John of the Cross, have bequeathed to us dramatic accounts of that miraculous work in the depth of the human psyche.

Love, then, is not merely a temporary high, a feeling of elation. It must be cultivated as a continuous spiritual disposition. We must love even when we feel slighted, hurt, angered, bored, or depressed—especially in those moments. Bhakti-Yoga is the steady application of our feeling capacity in all life situations. Even in our worst moments, we must extend our love, or fundamental respect, to all others. Even though life consists of peaks and valleys, our overall commitment must be to what is revealed in our brief spells on the peaks.

We are not expected to always walk around "happy," at least not while we are unenlightened. In fact, even enlightened beings can experience sorrow, but there is an underlying current of bliss that is always accessible to them, or even continuously present for them, regardless of their momentary states, which may include annoyance, anger, grief, as is clear from the classical descriptions as well as contemporary accounts.

Traditionally, Bhakti-Yoga harnesses a person's feeling-energy so that all his or her impulses get directed toward the Divine. For many of us, who have been brought up in a blatantly secular culture, this is difficult to understand and to do. We may find it easier to love concrete beings than what is likely to be a merely abstract God. Also, in the past, other beings have often been ignored and ill treated in the name of a false devotion to the Divine. We cannot reach the Divine over the maimed bodies, persecuted minds, or broken hearts of our fellow beings. Striving for enlightenment or God-realization must also not be an exclusive, selfish undertaking. The practice of love must be universal. We are obliged to love—not blindly but most profoundly.

There is, however, a certain danger in focusing our love on other conditional beings, and that is that we may confuse spirituality and love with "doing good," or exercising a merely social morality. If our loving of others is to be true, we must see in them, and respond to, that which is real and eternal, bright and blissful. As Sage Yājnavalkya instructed his students more than three thousand years ago: We do not love another for the sake of their wealth, personality, or beauty—but for the sake of the transcendental Self *(ātman)*, which is the same in all of us.

What does the practice of *bhakti* involve? First of all, it most certainly does not mean that we should love others *abstractly*. Love is not merely a wonderful feeling we have about others. It is not merely a benign or kind thought. We have every right to distrust a person who continually assures us of his or her love, but typically fails to express or manifest it to us and to others. To distrust someone, however, does not mean to reject him or her, or to be otherwise unloving ourselves.

Love is demonstrated in action. But more than being demonstrated in action, love is action. We can sit in our room for an entire lifetime and think loving thoughts about other people, but if we never express our love to them, if we never actively share our love with them, we will not have loved. Mother Teresa of Calcutta was someone in whom the spirit of Bhakti-Yoga was very much alive. Every day of her life, she actively shared her love with men, women, and children who were spurned by the larger society. Of course, we need not travel to Calcutta or treat lepers; yet, if we want to be *bhaktas*, or practitioners of love, we must certainly imbibe something of the spirit in which she conducted her life.

The fact is that we are not incapable of love but are only afraid to love. Our great fear is that we will not be loved in return, or that we will be outright rejected. There is of course no guarantee that our self-giving in love will evoke love in others, although love is infectious.

For our love not to crumble under the onslaught of the lovelessness around us, it must be a surplus in us, and it must be a steady force in our lives. Who can deny the lovelessness that surrounds us? It shows itself in a thoughtless remark, an inappropriate silence, a tasteless joke, an aggressive move, turning away from another's pain, the failure to really listen, the pursuit of orgasm at the expense of caring—all the many ways in which we unconsciously hurt one another, out of ignorance, inattention, or sheer unwillingness to make a relational gesture.

We must try to understand the robotic ways in which we block out love. We must become sensitive to our own habitual lovelessness, so that love can become an attractive force in our lives. If you imagine that you already love, examine your life more thoroughly. It is quite revealing how little we in fact love when we start paying attention to our actions and relationships. But unless we are realistic about our lack of love, we can never go beyond our present state.

We must love *concretely*, that is to say, we must give our love to *specific* beings. And we might as well start at home, with our spouse, our children, and not least our parents. What we will find is that sometimes loving them is easy, and at other times it is the hardest thing imaginable. To really love is a great discipline, because we must love stably and consistently and regardless of whether or not our love is returned. In other words, we must love despite our likes and dislikes—that is, despite our ego. We must simply *allow* love to be a transformative force in our lives. *Allowing* is the key. This the discipline of Bhakti-Yoga.

If we truly love, we discover that our love is concrete but not confined to specific beings. We must not confuse spiritual love with the feelings of affinity, friendship, or sexual attraction, or with being nice. Real love knows no content and boundaries. In a way, it is true to say that we are able either to love everyone or no one. *Bhakti* is all-inclusive. It shines through us and on to others without qualification. Its real "object" is the Divine itself, which is also its source. Love is thus unconditional. It is an intimate embrace of all beings and things in their entirety. As psychologist John Welwood commented:

> Whenever our heart opens to another person, we experience a moment of unconditional love. People commonly imagine that unconditional love is a high or distant ideal, one that is difficult, if not impossible, to realize. Yet though it may be hard to put into every day practice, its nature is quite simple and ordinary: opening and responding to another person's being without reservation.[4]

Love is not something we can "do." To say that we "make" love is a contradiction in terms. We only "make" our bodies mingle and our nervous systems fire. But love is either the case, or it is not. It is a state of being that is either true or not true of us. If it is true of us, we cannot help but love all and everyone, regardless of whether or not they offer us gratitude, friendship, or sexual fulfillment. Genuine love asks for nothing in return, though it always works toward duplicating itself in others. Thus, the greatest reward for a person who practices the discipline of love is that another being has become illumined by that love and is now carrying the gift to others.

Love, as I said earlier, has little to do with being nice. Rather, love is being present as a radiant force that comes from beyond the lesser self and reaches out toward that which is beyond the lesser self of others. When that radiance is true of us, we may feel moved to take actions that, by ordinary standards, are not particularly nice. As the French essayist Michel Eyquem Montaigne put it: "He loves little who loves by rule." This is an echo of Saint Augustine who said: "Love and do what thou wilt."

To be present as love does not, for instance, preclude the possibility of our feeling upset with someone, though in our anger we do not wish to obliterate the other, take revenge, or otherwise seek to further ourselves. Christians will remember the New Testament story of Jesus' stern handling of the money lenders in the temple of Jerusalem. Buddhists are well acquainted with the story of the famous Tibetan teacher Marpa, who was known for his fierce anger as well as his enlightenment. These two facts appear irreconcilable, unless one knows that Marpa's fierceness was for the sake of his disciples' enlightenment. He treated Milarepa and the other students so harshly only because he loved them and wanted to guide them to their own discovery of the ultimate Reality. Today, Milarepa is celebrated as one of Tibet's greatest *yogins*.

The love of the teacher for the student is a special form of the love the enlightened adept feels for all beings. When the disciple has awakened to the same intensity of love, the teacher has accomplished his or her task. But whether or not our spiritual practice is guided by a living master, we are always facing the same "impossible" demand: to be present *as* love in all circumstances. For a long time, all we will see is our failure to meet this demand. But this need not discourage us, because in every moment we have a new opportunity to practice that love. We must become fools who are willing to risk again and again that simple response of embracing the Divine in the form of specific beings and things.

❧ 60 ❧
Degrees of Love

IN BHAKTI-YOGA, only our love (*bhakti, preman*) for the Divine matters. Other beings, who also are creations of the Divine, are to be treated lovingly but never as exclusive love objects. God/Goddess must be what the Protestant theologian Paul Tillich called our "ultimate concern."

There are different degrees of love and devotion, and the ninth-century *Bhāgavata-Purāna* delineates nine stages. These have been formalized by Jīva Gosvāmin, the great sixteenth-century preceptor of Gaudīya Vaishnavism, in his *Shat-Sandarbha* ("Six Compositions") as follows:

1. Listening (*shravana*) to the names of the divine Person. Each of the hundreds of names highlights a distinct quality of God, and hearing them creates a devotional attitude in the receptive listener.
2. Chanting (*kīrtana*) praise songs in honor of the Lord. Such songs generally have a simple melody and are accompanied by musical instruments. Again, the singing is a form of meditative remembrance of the Divine and can lead to ecstatic breakthroughs.
3. Remembrance (*smarana*) of God, the loving and meditative recollection of the attributes of the divine Person, often in a human incarnation—for instance, as the beautiful cowherd Krishna.
4. "Service at the feet" (*pāda-sevana*) of the Lord, which is a part of ceremonial worship. The feet are traditionally considered a terminal of magical and spiritual power (*shakti*) and grace. In the case of one's living teacher, self-surrender is frequently expressed by bowing at the guru's feet. Service at the Lord's feet is understood metaphorically, as one's inner embrace of the Divine in all one's activities.
5. Ritual (*arcanā*), the performance of the prescribed religious rites, especially those involving the daily ceremony at the home altar on which the image (*mūrti*) of one's chosen deity (*ishta-devatā*) is installed.
6. Prostration (*vandana*) before the image of the Divine.

7. "Slavish devotion" (*dāsya*) to God, which is expressed in the devotee's intense yearning to be in the company of the Lord.

8. Feeling of friendship (*sākhya*) for the Divine, which is a more intimate, mystical form of associating with God.

9. "Self-offering" (*ātma-nivedana*), or ecstatic self-transcendence, through which the worshiper enters into the immortal body of the divine Person.

These nine stages also are lucidly explained in Rūpa Gosvāmin's *Bhakti-Rasa-Amrita-Sindhu* ("Ocean of the Immortal Essence of Devotion"). They form part of a ladder of continuous ascent to ever more fervent devotion and thus to union with the Divine. The practitioner on the path of love (*bhakti-mārga*) is always a devotee (*bhakta*), a lover, with the Divine as the beloved. This implies an unbridgeable gap between the imponderable vastness of God and the human soul (*jīva*), which is but a particle (*anu*) of the Divine—a notion reminiscent of the Christian mystical doctrine of the "soul spark."

At times, while treading the path of love, the aspirant may feel cut off from the Divine. In such moments, a deep longing provides the energy for ever-deepening love, which will overcome this temporary sense of separation (*viraha*). When love has become supreme love (*para-bhakti*), however, the soul particle does not feel itself to be isolated from the Divine or anything else; rather, it experiences everything as the Divine. Such mature love completely heals the sense of self-fragmentation that is the destiny of the ordinary ego-personality. Although the *bhakta* experiences the Divine as "other," this otherness is unlike anything we can experience at the level of conventional reality. The relationship between God/Goddess and devotee is analogous to the relationship between the ocean and its waves.

In Bhakti-Yoga, the devotee feels a growing passion (*rati*) for the Lord, and this helps to break down one artificial barrier after another between the human personality and the divine Person. Some schools of medieval Bhakti-Yoga, like the Christian love mystics, compared this passion to erotic love. Thus in Jayadeva's *Gītā-Govinda*, for instance, Krishna and the cowherd girls (*gopīs*) are portrayed as playful lovers who flirt, caress, kiss, and consummate their love.

The devotee's increasing love culminates in the vision of the cosmos penetrated, saturated, and sustained by the Divine. This is the kind of vision that overwhelmed and awed Prince Arjuna, as described in the famous eleventh chapter of the *Bhagavad-Gītā*. Witnessing the divine splendor of Lord Krishna, Arjuna in a state of ecstasy exclaimed:

> O God, in your Body I behold the deities and all the various kinds of beings, the Lord Brahma seated on the lotus throne, and all the seers and divine serpents! (11.15)
>
> Everywhere I behold you [who are] of endless Form, with many arms, bellies, mouths, and eyes. I can see no end, middle, or beginning in you, O All-Lord, All-Form! (11.16)
>
> I behold you with diadem, mace, and discus—a mass of brilliance, flaming all round. You are hard to see, for you are immeasurable, entirely a brilliant radiance of sun-fire. (11.17)
>
> Beholding that great Form of yours, with its many mouths and eyes, its many arms, thighs, feet, bellies, and formidable fangs, O strong-armed [Krishna], the worlds shudder, and so do I. (11.23)
>
> With flaming mouths, you lick up and devour all the worlds entirely. Filling the whole universe with your brilliance, your dread-inspiring rays blaze forth, O Vishnu. (11.30)
>
> Tell me who you of dread-inspiring Form are. Salutations to you! O foremost God, have mercy! I wish to know you [as you were] at first [in your human form], for I do not comprehend your [infinite] creativity (*pravritti*). (11.31)

Arjuna was not yet ready to let go of the stranglehold of the ego and merge with the Beloved—a merging that would have lifted him forever above his worldly cares and fulfilled his heart's deepest yearning. His unpurified mind and heart were unable to tolerate the freedom of living so close to the Source where *bhaktas* rejoice in surrendering completely to the divine will.

It was Arjuna's destiny to serve as an instrument of the Divine in a decisive moment in human history while simultaneously working out his own karma. His teacher, the God-man Krishna, lavished on him precious spiritual teachings to help him meet his fate and at the same time serve the divine purpose.

Speaking with the voice of God-realization, Krishna made this solemn promise to Arjuna and to all potential devotees:

> Be Me-minded, devoted to Me, sacrifice to Me, do obeisance to Me—thus you will come to Me. I promise you truly, because you are dear to Me. (*Bhagavad-Gītā* 18.65)

❧ 61 ❧
The Kriyā-Yoga of Patanjali

YOGA IS A KIND of technology or, if you prefer, counter-technology. It is the technology of consciousness transformation. This is, of course, true of all forms of genuine Yoga. But not every school or branch of the proliferating tradition of Yoga has such an elaborate theoretical underpinning as Patanjali's Classical Yoga.

For this reason, Patanjali's *Yoga-Sūtra* holds special significance for students of Yoga. This Sanskrit work, which is as old as the Christian gospels, defines important yogic concepts. Naturally, within the compass of this short tract, consisting of a mere 195 aphorisms (*sūtra*), one must not expect a complete exposition of the doctrinal structure of Classical Yoga. This was not Patanjali's purpose. His aphorisms were simply intended to aid the memory of initiates of Classical Yoga. Many things were not even mentioned, as is clear when we read the early commentaries on the *Yoga-Sūtra*, which fill some of the gaps. Modern students of the *Yoga-Sūtra* therefore have to be patient and diligent.

Patanjali's school is generally referred to as the "Yoga system" (*yoga-darshana*). It is also widely known as the "eight-limbed Yoga" (*ashta-anga-yoga*). However, as I have tried to show in various books, the section in the *Yoga-Sūtra* dealing with the eight "limbs" (*anga*) of the yogic path is very likely a quote from a previously existing *sūtra* composition. Patanjali's own teaching is more appropriately called *kriyā-yoga*. This expression is found in aphorism 2.1, which reads: "Asceticism, study, and devotion to the Lord [constitute] the Yoga of [ritual] action" (*tapah svādhyāya-īshvara-pranidhānāni kriyā-yogah*). Asceticism (*tapas*), study (*svādhyāya*), and devotion to the Lord (*īshvara-pranidhāna*) are the three principal means of Patanjali's Yoga.

These are sacred acts (*kriyā*) and fall under the category of "practice" (*abhyāsa*), with the complementary category being "dispassion" (*vairāgya*). Together, practice and dispassion provide the dynamic of spiritual life, as understood by Patanjali. The eight limbs are moral restraint (*yama*), self-restraint (*niyama*), posture (*asana*), breath control (*prānāyāma*), sensory inhibition (*pratyāhāra*), concentration (*dhāranā*), meditation (*dhyāna*), and ecstasy (*samādhi*). These can be considered as subcategories of asceticism, though study and devotion to the Lord also appear under self-restraint. For Patanjali, at any rate, they held special importance.

The objective of *kriyā-yoga*, as we learn from aphorism 2.2, is the cultivation of ecstasy (*samādhi*) and the attenuation of the "causes of suffering" (*klesha*). The ulterior motive for this psychotechnology is, according to aphorism 2.16, the prevention of future suffering (*duhkha*). For Patanjali, as for Gautama the Buddha, the source of all suffering is spiritual ignorance (*avidyā*). This is the primary *klesha*. From it spring the I-sense (*asmitā*), attachment (*rāga*), aversion (*dvesha*), and the will to live (*abhinivesha*). Patanjali explains these five *kleshas* as follows (2.5–9):

> Ignorance is seeing [that which is] eternal, pure, joyful, and the Self in [that which is] ephemeral, impure, sorrowful, and the nonself (*anātman*).

> "I-am-ness" (*asmitā*) is the identification as it were of the powers of vision [i.e., the mind] and "visioner" [i.e., the Self].

> Attachment is [that which] rests on pleasant [experiences].

> Aversion is [that which] rests on sorrowful [experiences].

> The will to live, flowing along by its own momentum, is rooted thus even in the sages.

These five causes of suffering furnish the dynamic of ordinary life. They are the motivational matrix of the unenlightened psyche. Kriyā-Yoga seeks to undermine this innate pattern so that the person can recover his or her authentic being, which is the Self. Self-realization is the only means of disrupting the cycle of repeated births and deaths to which the unenlightened being is subject.

The five *kleshas* urge the individual to feel, think, will, and act. These functions leave either positive or negative traces in the depths of the human psyche from where they instigate new activities and experiences that, in turn, generate further traces. This psychological model is central to Kriyā-Yoga. Long before modern psychology, Patanjali invented the significant concept of the "depth-mind," which he called *smriti* (literally "memory"). It is in this depth-mind that the psychic residue of one's actions and experiences is stored.

Like most other yogic concepts, the notion of the depth-mind is not merely a speculative construct. *Yogins* do not tend to indulge in philosophical flights, but their theorizing always has a definite and concrete purpose. Thus, the idea of the depth-mind is meant to explain and facilitate a very important aspect of the yogic process. The depth-mind can be understood as the total configuration of a person's psychic residue from past volitional activity. Any action, whether deliberate or involuntary, creates a corresponding disposition in the deepest recesses of the mind. These dispositions combine, presumably on the basis of association by similarity, to form complex chains and concatenations rather like crisscross tracks in the sand or snow. Of course, this three-dimensional picture is not entirely appropriate, because we are dealing here with immaterial realities rather than substances with spatial extension.

These configurations would be of no practical consequence if they were not the driving factors behind all our future volitional activity. Thus the depth-mind is not simply a bottomless ditch into which the content of our self-expression is dumped. But it is an active force, the nurturing ground that engenders new impulses toward self-expression.

This dynamic aspect of the depth-mind is captured in the Sanskrit term *samskāra*, which means literally "activator." Each unit of experience, or self-expression, creates a *samskāra* in the depth-mind. Patanjali does not tell us exactly how the subliminal activators determine our mental activity. He simply asserts that they do. His claim, however, can be verified very easily. We merely need to make an attempt to sit completely still and silence our thoughts and internal images. How many seconds are we able to do this exercise before thoughts and images intrude again? Even if we should succeed to curb our mind for ten seconds, with practice we would find that beneath the apparent stillness is a constant rumble of sensations and feelings. The depth-mind is constantly at work.

Before we know it, we are witnessing verbal fragments, images, thoughts, and sudden emotions bubbling up from below the surface of the mind: serious and funny ideas, blurred images and vivid panoramic flashbacks, feelings of guilt, shame, anger, or fear. We discover how very difficult it is merely to observe and not get involved in the drama that is being enacted on the stage of our inner theater. As we watch the play we tend to become gradually and imperceptibly more involved until we have completely lost our original stance of a detached witness. All of a sudden, we identify with the drama.

The mind is a billowy sea with numerous whirlpools in which we continually lose our true identity as the Self (*purusha*). It is by force of habit that we cannot remain observers for very long. And "habit" is merely another word for the *samskāra* chains that form the lattice of the depth-mind. Patanjali employs the term *vāsanā* (trait) for these subliminal configurations composed of a series of similar *samskāras*. He also refers to them collectively as "karmic deposit" (*karma-āshaya*).

Patanjali's model reminds one of certain modern theories of learning, conditioning, and habit formation. However, there is one all-important difference between these contemporary theories and Patanjali's formulations. According to Patanjali, only a very small segment of the total network of subliminal traits is the product of the present life's mental activity. The larger part of the depth-mind was in existence before our present birth and was indeed instrumental to our assumption of a new body. The depth-mind is the crystallization of a person's untold past existences, and it is the medium that regulates the entire process of re-embodiment. The doctrine of rebirth, or *punar-janman*, is one of the fundamental axioms of Yoga philosophy.

The practical implications of this belief are enormous. On the one side, it is intended to account for the fact that people are endowed with different mental capacities and that their lives proceed along idiosyncratic lines that cannot be satisfactorily explained in terms of environmental or other external factors. On the other side, far from relieving a person from all responsibility, the teaching of reincarnation constitutes a challenge to actively determine his or her future lot. Nothing would be more wrong and destructive than to regard the doctrine of repeated births as a convenient excuse for a fatalistic attitude. Rather it should be seen as urging us to accept our individual "starting point," however disadvantageous it may seem, as the direct outcome of our previous mental activities, and to make the best of our life within the given parameters.

Although the "gravity pull" of the subliminal deposits is exceedingly powerful—"old habits die hard"—the yogic adepts assure us that we can overcome it through conscious work on ourselves. In fact, Patanjali insists that we can completely transcend the forces of destiny, and this optimistic assumption underlies all forms of Yoga. We can outwit *karma* by assuming the position of the witnessing Self, by disidentifying with the body-mind that is the karmic fruit of previous lives and of present volitional activities.

As a product of the cosmos (*prakriti*), the body-mind—which includes individuated consciousness (*citta*)—has no awareness of its own. It is rather like a clock that ticks until the wound-up spring is unwound. This mechanical imagery is not at all inappropriate here. The dualist metaphysics of Classical Yoga correspond to the materialist view proposed in the eighteenth century by Descartes, who regarded the body as a machine. So long as we identify with the body-mind, we are also subject to its laws. However, the moment we identify with the Self, the transcendental principle of Awareness (*cit, citi*), we become disentangled from the fate of the body-mind.

Although Patanjali does not discuss the philosophical issue of free will in his *Yoga-Sūtra*, his yogic technology implies that we can determine our future. We can choose to live either as the body-mind or as the Self. Different destinies follow from this choice. Already in the pre-Christian *Bhagavad-Gītā* (16.6), the God-man Krishna speaks of "divine" (*daiva*) and "demonic" (*āsura*) destinies, which depend on whether we place our attention on spiritual matters or on worldly concerns. In aphorism 4.7, Patanjali distinguishes between the "black," the "white," and the "mixed" *karma* of ordinary mortals, contrasting it with the *karma* of *yogins*, which is neither black nor white nor mixed because it tends toward Self-realization and thus toward the end of all future suffering in repeated births and deaths.

But the exercise of free will in favor of Self-realization, or enlightenment, must not remain a mere good intention: it must be expressed in a definite course of action. This action (*kriyā*) must countermand the production of subliminal activators (*samskāra*) and delimit their sphere of influence. Patanjali recognizes different stages in this process of control over the incessantly active depth-mind. According to aphorism 2.4, the causes of suffering can be fully operative (*udāra*), dormant (*prasupta*), intercepted (*vicchinna*), or attenuated (*tanu*). The *yogin's* goal is the attenuation and, finally, the utter cessation of their functioning.

It is to this end that the practitioner of Yoga employs the various yogic "limbs," notably the practice of ecstasy. This use of techniques of ecstatic self-transcendence significantly distinguishes Yoga from psychoanalysis, which also works with the depth-mind. Psychoanalysts assume that the depth-mind, the so-called unconscious, can be positively influenced and moderately controlled by means of intellectual insight into the causes of unconscious automaticities (neuroses, psychoses, etc.). The masters of Yoga, however, have long understood that insight is necessary but not sufficient to transcend the powers of the "unconscious."

Even insight produces subliminal activators, which fuel the depth-mind. The *yogin* is not satisfied with generating better *samskāras*. He wants to generate none at all and, more than that, dissolve the rest. According to Patanjali, this is possible only in the fire of ecstatic transcendence in *asamprajnāta-samādhi*. This "supraconscious" ecstasy does not involve the powerful ego-habit and therefore generates a counter-*samskāra* based on enlightenment, which slowly dissolves all the other *samskāras*. In other words, as we make a habit out of Self-identification by regularly ascending into supraconscious ecstasy, we weaken the habit of self-identification, or ego-consciousness, when we return to the ordinary state of mind. In the end, the ordinary consciousness is what is extraordinary, because the advanced practitioner identifies less and less with the body-mind, until he or she permanently abides as the Self.

The eight "limbs" of Yoga are aids in this progressive shift away from the egoic identity. Yet, in the final analysis, the causes of suffering (*klesha*) are overcome not through any specific exercise but solely by the act of disidentifying with the body-mind. As Patanjali states in aphorism 2.17:

> The correlation between the "seer" [i.e., the Self] and the "seen" [i.e., the body-mind] is the cause of [that which is] to be overcome [i.e., future suffering].

The "correlation" *(samyoga)* between the body-mind and the transcendental Self *(purusha)*, which is pure Awareness, is said to be beginningless. Yet it can be terminated. Yoga is in fact a graduated process of severing that connection through gnosis (*vidyā*), through awakening as the Self beyond spiritual ignorance and suffering. Such Self-realization is liberation, freedom, or what Patanjali calls "aloneness" (*kaivalya*). The Self is "solitary" (*kevala*) not because it is a windowless monad but because it transcends the mechanics of the cosmos, whether visible or invisible. It is unaffected by *karma*, the law of action and reaction. It is merely witnessing the events unfolding at the various levels of cosmic existence.

As King Bhoja, a tenth-century commentator on the *Yoga-Sūtra*, rightly noted, *yoga* is not so much "union" (*samyoga*) as "separation" (*viyoga*). It entails a process of sifting out the nonself from the Self, the unreal from the Real. The Real is the transcendental Self *(purusha)*, which shines forth in its solitary splendor when we have successfully overcome our illusions about reality. However, we must not think of the solitary Self as being lonely. Emotions belong to the body-mind, not the Self. Yet, in aphorism 2.5, Patanjali implies that the Self is joyful (*sukha*). This corresponds to the description of the Self as pure bliss (*ānanda*) in the tradition of Vedānta. But the Self's delight is not an emotional condition. Rather, like the Self's eternal nature or its intrinsic Awareness, that delight is an inalienable quality of Reality.

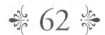

62

Faith and Surrender
A New Look at the Eightfold Path

RIGHTLY OR WRONGLY, the eight "limbs" (*anga*) of Yoga have come to stand for the Yoga taught by Patanjali in his *Yoga-Sūtra*. Generally, they are conceived as a series of stages that the spiritual practitioner ascends, rather like a staircase, to the ideal of liberation or Self-realization. This popular "vertical" interpretation of the eight limbs is not entirely convincing; for, clearly, some of them are to be practiced simultaneously. But the underlying idea of these limbs as a kind of organic whole is unchallengeable.

What is rarely considered, though, is the question of what exactly links together all these limbs to give one the impression of such unity. To say that they are all essential parts of the yogic enterprise would be the obvious answer. What do they all have in common at the deepest level, so that we can recognize them to be integral components of Yoga? I would like to propose that this "missing link" is the practice of surrender and faith, which have nothing to do with quasi-religious emotionalism but, rather, are profound attitudes without which spiritual growth cannot occur. Before I go on to illustrate this point with regard to each constituent practice of the eightfold path, I would like to further explain what I mean by these two terms.

Linguistically, the word *surrender* is composed of the prefix *sur* and the verb *render*, meaning "to deliver over, to yield up, to render unto." The word is used in a variety of ways: to relinquish an office or entitlement, to offer up for sale an insurance policy, to capitulate to the enemy, to give oneself up to the authorities, or to succumb to despair. In each case the act involved is one of making over, or handing over, something.

In Yoga, as in all other forms of spirituality, this surrender consists not so much in any external transaction but primarily in an inner attitude or response. This attitude is one of "standing back" from oneself, a deliberate relaxation of the boundaries of the ego. What this involves is best indicated by the act of emotional and physical surrender between lovers—a further important usage of the word. In fact, once when I spoke on this subject to a group of Yoga enthusiasts, this was their first and foremost association. Nor was the group's association of surrender with the act of yielding between lovers entirely positive. There was a feeling that such sexual-emotional surrender is usually a unilateral affair, that it is expected of the woman but that it does not match the masculine "aggressive" self-image of the male lover. Undoubtedly, women have widely been and still are exploited sexually, and an ideology of surrender would fit the bill of the male chauvinists perfectly. However, the present consideration does not focus on these social patterns.

Here we are interested in the dynamics of a *true* loving relationship between sexual partners. They are by definition "equal," for their surrender must be mutual. Of course, such mutual surrender presupposes great individual maturity. Starry-eyed teenagers who have "fallen" in love are incapable of this act, although to outsiders and to themselves, they may seem to be completely absorbed in one another; in fact, their "love" is a subconscious projection of themselves onto the partner. Strictly speaking, they love themselves in the other. Hence, when reality hits, they "fall out of" love again. That not only teenagers but also so-called adults succumb to this "falling in and out of" love is a commentary on their level of maturity.

I am making so much of this because in *spiritual* surrender, the element of mature love is present as well. When the lover surrenders "body and soul" to the beloved, really what she or he yields up is the usual self-identification with the body and with bodily and emotional and even mental processes. There is a melting away of conventional propriety, shame, and guilt. Indeed, lovers delight in pouring their hearts out to one another, in confiding long-kept secrets or long-cherished hopes, and in "daring" each other to demonstrate their love by overcoming inhibitions and taboos.

They are self-forgetful—or so it seems. At least they are on the way to being self-forgetful. That they never quite succeed is as obvious as it is subtle. Their surrender is necessarily incomplete, because their love is imperfect. This lies in the nature of ordinary human love, however extraordinary it may be by conventional standards.

Perfect love is possible only with regard to a perfect "object" or, to be more precise, when love is without a specific object but includes all possible objects, the whole universe. This, again, means that perfect love is possible only when there is no ego to create the usual barrier—however tenuous—between an experiencing subject and an experienced object. A genuine loving relationship, especially at the height of its sexual expression, approximates this condition of subject-object transcendence. But it only *approximates* it. For this condition of near-genuine love to turn into genuine love, the lovers' images of each other (and of themselves) would have to be sacrificed. In other words, it is only when they come to love the whole person that they love perfectly. Here "whole person" refers to the human being in his or her entirety, comprising both the visible aspects and the invisible dimension; as a manifestation of the Whole (or God) and as that unmanifest Whole itself.

To put it in Hindu terms, perfect love is the love between Shiva and Shakti, between the tranquil, abiding aspect of the Whole (conceived as masculine) and its dynamic counterpart (conceived as feminine). God Shiva and Goddess Shakti—there is much instruction to be found in this kind of mythological imagery—are eternally in blissful embrace or surrender to one another. That is to say, the Absolute or Divine Reality is its own sacrifice: It is both Being *and* Becoming, State *and* Process.

It is in this transcendental condition that we have the key to the surrender that spiritual seekers cultivate. They adopt and follow a path that attempts to reverse such normal human values and attitudes as greed, hatred, envy, jealousy, or fearful avoidance. Through this yogic or spiritual reversal (*parāvritti*), they create for themselves a life that is analogous to the transcendental state of being. Their entire life is modeled on the nonordinary, nonhuman Reality. It becomes an imitation (in the best sense of the word) of the milieu of Reality. This is exactly what is implied in Jesus' well-known admonition: "Be perfect, therefore, as your heavenly Father is perfect" (Matthew 5:48). In the same spirit, Saint Paul said: "I have been crucified with Christ, and it is no longer I who live but it is Christ who lives in me" (Galatians 2:20).

Yoga practitioners, then, surrender their "usualness." The more complete and unquestioning this surrender becomes, the nearer they draw to, or rather the more they participate in, the dimension of absolute Reality. Ultimately, they hope to fully and permanently realize their authentic Being, which is the Self (*ātman*).

Next, I intend to briefly examine the second focus of this essay: faith. The word itself is derived from the Latin term *fides*, which means "trust" or "certainty." The first observation to be made is that faith and belief, though frequently thrown into the same pot, denote essentially distinct inner processes. "I believe in God (or the abominable snowman)" means something quite different from "I have faith in God (but not in the Yeti)." Belief is the intellectual judgment that something is such and such. It can range from a hypothetical opinion to a deeply held conviction.

Faith is more than that. It is a *radical openness* to something that (or someone whom) we consider of superlative personal significance. One of the great Protestant theologians of our time, Paul Tillich, described faith as "the state of being grasped by an ultimate concern."[1] In this sense, faith is part of daily life. There is no one who has no faith. True, the object of a person's faith—his or her "ultimate concern"—may be a most unworthy thing, as when a blindly loving wife "worships" a husband who chronically mistreats her.

Faith has to do with the very depths of our being. It is the mainspring of our will to live, our primary inspiration. Therefore when we are in the throes of a crisis of faith, we experience a profound disorientation and even fear of annihilation. Like love, as understood above, faith is not simply an emotion; rather it is a kind of basic orientation within us, a person's "trajectory," which can become associated with different emotions. Love, again, is a movement of one's whole being toward overcoming the separation between beings.[2]

The spiritual significance of faith and surrender, then, is that both are deeply felt *responses* to something that (or someone who) exceeds our personal life. They well up within us and pull us toward that something or someone.

In the following paragraphs I will show how faith and surrender are present in the practice of all the limbs of Yoga. The foundation of any authentic yogic approach is moral discipline or *yama* (restraint or control). This is meant to regulate the social behavior of spiritual practitioners. Moral integrity is a must for the *yogins* and *yoginīs* who do not wish to fall prey to any attitudes and habits that countermand their spiritual aspirations. Through the universal application of the rules of *yama*, they ensure that they will never abuse the power—whether psychic or social—that is acquired in Yoga.

There are five such rules. The root of all of them is said to be nonharming (*ahimsā*). This Sanskrit word is also frequently translated as "nonviolence." It consists in unconditional nonmaliciousness toward all beings at all times and in all situations. *Ahimsā* has to be practiced not only in deed, but also in word and in thought. Thus it includes refraining from gossip and even thinking ill of a person, a whole group of people (e.g., xenophobia, racism, etc.), or even animate beings in general (i.e., speciesism). This presupposes a considerable degree of detachment or dispassion (*vairāgya*), which, as readers of the *Yoga-Sūtra* will know, is one of the two poles of Yoga—the other pole being constant application (*abhyāsa*) to the practical disciplines.

How can *ahimsā* be said to be an expression of surrender and faith? The faith component in it is found in the recognition that our authentic Being, the Self, is beyond hurt (*ahimsā*), beyond ill (*anāmaya*), beyond sorrow (*aduhkha*), beyond pain (*aklesha*). We may surrender to it by acknowledging that our own authentic Being also is the authentic Being, or Self, in all other creatures and by treating them not as potential or actual enemies but as that universal benign Self. The virtue of nonharming, then, is grounded in the recognition that there is no cause for fear with regard to anybody or anything, since everyone and everything is that same Reality, or Singularity. Once we have overcome this fundamental fear, which is conjured up by the ego experiencing itself as an island apart from others, we also will be able to practice nonharming with consummate skill.

The second constituent of the category of *yama* is truthfulness (*satya*). Here the traditional scriptures again demand of us that we cultivate this virtue in action, speech, and thought. The *yogins* or *yoginīs* who practice truthfulness in this way cannot possibly be prone to lying, hypocrisy, or deception. It is easy to see how this virtue is rooted in the moral principle of nonharming. Our faith in truthfulness is our faith in Truth, also called *satya*. And Truth is another name for the transcendental Reality, the Self. The Self is that in which there is not a single trace of falsehood; it is the Real. The sages also refer to it as *tattva* (thatness) and *tathatā* (thusness).

In surrendering to this Truth, we are capable of casting off all the needless ballast of little or big deceptions that we tend to carry around with us all our lives. Again, there is an element of fearlessness involved in this commitment to Truth (and specific truths). Even when we have just started to cultivate this virtue, we quickly realize to what extent our whole civilization is operating on the reverse principle of untruth: from advertising and political campaigning (both of which are almost wholly institutionalized forms of lying), to the manipulation of the law and of "facts" by lawyers, as well as all the myriads of techniques employed by people in order to preserve face or to remain one up.

The third component of *yama* is nonstealing (*asteya*). Once again, this is to be understood in a very comprehensive sense. As a form of dispassion it is the abstention—in deed, word, and thought—from grasping after another's property. Even merely coveting our neighbor's strawberries, let alone his wife or her husband (who is of course not property), constitutes an infringement of this moral commandment.

This virtue is connected on the one hand with nongrasping (*aparigraha*) and on the other hand with contentment (*samtosha*), which will be discussed below. Where does faith come into play in this case? The Yoga practitioner's faith is placed in the Self as the inexhaustible Fullness (*pūrnatva*) that, once it has been realized, leaves nothing to be desired. Our external grasping after, or seizing of, things (and also relationships) is an expression of the ego's strategy to overcome its basic fearfulness created by its self-isolation (or separation from the Self). But in this endeavor to extend its radius, the ego necessarily encroaches on the life-space of others, and this violates the first law of nonharming. Through surrender to the Self as the absolutely self-sufficient Reality, the ego's harmful activity is gradually neutralized.

The *yogins* or *yoginīs* who live this ideal are no longer at war with the world or themselves.

The next element of *yama* is chastity (*brahmacarya*). The literal meaning of this old Sanskrit word is "brahmic conduct," that is, the "behavior of a *brahmin*" or "mode of the Absolute." Here the principle of reversal, spoken of above as the very essence of the yogic process, is most clearly expressed. To behave like the Absolute means to model one's life on the ideal condition of the genderless Absolute. This is the underlying idea of chastity. Our ordinary experience of the world is always framed in terms of male and female (and occasionally neuter). "Chastity" is, first of all, the attempt to break away from this binary compartmentalization of life. True continence begins in the mind.

Spiritual practitioners who have mastered this virtue regard all people as the same (*sama*), irrespective of their sex. On the physical level, chastity involves the abstinence from sexual activity. Some schools make this an unqualified condition, whereas others hold a more lenient view. The latter apply the principle of moderation to this aspect of one's personal life, but also have rather definite notions about what is to be considered as legitimate sex. Sexual exploitation between men and women, which is often what today's sexual revolution is about, is in yogic terms not only a waste of precious vital energy (*ojas*), but also a kind of violence, theft, and deception. Certain that the eternal Self not only transcends all bodily distinctions but also is inherently blissful (*ānanda*), Yoga practitioners are able to surrender their desire for the transient pleasure afforded through sexual activity.[3]

The fifth and last member of *yama* is nongrasping or greedlessness (*aparigraha*). In a way, this is the perfect form of nonstealing. When everything has been recognized as being alien to one's true nature (i.e., the Spirit), then all expressions of self-assertion, however subtle, become theft. Roughly speaking, people fall into two psychological types. There are those who have what is called "belonging identity" and those who have "awareness identity."[4] To the former, the Yoga practitioner's total disinterest in worldly things (including titles, positions, etc.) will seem either perfectly insane or very frightening. To the latter, however, the yogic way of life will make sense more readily. The practitioners of Yoga themselves belong to this second category. Travelers on the yogic path place their faith in the Self, the ultimate unit of Awareness, which is without properties or qualifications and which is yet the foundation of all things. If they can surrender to it, all avarice will automatically fall away from them.

We now come to the second limb (*anga*), the fivefold category of self-restraint (*niyama*). Whereas the rules of *yama* are designed primarily to harmonize the Yoga practitioner's social relationships, the disciplines of *niyama* serve to deepen his or her orientation toward the ultimate Reality.

The first component of *niyama* is purity (*shauca*). Often interpreted as mere bodily cleanliness, this practice actually entails much more. From one point of view, the whole yogic path is an extensive process of purification or catharsis (*shodhana*). To paraphrase one of Patanjali's aphorisms (viz., *Yoga-Sūtra* 3.55): When the deepest level of the mind (i.e., the principle of *sattva*) is as translucent as the Self, this is equivalent to the condition of liberation. According to Yoga philosophy, the ordinary person lives in a state of corruption or impurity caused by the delusion that he or she is other than the Self, that he or she is a particular body-mind dissociated from the universal superconscious Ground of all things, which is simple and devoid of defects. *Shauca* is the gradual retrieval of that essential purity at the innermost core of our being and of the world at large.

Shauca comprises physical cleansing techniques, which came to be especially developed in Hatha-Yoga, but also internal practices intended to remove the cobwebs of the mind. Through *shauca*, so Patanjali tells us (viz., 2.40), we acquire a sense of distance from the body. This is the attitude of dispassion applied to our most immediate environment, the body-mind. The Yoga student's faith is in the Self as the eternally pure principle beyond all defects and blemishes. On surrendering to That, he or she finds the inner strength to cease polluting the environment, the microcosm, with spiritually marred and hence impure actions, words, and thoughts.

The next constituent of *niyama* is contentment (*samtosha*). Vyāsa, in his commentary on the *Yoga-Sūtra* (11–32), explains that this is the "non-hankering after more than is at hand through one's spiritual practice." The attitude behind this is identical with the message contained in the saying attributed to Jesus: "Behold the birds of the air; they neither sow nor reap nor gather into barns, and yet your heavenly Father feeds them" (Matthew 6:26).

In other words, Yoga practitioners "seek first the Kingdom of Heaven" and put their trust in the plenitude of the omnipresent Reality. They surrender their fear that, unless they seize and hoard things, they will not survive. Some of the greatest masters have demonstrated the viability of this principle of contentment by living the simplest life imaginable, while happily passing on to others the wealth and property gifted to them by their disciples.

Austerity (*tapas*), the next member of *niyama*, consists in special practices that are meant to test and strengthen our will. Typical exercises are fasting, prolonged sitting, and observing silence. The word *tapas* means literally "heat" or "glow." All *tapas* is a symbolic re-enactment of the austerity involved in the creation of the universe. For, according to Hindu mythology (and many other mythologies), the Creator heated himself and sweated out the world. The yogic *tapas*, however, is practiced for the opposite purpose, namely to resolve the personal universe, our microcosm, back into the single Reality. *Tapas* is thus the surrender or sacrifice of our continual out-flowing tendency, and is founded in our faith in the Absolute as the supreme Power, the ultimate Light.

The fourth element of *niyama* is self-study (*svādhyāya*), in the sense of both "study of oneself" and "studying by oneself." Vyāsa defined it in this way: "*Svādhyāya* is the study of the sciences of liberation, and it is [also] the recitation of the *pranava* [i.e., the sacred syllable *om*]." From this explanation it is clear that study does not stand for just any kind of learning. It refers specifically to the Yoga practitioner's consideration of the spiritual heritage of his or her tradition. Perhaps a still more liberal view would be to include *all* traditions and, indeed, all forms of knowledge, on the basis that the truly committed Yoga practitioner will be able to extract important lessons from any kind of knowledge, secular and sacred. The meditative recitation of *om* or other similar words of power (*mantra*) also leads to spiritually important experiences and insights about the structure of the body-mind. Any form of meditation, in the last analysis, is a means of such self-study.

Where do we find a place for faith and surrender in this practice? Here spiritual practitioners sacrifice the mind's natural penchant for spiritually insignificant thoughts and subjects, all the futile learning for the mere sake of it. They discipline themselves by resorting to a careful diet of wholesome intellectual "food." Their trust is in the Self as the all-knowing Reality, which is the foundation of all information and which yet transcends all information.

The last component of *niyama* to be explained is devotion to the Lord (*īshvara-pranidhāna*). While the previous practice addressed our mental capacity, devotion to the Lord is a matter of the heart, or feeling. There is no need to interpret this requirement in a narrowly theistic sense. In Classical Yoga, the concept of the Lord (*īshvara*) is anyway somewhat peculiar and problematic. Perhaps the least complicated way of understanding the present practice is by regarding it as a radical opening up of oneself toward that which is sensed to be greater than oneself. It is not necessary to think of this Something or Someone in terms of a Creator God. So, even self-styled atheists, provided they appreciate the fact of their own relative insignificance and dependence on the cosmos at large, can fruitfully embark on this opening-up. Ultimately, this is what has to happen anyway, if the personality is to be transmuted and the ego transcended. The surrender and faith aspects in this practice or attitude are self-evident.

We have now reached the third limb of the eightfold path, the one with which Western students are most familiar, namely posture (*āsana*). The surrender element in this practice is apparent from Patanjali's instruction (viz., 2.47) that posture, in addition to being stable and easeful, should be accompanied by the "relaxation of tension" (*prayatna-shaithilya*) as well as "(mental) coinciding with the infinite" (*ananta-samāpatti*). Posture is thus a letting-go, a loosening-up of the naturally contracted condition of the body-mind. When performed properly, any *āsana* turns into a bodily and mental act of expansion. In performing an *āsana*, practitioners surrender their egoic image and experience of the body as something solid with definite boundaries. Thereby they overcome their mistaken notion that the body-mind (in its contracted state) is their authentic nature. The faith expressed in this technique is their trust in the incorporeal (*asharīra*) Self that is nonetheless omnipresent.

By means of breath control (*prānāyāma*), the fourth limb, students of Yoga further experience the body as nonsolid, an energy field. *Prāna* is the life energy whose physical manifestation is the breath. *Āyāma* means literally "extension," so that *prānāyāma* signifies the "extension of the life energy" by way of controlling and regulating its flow in the body. In aphorism 2.52, Patanjali states that through this exercise, the coverings (*āvarana*) concealing the inner Light are removed. In this practice, Yoga practitioners place their trust in the universal principle of life, the Self. What they surrender is the ego-bound, disharmonious "energy field," which is their contracted body.

The fifth limb of the eightfold path is sense-withdrawal (*pratyāhāra*). This is the abstraction of the senses from the external world. It is an important phase in the cultivation of inwardness leading to concentration and meditation proper, because in this exercise the habitual centrifugal tendency of consciousness is checked. The attractions of sights and sounds are neutralized in order to develop inner seeing and hearing. The classical texts employ the simile of a tortoise that draws its limbs back into the shell. *Pratyāhāra* is on the sensory level what nongrasping is on the ethical level. In *pratyāhāra*, the spiritual practitioners sacrifice their craving for multiplicity, so that they may come to realize the One that underlies everything. Their faith is directed to the immortal Self, which is the Self of all beings and which, in the words of the *Shvetāshvatara-Upanishad* (3.19), "sees without eyes, hears without ears."

With concentration (*dhāranā*), Yoga practitioners move out of the sphere of the so-called outer limbs *(bahir-anga)* into the sphere of the inner limbs (*antar-anga*) of the eightfold path. Concentration is *āsana* applied to the mind. It is a firm, steady focusing of our attention upon a particular internal object or locus within the body. It is the flip side of "sense-withdrawal." Another name for it is "one-pointedness" (*ekāgratā*). In this practice, spiritual practitioners surrender their usual identification with the mind's hectic activity. This is expressive of their faith in the Self as that which is beyond the pale of thought and which is yet the basis of all thinking.

The seventh limb of the classical yogic path is meditation (*dhyāna*). This is a deepened state of concentration in which the same object is held unwaveringly for a long period. It is a more complete form of surrendering the mind. It is no longer a mental effort, but a state of reposing in a noncontracted condition of the body-mind. This condition is beautifully described in a passage in the ancient *Chāndogya-Upanishad* (7.6.1) where we can read: "Meditation certainly is more than thought (*citta*). The Earth meditates as it were; the atmosphere meditates as it were . . ." That is to say, meditation is abiding in the natural state, without mental complications. The practitioners of Yoga surrender the mind's tendency to appropriate different objects, whether external or internal. Instead they trust in the Self as the Experiencer of all, the unfailing Continuity behind the incessant change of the finite world.

The last limb of Patanjali's eightfold path is *samādhi*, which is generally rendered as "ecstasy." The world-renowned historian of religion Mircea Eliade proffered an alternative rendering—*enstasy*. This coinage takes into account that *samādhi* is not so much a state of exuberance, as suggested by the word "ecstasy," but a condition of great stillness and focusedness in which we "stand in" (*en stasis*) our true nature. Eliade's coinage, however, has not

achieved wide currency, and therefore, after using it in several of my publications, I reverted to the more common term "ecstasy."

The previously described techniques of concentration and meditation
cause a slowing down of the movement within the mental world. In the state
of *samādhi*, our inner architecture can be said to collapse altogether. For
the practitioner surrenders the characteristic feature of human consciousness, which is its bipolar nature, its tension between subject and object. In
samādhi, the experiencing subject *becomes* the contemplated object. At the
highest level of this paradoxical condition, the experiencing subject awakens as the transcendental Self, realizing that he or she has never been anything else but the Self. According to Patanjali's dualistic system, there is a
radical distinction between the Self (*purusha*) and the cosmos (*prakriti*),
and the highest form of *samādhi* necessarily implies a radical transcendence of the cosmos at all levels. The faith element in the ecstatic process
can be said to be the Yoga practitioner's complete trust in the ultimate Subject as pure Being-Awareness.

It is important to understand that the abolition of the ordinary consciousness does not signal a state of unconsciousness or stupor. On the contrary, the
Reality revealed in the highest degree of *samādhi* is pure Awareness (*citi*). In
the language of nondualist Yoga, that Reality is Being-Consciousness-Bliss
(*sat-cid-ānanda*). The recovery of the ultimate Reality, or Self-realization, is
the fulfillment of the practitioner's consistently cultivated disposition of faith
and surrender. From another perspective, this Self-remembering is perfect
self-forgetfulness, which transcends all categories of the mind, including
faith and surrender. Faith and surrender call for an object, but for the person
who has awakened *as* the Self, there is no outside and no object, just as there
is no inside and no self. Hence Janaka, upon having been granted the vision
of the Absolute by the grace of the enlightened adept Ashtāvakra, exclaimed
in ecstasy:

> Oh, even among a multitude of people, I see no duality. [Everything is
> singular] like an enclosed forest. Upon what should I fix my desire?

> Marvelous! In me, the unbounded ocean, [countless] waves of being
> (*jīva*) come in conflict, play, and merge according to their nature.[5]

Giving testimony to his own realization, Sage Ashtāvakra said:

> I am boundless like space; the created universe is like a jar [filled
> and surrounded by space]. Hence there is no [need for] relinquishing,

accepting, or dissolving this [world]. Such is wisdom (*jnāna*). Where is darkness or light, where cessation? Indeed, where is anything at all for the sage who is ever immutable and untroubled?

There is no heaven and no hell, not even living liberation (*jīvanmukti*). In brief, nothing [that could be grasped by the mind presents itself] to the yogic vision.[6]

That which is left when the mind has been stripped of all erroneous ideas about reality is indescribable. It is not a mere void, and, as Ashtāvakra and all the other sages vouchsafe, "It" is incomparably blissful.

63

Mantra-Yoga
Sounding Out the Depth Within

THE VIBRATORY UNIVERSE

According to Kashmiri Shaivism, a sophisticated branch of Tantra, the Ultimate Reality is both Consciousness/Awareness and Energy—Shiva and Shakti. This polar nature is captured in the idea that Reality itself is *parinispandana*, or, in David Bohm's terms, a "holo movement." Creation happens when this transcendental movement becomes specific, manifesting first space and time and then all the countless forms of the cosmos. Thus vibration (*spanda*) is the essence of cosmic existence. Put differently, the universe is an ocean of energy, which is also what contemporary physics is telling us.

In the individual human body, this infinite energy is contained in the form of the serpent power (*kundalinī-shakti*). As the *Shāradā-Tilaka-Tantra* (1.108) states, the *kundalinī* is the sonic Absolute (*shabda-brahman*). The sonic Absolute is the stepped-down version of the soundless Absolute (*ashabda-brahman*). The *kundalinī* is the power of Consciousness (*cit-shakti*), and as such is the superintelligent force sustaining the body and the mind through the mediating agency of the life force (*prāna*), which is directly related to and accessible through the breath.

MANTRIC SCIENCE

According to an esoteric explanation, the Sanskrit term *mantra* signifies "that which protects (*trāna*) the mind (*manas*). Specifically, mantra is a sound (letter, syllable, word, or phrase) that is charged with transformative power, such as the letter *a*, the sacred syllable *om*, the word *hamsa*, or the phrase *om mani padme hūm*. Thus a mantra could be explained as a potentized sound by which specific effects in consciousness can be produced. Most high-minded practitioners are reluctant to use mantras for anything other than the greatest human goal (*purusha-artha*, written *purushārtha*), which is liberation. In Tantric rituals, mantras are used to purify the altar, one's seat, implements such as vessels and offering spoons, or the offerings themselves (e.g., flowers, water, food), or to invoke deities, protectors, and so on. Yet, the science of sacred sound (*mantra-shāstra*) has since ancient times been widely put to secular use as well. In this case, mantras assume the character of magical spells rather than sacred vibrations in the service of self-transformation and self-transcendence.

The serpent energy hidden in the body is associated with the Sanskrit alphabet constituted of fifty basic letters, or sound vibrations, which go into the making of mantras. In contrast to ordinary words, however, mantras most often do not have a particular meaning, and their potency is tapped into through frequent repetition, whether mentally, whispered, or aloud.

It is not commonly understood that for a sound to be a mantra, it must have been given in the context of initiation (*dīkshā*), whether formally or informally. Only then does the mantra have truly transformative power. For a mantra to become "active" or "awakened," it must be recited at least 100,000 times. A mantra lacking in "consciousness" is just like any other sound. As the *Kula-Arnava-Tantra* (15.61–64) states:

> *Mantras* without consciousness are said to be mere letters. They yield no result even after a trillion recitations.

> The state that manifests promptly when the *mantra* is recited [with "consciousness"], that result is not [to be gained] from a hundred, a thousand, a hundred thousand, or ten million recitations.

> O Kuleshvarī, the knots at the heart and throat are pierced, all the limbs are invigorated, tears of joy, gooseflesh, bodily ecstasy, and tremulous speech suddenly occur for sure . . .

> . . . when a *mantra* endowed with consciousness is uttered even once. Where such signs are seen, that [*mantra*] is said to be according to tradition.

Mantras of concentrated potency are known as "seed syllables" (*bīja*). *Om* is the original seed syllable, the source of all others. The *Mantra-Yoga-Samhitā* (71) calls it the "best of all *mantras*," adding that all other mantras receive their power from it. Thus *om* is prefixed or sometimes also suffixed to numerous mantras, such as *om namah shivāya* (Om. Salutation to Shiva) or *om namo bhagavate* (Om. Salutation to Lord [Krishna or Vishnu]).

Over many centuries, the Vedic and Tantric masters have conceived, or rather envisioned, numerous other primary power sounds besides *om*. These seed syllables (*bīja*), as they are called, can be used on their own or, more commonly, in conjunction with other power sounds forming a mantric phrase. According to the *Mantra-Yoga-Samhitā* (71), there are eight primary *bīja-mantras*, which are helpful in all kinds of circumstances but which yield their deeper mystery only to the *yogin:*

1. *aim* (pronounced "I'm")—*guru-bīja* (seed syllable of the teacher), also called *vahni-jāyā* (Agni's wife)
2. *hrīm*—*shakti-bīja* (seed syllable of Shakti), also called *māyā-bīja*
3. *klīm*—*kāma-bīja* (seed syllable of desire)
4. *krīm*—*yoga-bīja* (seed syllable of union), also called *kāli-bīja*
5. *shrīm*—*ramā-bīja* (seed syllable of delight); Ramā is another name for Lakshmī, the Goddess of Fortune; hence this seed syllable is also known as *lakshmī-bīja*
6. *trīm*—*teja-bīja* (seed syllable of fire)
7. *strīm*—*shānti-bīja* (seed syllable of peace)
8. *hlīm*—*rakshā-bīja* (seed syllable of protection)

All this implies that only an adept in whom the *kundalinī* is awake can empower a sound—*any* sound—so that it is transmuted into a mantra. Mantras are the gift of masters of Yoga, great sages (*muni*), and seers (*rishi*), and as such they should be treated with respect and with the understanding that they are indeed potent tools of self-transformation.

❧ 64 ❧
The Gāyatrī-Mantra

IF ONE WERE TO ask a practicing Hindu which of all the single-syllable mantras is the most sacred, he or she would undoubtedly reply: *om*. If one were to ask which composite *mantra* is the most precious or sacred, he or she would name the *gāyatrī-mantra*. Every day, at dawn, millions of Hindus recite this mantra as part of their morning ablutions. Specifically, *samdhyā* (juncture) must be observed just prior to sunrise until the solar orb is fully visible above the horizon. The scriptures recommend that one should recite the *gāyatrī* as often as possible during this short period in order to attain a long and auspicious life as well as spiritual understanding. Typically, a brahmin holds water in his right hand and, bringing it close to his nose, blows on the water first through the right and then the left nostril, repeating the *gāyatrī* three times before pouring the water out.

The mantra gets its name from the poetic meter, which consists of three feet (*pāda*) of eight syllables each. The first four syllables are unfixed, while the last four have a prescribed cadence. The word *gāyatrī* is derived from the verbal root *gā/gai* "to sing, chant" to which is added the suffix *trī*. The same root produces *gītā* (sung, i.e., song), which is the past participle of *gāya* (singing). An esoteric interpretation is furnished in the *Brihad-Āranyaka-Upanishad* (5.14.4), which states that it acquired its name because it protects (*trā*) one's wealth (*gaya*), presumably both material and spiritual. The *Chāndogya-Upanishad* (3.12.1) declares:

> The *gāyatrī* is speech, for speech sings (*gāyati*) and protects (*trāyati*) the whole world.

The true power of the *gāyatrī* is thought to lie in its fourth foot, which transcends grammar and is the blazing Sun itself (see *Brihad-Āranyaka-Upanishad* 5.14.3). The "Fourth" (*caturtha* or *turīya*) is an important metaphysical concept of the *Upanishads*: It stands for that part in us that exceeds waking, dreaming, and sleeping. It is the ever-wakeful transcendental Self (*ātman*) symbolized by the Sun. Hence the *Brihad-Āranyaka-Upanishad* (5.14.7) contains the verse:

Salutation to your fourth foot (*pāda*) visible beyond the sky.

The *gāyatrī-* or *sārasvatī-mantra* has been recited daily since Vedic times. It was first recorded in the *Rig-Veda* (3.62.10), the receptacle of India's most ancient wisdom that subsequently led to Hinduism. According to this Vedic hymnody, the *gāyatrī-mantra* runs:

> *tat savitur varenyam*
> *bhargo devasya dhīmahi*
> *dhiyo yo nah pracodayāt*

To this verse are usually prefixed the *om* sound and what are called the three *vyāhritis* (utterances) consisting of *bhūh, bhuvas, svah,* namely "Earth," "Mid-heaven," and "Heaven." In the *Brihad-Āranyaka-Upanishad* (5.5.3–4), these three are respectively correlated with the head, the arms, and the feet of the person. Curiously, the head is connected not with Heaven, as one might expect, but with Earth, while the feet are connected with Heaven. This hints at an archaic teaching about the human being springing from Heaven (involution) rather than from an earthly womb (evolution). The work of Yoga consists in finding our feet, or roots, in Heaven.

Also, there is a string of *mantras* often preceding the three *vyāhritis* that is known as *shiras* (head); it consists of *om āpo jyotī raso'mritam brahma* (*om*, water, light, essence, immortality, the Absolute). Thus the full text of the *gāyatrī* runs:

> *om āpo jyotī raso'mritam brahma*
> *om bhūr bhuvah svah [or suvah]*
> *tat savitur varenyam*
> *bhargo devasya dhīmahi*
> *dhiyo yo nah pracodayāt*

Om. Water. Light. Essence. Immortality. The Absolute.
Om. Earth. Mid-heaven. Heaven.
Let us contemplate the most excellent splendor of God
Savitri, so that He may inspire our contemplations.

The *Amrita-Bindu-Upanishad*, an early medieval Yoga scripture, defines breath control (*prānāyāma*) as consisting of the threefold repetition of the *gāyatrī* along with the three *vyāhritis* and the *shiras* in a single breath.

The *gāyatrī-mantra* invokes the Solar Spirit, whose body is our Sun. The most ancient Yoga was a solar Yoga, and this tradition still lies at the heart of much of Hindu Yoga. Without the Sun, there would be no life on Earth. Thus the Hindus celebrate and worship the Solar Spirit as life-giver and also the principle that illuminates the mind.

The *gāyatrī* is explained in many places in the Sanskrit literature. For instance, the *Tripurā-Tāpanī-Upanishad*, a fairly late work belonging to the Shākta tradition, connects this mantra with the worship of the Goddess Tripurā. She is celebrated as the great Power (Shakti) behind all manifestation.

In that scripture, we learn that the Sanskrit word *tat* ("that") refers to the eternal, unconditioned Absolute (*brahman*), the transcendental Reality out of which the world in all its many layers has evolved.

Savitur (or Savitri), the *Upanishad* further tells us, refers to the primal power of the Goddess Tripurā, even though the Sanskrit name *Savitri* is a masculine word standing for the "Impeller," that is, the Sun or Solar Spirit. Savitri must not be confused with the Goddess Savitrī, who presides over all learning but also over the mighty river by the same name that once flowed from the Himalayas to the Indian Ocean. The name *Savitri* derives from the verbal root *su* meaning "to urge, instigate, impel," which is closely related to the second connotation of this root, namely "to extract, press." What Savitri extracts out of himself are two closely connected things: life-giving light and warmth.

Varenyam means "most excellent" or "most beautiful," designating that which has no superior. This word qualifies the term *bhargas*.

Bhargo (from *bhargas* or "splendor") is said to be the transcendental aspect of Savitri, which strikes us with awe—a splendor that cannot be seen with human eyes but that discloses itself only to the inner vision of the great Yoga adept.

Devasya (from *deva*) means "of God," that is, "of Savitri."

Dhīmahi means "let us contemplate" and implies a heartfelt desire to focus the mind on the ultimate Reality through the medium of contemplation (*dhī*). In the *Rig-Veda*, the archaic term *dhī* stands for the later term *dhyāna*, which means "meditation/contemplation."

Dhiyo (from *dhiyas*) is the plural of *dhī*. Repeatedly the ancient sages fixed their minds on that One, and contemporary *yogins* still follow the same age-old practice. As their contemplations deepen, Savitri increasingly illuminates the mind.

Yo (from *yah*) is simply the relative pronoun "who," which here refers to God Savitri.

Nah means "us/our" and qualifies the contemplations of the sages.

Pracodayāt is derived from the verb *pracodaya* (meaning "to cause to be inspired").

Without Savitri, the masters of yore felt, their contemplations lacked inspiration. Only Savitri could inspire or illuminate their inner world, just as he illuminates the Earth through his radiant physical body (the visible solar orb).

The Sacred Syllable Om

THE MEANING OF OM

There is no question that *om* is the oldest mantra, or sound of numinous power, known to the sages of India. Its origin, however, is somewhat obscure. A century ago, the German scholar Max Müller, editor and translator of the *Rig-Veda*, had the idea that *om* might be a contraction of the word *avam*, "a prehistoric pronominal stem, pointing to distant objects, while *ayam* pointed to nearer objects."[1] He continued, "*Avam* may have become the affirmative particle *om*, just as the French *oui* arose from *hoc illud*."[2] This obscure comment refers to the fact that *om*, in addition to its sacred significance, came to be used in the prosaic sense of "Yes, I agree." Müller's interesting philological speculation remains unsubstantiated, however.

More recently, a different approach was taken by Swami Sankarananda, who proposed that *om* derives from the Vedic word *soma*.[3] Through the influence of the Persians, who did not pronounce the letter *s*, the word *soma* was changed to *homa* and subsequently was shortened to *om*. Like Müller's derivation, this is pure conjecture, but is nonetheless intriguing, as it brings out the traditionally accepted relationship between *soma* and *om*.

Soma is the sacred substance used in the principal Vedic sacrifice. It has been characterized as an intoxicant, and various scholars have, in my opinion, wrongly identified it as a concoction prepared from the fly agaric mushroom. In the Vedic literature, *soma* is always described as a creeper, which cannot be said to apply to a mushroom. Be that as it may, the real *soma* was not a plant or plant extract but a spiritual "elixir," or illuminating experience, as is evident from certain hymns of the *Rig-Veda* (e.g., 10.85.3). In this sense, we also encounter it in later Tantra, where *soma* stands for an inner process or esoteric phenomenon: the nectar of immortality said to ooze from the "Moon" at the *tālu-cakra* (palate wheel) in the head, dripping into the "Sun" stationed at the *nābhi-cakra* (navel wheel). On the physical level, it corresponds to the saliva, which is known to have antiseptic, healing properties.

Swami Sankarananda believed that, like *soma*, the sacred syllable *om* represents the Sun. This seems to be confirmed by the *Aitareya-Brāhmana* (5.32): *om ity asau yo'sau [sūryah] tapati*, "That which glows [i.e., the Sun] is *om*." The Sun was indeed central to the Vedic spirituality, and the Vedic sages looked upon the Sun not merely as a star that supplies our planet with the necessary light and warmth but as a multidimensional entity of which the visible stellar body is merely its outermost material shell.

The esteemed Swami's conjecture is worthy of deeper consideration. However, most spiritual authorities regard *om* as the vocalization of an actual "sound," or vibration, which pervades the entire universe and is audible to *yogins* in higher states of consciousness. In the Western hermetic tradition, this is known as "the music of the spheres." The Indian sages also speak of it as the *shabda-brahman* or "sonic Absolute," which, in the words of the *Chāndogya-Upanishad* (2.23.3), is "all this (*idam sarvam*)." What this means is that *om* is the universe as a totality, not a conglomerate of individual parts, as we experience it in our ordinary state of consciousness. Thus *om* is the primordial sound that reveals itself to the inner ear of the adept who has controlled the mind and the senses.

Vihari-Lala Mitra, in the introduction to his translation of the *Yoga-Vāsishtha*, equated the Greek word *on* ("being") with *om*.[4] While this is linguistically unsustainable, philosophically the connection is valid, as *om* is the symbol of That Which Is, or *brahman*. He also made the link between *om* and *Amen* to which the same strictures apply.[5]

THE EARLY HISTORY OF THE SACRED SYLLABLE

Significantly, the syllable *om* is not mentioned in the ancient *Rig-Veda*, which has recently been dated back to the third millennium B.C.E. and earlier still.[6] However, a veiled reference to it may be present in one of the hymns (1.164.39), which speaks of the syllable (*akshara*) that exists in the supreme space in which all the deities reside. "What," asks the composer of this hymn, "can one who does not know this do with the chant?" He adds, "Only those who know it sit together here." That is, only initiates gather to delight in the mystery of the sacred syllable and the company of the deities.

The word *akshara* means literally "immutable" or "imperishable." This designation is most appropriate, since grammatically syllables are stable parts that make up words. In the case of the mantric *om*, this monosyllable came to represent the ultimate One, which is eternally unchanging (*akshara, acala*). The term *akshara* is used as a synonym for *om* in many scriptures, including the *Bhagavad-Gītā* (10.25), which has Krishna say, "Of utterances I am the single syllable."

In light of the early prominence given to *om* as the primordial seed sound, there is no good reason for assuming that the sagely composers of the Vedic hymns were ignorant of the sacred syllable *om*. Indeed, they were great masters of Mantra-Yoga, and the Vedic hymnodies are the astounding creation of their mantric competence. Possibly, *om* was considered so sacred that it could not be mentioned outside the actual context of the Vedic sacrifices. In that case, it would have been passed on from teacher to student by word of mouth in strictest confidence. There would therefore have been no need to mention *om* in the sacred hymns. All initiates would have known it and also understood its sublime meaning. In any case, for countless generations, any recitation of the Vedic hymns has begun with the syllable *om*. The *Atharva-Veda* (10.8.10) seems to hint at this with the following riddle:

> What is joined to the front and to the back and is joined all around and everywhere, and by which the sacrifice proceeds? That praise (*ric*) I ask of you.

The syllable *om* is often appended to longer mantric utterances, both introducing and concluding them, and this practice is very old indeed. As time went by, the ban on uttering the sacred syllable or even writing it down outside the sacrificial rituals was relaxed. Thus the sacred syllable is first mentioned by name in the opening hymn of the *Shukla-Yajur-Veda* (1.1), the "white" recension of the Vedic hymnody dealing strictly with the performance of the sacrifices (*yajus*). This could be a later addition, however. For the *Taittirīya-Samhitā* (5.2.8), which is appended to the *Yajur-Veda*, still cryptically speaks of the "divine sign" (*deva-lakshana*) that is written threefold (*try-alikhita*). Some scholars have seen this as a reference to the three constituent parts of the syllable *om*, as written in Sanskrit: *a* + *u* + *m*. The three constituents of *om* are referred to, for instance, in the *Prashna-Upanishad* (v. 5). The symbolic elaboration of this is found in the *Māndūkya-Upanishad*, as we will see later.

That the sacred syllable was written down early on is clear from the fact that it had to be traced in sand or water during certain of the ancient rituals. This is also a significant piece of evidence in favor of writing at least in the late Vedic era, which is generally denied by historians. However, today we appreciate that ancient Indian history needs to be completely rewritten.

The long-held belief that the Vedic people invaded India between 1200 and 1500 B.C.E. has been shown to be unfounded. In fact, all the evidence points to the identity between the Vedic people and the builders of the great cities along the banks of the Indus River. Since inscribed artifacts have been found in the Indus cities, the question of whether or not the Vedic people knew writing can be conclusively answered in the affirmative.

It is true, though, that the Vedic hymnodies were in all probability never written down until comparatively recently. Yet, the *brahmins* had devised an ingenious system of memorization to guarantee that the *Vedas* were preserved with utmost fidelity. It appears that they have been successful in this, thanks to the prodigious memories of the Vedic specialists. Other cultures, which held their sacred tradition in a similar high regard, sought to preserve it by memorization rather than writing it down on impermanent materials that, moreover, might fall into the wrong hands. However, nowhere has the art of memorization reached the sophistication that it did in India.

Over many generations, *om* was not uttered outside the sacred context of ritual worship. It was a secret sound communicated by word of mouth from teacher to disciple, that is, originally from father to son. Even the early *Upanishads* (which have recently been dated back to the second millennium B.C.E.) often still refer to it only indirectly as the *udgītha* (up sound) and the *pranava* (pronouncing). The former word hints at the nasalized way in which *om* is sounded out, with the sound vibrating at the psychoenergetic center located between and behind the eyebrows (i.e., the *ājnā-cakra*). The term *pranava* is derived from the prefix *pra* (etymologically related to the Latin "pro") and the stem *nava* (derived from the verbal root *nu* meaning "to call out" and "to exult"). It is used, for instance, in the *Yoga-Sūtra* (1.27), where it is called the symbol (*vācaka*) of the Lord (*īshvara*). Patanjali further states (in 1.28) that in order to realize the mystery of the Lord, the *om* sound should be recited *and* contemplated.

Another, later term for *om* is *tāra*, which is derived from the verbal root *trī*, meaning "to cross, traverse." This is a reference to the liberating function of the *om* sound, which safely transports the *yogin* across the ocean of existence (*bhāva-sāra*) to the "other shore." Through recitation, which is mindful repetition of the *om* sound, the *yogin* can transcend the mind itself and thus is freed from the illusion of being an insular being separate from everything else. The *om* sound is truly liberating because it expands the reciter beyond the physical boundary of the skin and beyond the metaphorical boundary of preconceptions, thus restoring the recognition of the universal Self as his or her true identity.

In the earliest *Upanishads*, such as the *Brihad-Āranyaka, Chāndogya,* and *Taittirīya*, the sacred syllable *om* is mentioned many times by name, both as *om* (or *aum*) and *om-kāra* (*om* making, meaning the letter *om*). However, *udgītha* is more common. It is the *Chāndogya* that first clearly spells out the equation between the words *udgītha* and *pranava* (a term not found in the *Brihad-Āranyaka*). Perhaps these two terms came in vogue because for un-known reasons *om* had, by that time, spread beyond the sacred domain and begun to be used in the sense of "Yes, I agree." The first record of this usage is in the *Brihad-Āranyaka-Upanishad* (3.9.1) itself, where *om* is employed seven times in this manner. Indeed, the *Chāndogya-Upanishad* (1.1.8) clearly states: "That syllable is a syllable of assent, for whenever we assent to anything we say *aum* [= *om*]." Max Müller commented on this as follows:

> If, then, *om* meant originally *that* and *yes*, we can understand that, like Amen, it may have assumed a more general meaning, something like *tat sat*, and that it may have been used as representing all that human lan-guage can express.[7]

The *Chāndogya-Upanishad* (1.1.9) also has this relevant passage:

> By this the threefold knowledge proceeds. To honor this syllable, *aum* is recited, *aum* is exclaimed, *aum* is chanted, with its greatness and essence.

Interestingly, in his commentary on this *Upanishad*, Shankara takes this passage to refer to the *soma* sacrifice, which again affirms the connection between *om* and *soma* mentioned above. He states that the *soma* ritual is performed to celebrate, or honor, the sacred syllable, which is the symbol of the Divine. This sacrifice, he further explains, maintains the Sun from which proceeds all life and nourishment by means of warmth and rain.

The *Chāndogya-Upanishad* (1.9.4) also quotes Atidhanvan Shaunaka, the teacher of Udara Shāndilya, as saying, "So long as your descendants will know this *udgītha*, their life in this world will be the highest and best." This expresses the idea that the sacred syllable is a blessing for those who utter it. For this reason it is worthy of being held in the highest esteem, as this and other scriptures emphasize.

According to the concluding verses of the *Brihat-Samnyāsa-Upanishad* —a text of the medieval period—twelve thousand recitations of *om* remove all sins, while twelve thousand recitations daily for a period of one year bring realization of the Absolute (*brahman*). What greater blessing can there be than this?

FROM OM TO AUM

At least two millennia after the sacred syllable *om* was discovered by the Vedic seers (*rishis*), the anonymous sage who composed the brief *Māndūkya-Upanishad* utilized this age-old mantra to expound the metaphysics of Advaita Vedānta. Thus he explained the three constituent parts (*mātrā*) of the syllable—namely *a* + *u* + *m*—as symbolizing past, present, and future, as well as waking, dreaming, and deep sleep. He also spoke of a fourth part that transcends the other three and concluded his esoteric observations with the statement that *om* is the Self (*ātman*), saying, "He who knows this enters the Self with the self—indeed, he who knows this!"

The importance of the *Māndūkya-Upanishad* can be gauged from the fact that the venerable sage Gaudapāda wrote his celebrated commentary entitled *Māndūkya-Kārikā* on it, which was subsequently commented on at length by Shankara, the great preceptor of the school of nondualism (*advaita*). Gaudapāda was the teacher of Govindapāda, Shankara's *guru*.

Another scripture, given exclusively to explaining the sacred syllable *om* is the *Atharva-Shikhā-Upanishad*. This scripture begins with the question: What should one meditate on? The answer is: the syllable *om*, which symbolizes the supreme Absolute (*brahman*). The text speaks of four constituent parts of this mantra, each having its own symbolic correlations as follows:

1. The sound *a*: earth—*ric* (hymn of praise)—*Rig-Veda*—Brahman—Vasus (a class of eight deities)—*gāyatrī* meter—*gārhapatya* fire—red—dedicated to Brahman.
2. The sound *u*: atmosphere—*yajus* (sacrificial formula)—*Yajur-Veda*—Vishnu—Rudras (deities governing the region between earth and heaven)—*trishtubh* meter—*dakshina* fire—bright—dedicated to Rudra.
3. The sound *m*: heaven—*sāman* (sacred chants)—*Sāma-Veda*—Vishnu—Ādityas (deities connected with the Goddess Aditi, symbolizing primordial infinity)—*jagatī* meter—*āhavanīya* fire—black—dedicated to Vishnu.
4. "Half-part" (*ardha-mātra*): Atharvan songs—*Atharva-Veda*—fire of universal destruction—Maruts (deities of the mid-region who are especially associated with the wind)—Virāt—lightning-like and multicolored—dedicated to Purusha.

The most important part is the nasalized "half-part" sound *m*, which brings its own illumination and causes the life force (*prāna*) in the body to rush upward into the head. This *Upanishad* further states that the *om* sound is called *om-kāra* because it sends the currents of the life force upward (*ūrdhvam utkrāmayati*) and that it is called *pranava* because it makes all the life currents bow down (*pranāmayati*) before it. The text concludes by stating that the *om* sound is Shiva.

Interestingly, in Tantra-Yoga, the serpent power (*kundalinī-shakti*) resting in the psychoenergetic center (*cakra*) at the base of the spine, is said to be coiled up three and a half times. Very likely, this captures the same idea as in the notion of the three and a half units of the *om* sound. The *Tantras* would presumably modify the *Upanishad's* final claim to replace Shiva with Shakti, which in the form of the *kundalinī* rises upward and while doing so assimilates the life currents. In fact, the ascent of the serpent power is accompanied by manifestations of ever more subtle sound.

According to the *Amrita-Bindu-Upanishad* (4), only the silent part of the sound *m* leads to the soundless, invisible Abode, the ultimate Reality. This scripture explains breath control (*prānāyāma*), a very important aspect of yogic discipline, as the recitation of the *gāyatrī-mantra: tat savitur varenyam bhargo devasya dhīmahi dhiyo yo nah pracodayāt*. This mantra is to be recited together with the *pranava* and the *vyāhritis* (formulaic utterances, notably the words *bhūh bhuvah svah*, standing for earth, mid-region, and heaven respectively). This sacred mantra should be recited three times in a single breath.

The *Amrita-Nāda-Upanishad* (2ff.) recommends that one should mount the "chariot of the *om* sound," make Vishnu one's charioteer, and steer steadily toward the ultimate Reality. As one approaches the supreme Self, one should abandon the chariot and enter the splendor of the Self by means of the unsounded letter *m*. This is the silent, subtle part of *om*.

This *Upanishad* prescribes breath control, especially retention of the breath, as a means of controlling the senses and focusing the mind upon the inner world. It defines Yoga as the state of restraint over a period of twelve units or measures (*mātrā*), that is, twelve recitations of *om*. It promises the dawning of wisdom within three months of diligent and continuous practice, an inner vision of the deities within four months, and final liberation within a mere six months. Of course, one must be able to sustain unwavering concentration for that span of time in order to succeed. For most people, this is an impossibility. For, as one Vedic seer-bard (*rishi*) complained in the *Rig-Veda* (10.33.2), "My mind flutters here and there like a bird."

According to the *Dhyāna-Bindu-Upanishad* (15), the *pranava* is the bow, oneself is the arrow, and the Absolute is the target. This metaphor is first found in the *Mundaka-Upanishad* (2.2.3–4). It also calls the *pranava* imperishable and states that its "fine end" cannot be expressed. Another favorite metaphor, also recapitulated in the *Dhyāna-Bindu-Upanishad* (22), is that of oneself as the lower churning stick (*arani*) and the *om* sound as the upper churning stick. By practicing it, one can restrain one's breath and dissolve the subtle sound (*nāda*).

Through constant cultivation of the subtle inner sound, declares the *Nāda-Bindu-Upanishad* (49), the karmic imprints (*vāsanā*) left by our past volitional activity are eradicated. This leads to the merging of mind and life force. When the mind and the life force are motionless, the person abides as the subtle sound known as *brahma-tāra-antara-nāda*, which can be translated as the "innermost sound that is the brahmic liberator (*tāra*)."

A fascinating account of the sacred syllable is given in the *Nārada-Parivrājaka-Upanishad* (8.1ff.), a medieval scripture. Here *om* is said to be threefold: the destructive *om*, the creative *om*, and the internal-and-external *om* (comprising the two former types). Another threefold division is: the brahmic *om*, the internal *om*, and the practical *om*. Then the text mentions two more sets: the external *om*, the *om* of the seers (*rishi*), and the *virāt om* (consisting of the former two), as well as the destructive *om*, the Brahma *om*, and the *om* of the half-measure (*ardha-mātrā*).

This *Upanishad* goes on to explain these various forms of *om* as follows: The internal *om* is the single syllable *om*, which has eight parts—*a, u, m, ardha-mātrā, nāda, bindu, kalā,* and *shakti*. The phoneme *a* is said to consist of ten thousand parts, the phoneme *u* of one thousand parts, the phoneme *m* of one hundred parts, and the *ardha-mātrā* of an infinite number of parts. The creative *om* is described as having qualities and the destructive *om* as having none. The *virāt om* is said to consist of sixteen units (*morae*). In addition to the above-mentioned eight parts (which are explained below), the sacred syllable also has *kalā-atīta, shānti, shānti-atita* (written *shāntyatīta*), *unmanī, mana-unmanī* (written *manomanī*), *purī, madhyamā, pashyantī,* and *parā*. This text also refers to 64 and 128 parts of the sacred syllable, but it makes the point that ultimately its designated object—the Absolute—is singular.

THE SACRED SYLLABLE OM IN THE TANTRAS

The above Upanishadic ideas lead to the speculations about *om* in the Tantric literature where concepts like *nāda, bindu, kalā, shakti,* and so forth, abound. The *Shāradā-Tilaka-Tantra* (1.108) describes the cosmogonic process in terms of the production of sound as follows: From the supreme Shakti—pure Consciousness combined with the factor of lucidity (*sattva*)—comes the most subtle sound (*dhvani*), which is marked by a pre-eminence of the factors of lucidity and dynamism (*rajas*). Out of the *dhvani* develops the subtle sound (*nāda*), characterized by a mixture of the factors of lucidity, dynamism, and inertia (*tamas*). This subtle sound, in turn, gives rise to the energy of restriction (*nirodhikā*), which has an excess of the factor of inertia. This ontic principle emanates the "half-moon" (*ardha-indu*, written *ardhendu*), which at this lower level again shows a predominance of the factor of lucidity. Out of it comes the vibratory source point (*bindu*), the immediate source of all letters and words. These form mantras, which are thus manifestations or vehicles of Shakti.

This scripture (1.8) further explains that the *bindu* is itself composed of three parts, namely, *nāda*, *bindu*, and *bīja* (seed). The first part has a pre-dominance of Consciousness (i.e., Shiva), the second a preponderance of Energy (i.e., Shakti), and the third an equal presence of Consciousness and Energy. Such esoteric accounts of the evolution of sound remain relatively unintelligible outside of Tantric practice; however, they become increasingly meaningful as the practitioner makes progress on the path of *mantra-vidyā* or "mantric science."

The primordial sound is uncaused. In the language of Kashmiri Tantrism, it is pure vibration (*spanda*). According to the *Kirana-Tantra* (copied in 924 C.E.), *om* resides in the throat of Shiva and is the Divine itself. This scripture also describes it as the root of all mantras, stating that upon articulation it becomes *vāc* (speech), corresponding to the Greek concept of *logos*.

As we get higher up the ladder of ontic unfoldment (i.e., creation), we encounter ever more subtle energies. Thus the *mātrikās* ("matrices" or "little mothers") are the subtle alphabetic counterpart to their corresponding audible sounds; the *bindu* is subtler than the *mātrikās*, and the *nāda* is still more subtle. As the *Yoga-Shikhā-Upanishad* (2.21) states, "There is no *mantra* higher than the *nāda*." In old graphic representations of the *om-kāra*, the *nāda* symbol is drawn or painted as an inverted crescent *above* the *bindu*, which suggests that the *nāda* is prior to the *bindu*. Later the crescent placed *below* the *bindu* emphasized that the *nāda* contains the *bindu*. Both graphic representations make the same point, however.

The *nāda* itself has various levels of subtle manifestation. According to the *Hamsa-Upanishad* (16) it manifests in ten different ways. First there is the sound *cini*, then *cini-cini*. The third sounds like a bell, the fourth like the blast of a conch, whereas the fifth has the quality of a harp sound. The sixth through the ninth respectively resemble the sounds of cymbals, flute, kettle drum, and tabor. Only the tenth type, which is like a thunder clap, should be cultivated. Various physiological symptoms are said to accompany these sounds. Thus when the fourth sound is heard (in the right ear), one's head begins to shake, while the fifth sound causes the subtle center at the root of the palate to stream with the lunar ambrosia, and so on. The final sound alone is accompanied by identification with the supreme Absolute (*para-brahman*).

Some *Tantras* differentiate between *mahā-nāda* (also called *nāda-anta*) and *nirodhinī*, which is transmuted into *bindu*. This is also called *tri-bindu* because it is subdivided into *nāda, bindu,* and *bīja.* In this case, the *nāda* is correlated with *shiva,* the *bindu* with *shakti,* and the *bīja* with both Shiva and Shakti. The ultimate Reality itself can be viewed as a point origin, and as such is sometimes referred to as *para-bindu* or transcendental germinal point.

Om is the ultimate *bīja-mantra.* The idea of *om* being the root of other *mantras* may actually have given rise to the whole idea of *bīja-mantras,* which are root sounds associated with particular deities. They are special high-potency sounds or vibrations giving direct access to the spiritual realities for which they stand. Thus *om* is prefixed or suffixed to numerous *mantras:*

Om namah shivāya. "*Om.* Salutation to Shiva."
Om namo bhagavate. "*Om.* Salutation to the Lord [i.e., Krishna or Vishnu]."
Om namo ganeshāya. "*Om.* Salutation to [the elephant-headed] Ganesha."
Om namo nārāyanāya. "*Om.* Salutation to Nārāyana [Vishnu]."
Om shānte prashānte sarva-krodha-upashamani svāhā. "*Om.* At peace! Pacifying! All anger be subdued! Hail!" (Note pronunciation: *sarva-krodhopashamani*)
Om sac-cid-ekam brahma. "*Om.* The singular Being-Consciousness, the Absolute."

The *Mahānirvāna-Tantra* (3.13) calls the last-mentioned *brahma-mantra* the most excellent of all *mantras,* which promptly bestows not only liberation but also virtue, wealth, and pleasure. The *para-bindu* mentioned above is said to have a masculine and a feminine side, which are respectively called *ham* and *sa,* thus yielding the sound or word *hamsa,* meaning "swan," but signifying the sound of the breath and indeed the breath itself as it enters and leaves the body. This natural motion of breathing, which is calculated to occur 21,600 times every day, is called spontaneous recitation (*sahaja-japa*) or unrecited recitation (*ajapa-japa*).

The *hamsa* also stands for the psyche (*jīva*), which lives through the breath. This spontaneous *mantra* is understood as *so'ham* or "I am he," that is, "I am Shiva, the ultimate Reality." But ignorance prevents us from realizing this; hence the need for spiritual practice. The *Yoga-Bīja* (156), a comparatively late Hatha-Yoga text, states that when the *prāna* enters the central channel, the natural *mantra* reverses itself from *hamsa* to *so'ham*. Experientially, however, this is not different from the primordial *om*, the root *mantra* that reverberates through the entire cosmos. The *Mantra-Yoga-Samhitā* (73) has this stanza:

> When people hear the *pranava* they hear the Absolute itself.
> When they utter the *pranava* they go to the abode of the
>   Absolute.
> He who perceives the *pranava* sees the state of the Absolute.
> He who always has the *pranava* in his mind has the form of
>   the Absolute.

CONCLUSION

This brief discourse on the history and nature of the sacred syllable *om* is meant to give the reader a better appreciation of the metaphysical complexities surrounding this age-old mantra and of some of the profound spiritual practices associated with it. It would be possible to write several volumes on this subject, just as it would be possible to provide an overview of India's spiritual traditions based solely on the theory and practice of the *om* sound. What has been presented here is but a minute fraction of the teachings about *om* developed over a span of five millennia.

The Yoga tradition is very rich and immensely sophisticated; yet its various schools and their respective paths are at core very simple, and in their simplicity they have many features in common. Above all, they lead to the same goal, which is the transcendence of the ego-personality, however this may be conceived and expressed in words. As the *Rig-Veda* (1.164.46) declared five millennia or more ago, "There is a single Truth but the wise call it by different names."

❧ 66 ❧

Mudrās

Gestures of Wholeness

In Yoga, MUDRĀS are primarily special hand gestures that are used to conduct the body's subtle energy or life force (*prāna*) in specific ways.[1] They are employed during meditation, visualization, breath control, and rituals of worship, as well as for therapeutic purposes in Tantric medicine. The most common *mudrā* is the *anjali* gesture, which is used in India to greet others by bringing the palms of the hands together in front of the heart, with the extended fingers pointing upward.

The Sanskrit term *mudrā*—which means literally "seal"—also is associated with other yogic practices that are intended to contain, direct, or augment the life force. Thus this technical term is applied to certain gestures involving the tongue (i.e., *khecārī-mudrā*), the eyes (i.e., *shāmbhavī-mudrā*), the openings of the head (i.e., *shan-mukhī-mudrā*), the genitals (i.e., *vajrolī-mudrā* and *yoni-mudrā*), the anus (i.e., *ashvinī-mudrā*), and the body as a whole (i.e., *viparīta-karanī-mudrā*, otherwise known as the shoulder stand or headstand). According to esoteric explanations, the word *mudrā* is to be derived from the verbal root *mud*, meaning "to gladden, delight." Thus a *mudrā* is a practice that brings delight (*mudā*) to the deities while causing the dissolution (*drava*), or transcendence, of the mind.

A wide range of *mudrās* of the hands, arms, legs, head, and trunk also are employed in Indian dance, and over the centuries Indian dance and Yoga (especially Tantra-Yoga) very likely crossfertilized each other. But the origin of the yogic *mudrās* undoubtedly lies in ritual. The *Brāhmanas* contain descriptions of correct hand gestures for pouring ghee, honey, or *soma* into the fire as an offering to the deities. Conceivably, this "body magic" originated much earlier in prehistoric shamanism. It is very probable that *mudrās* were originally discovered spontaneously in states of psychoenergetic awakening, such as meditation (see, e.g., Kshemarāja's *Vimarshinī* commentary on the *Shiva-Sūtra* 3.26). Even today, practitioners who are deeply immersed in Tantric practice, can experience spontaneous *mudrās*, some of which are exact replicas of traditional seals while others are absolutely unique to the person. Each is accompanied and presumably the expression of a specific kind of psychic energy.

Mudrās came to play a significant role in Tantra, which gained prominence in the early centuries of the Common Era and achieved its classical form about 1000 C.E. *Mudrās* are utilized in the Tantric schools of Hinduism, Buddhism, and Jainism. In the *Mudrā-Avadhi*, a Jaina scripture, 114 seals are named, and the Buddhist *Manjushrī-Mūla-Kalpa* (chapter 35), mentions 108, stating that 55 are in common use. The Hindu *Jayākhyā-Samhitā* (chapter 8) mentions 58 *mudrās*. Swami Gitananda claimed that there are a total of 729 *mudrās*, all of which he taught.[2]

"Your brain," observed Swami Gitananda, "is a giant super computer, but without input or programming 99.9 per cent of its cellular area. When you use the Mudras, you programme the brain, which then increases your efficiency considerably and your sense of awareness as well."[3]

In Hindu Tantra, *mudrā* also is counted among the "Five Ms" (*panca-makāra*), where it stands for parched grain—an item to be ingested as part of the left-hand ritual and thought to be an aphrodisiac. In Hatha-Yoga, which is an offshoot of Tantra, *mudrā* also stands for certain bodily postures, such as *viparīta-karanī-mudrā*, or inversion pose. In Buddhist Tantra-Yoga (i.e., Vajrayāna), *mudrā* has an important additional meaning, signifying the Tantric partner. *Mudrā*, then, is a very important yogic concept, which most Western practitioners still have to discover.

❧ 67 ❧

Tāraka -Yoga
Seeing the Light

THE VAST TREASURE-HOUSE of Indian esoteric knowledge has hardly been tapped as yet. What are a mere two hundred years of piecemeal scholarship compared to three millennia of experimentation and development? For this is the considerable space of time that Yoga has taken to reach its present shape. Considering the persistent stepmotherly treatment of Indian esoteric lore at the hand of Western scholars, it is not really surprising that there are still innumerable gaps in our knowledge and understanding of Yoga. Many of its more obscure aspects have escaped the notice of the historians of religion. One of these gaps concerns the mysterious Tāraka-Yoga.

The Sanskrit word *tāraka* means "that which delivers" and in this particular school of Yoga the term stands for a definite set of yogic experiences. These are thought to conduct the *yogin* across the threshold of the finite world into the realm of the Unconditioned, the Real. Nothing is known about the history of this school except that it was probably established in the heyday of Tantra in the opening centuries of the second millennium C.E. It is quite possible that at one time Tāraka-Yoga attracted a large following from among the hundreds of thousands of spiritual seekers of medieval India.

Two Sanskrit texts setting forth this tradition have come down to our age, namely, the *Advaya-Tāraka-Upanishad* and the *Mandala-Brāhmana-Upanishad*. The former consists of nineteen verses, while the latter is a more elaborate version comprising ninety-one sections. Both scriptures belong to the medieval period, though their exact age is unknown.

Tāraka-Yoga is based on the nondualist philosophy of Advaita Vedānta. A fairly intricate system of thought formulated in its classical form by the renowned Shankara Ācārya, who lived in the seventh or eighth century C.E., Advaita Vedānta can be said to constitute the mainstream of contemporary Indian philosophy. Despite its considerable complexity, the principal axioms of this school can easily be grasped. In the *Viveka-Cūdāmani* (Crest-jewel of Discernment), a popular work of spiritual edification, the doctrine is put in a nutshell thus:

> This entire universe, which through our spiritual blindness assumes manifold forms, is really nothing but *brahman* utterly free of any defects. (227)

> A pot, though a product of clay, is not anything different from it. For the pot is essentially the same as the clay. Why then call it a pot? It is a fictitious, constructed name merely. (228)

> Similarly, the whole world, being the effect of the real *brahman*, is nothing but that *brahman*. He who says it is something other than *brahman* babbles like one who is asleep. (230)

> Hence whatever is manifested as this world is the supreme *brahman* only, [which is] real, nondual, pure, of the essence of Awareness, taintless, tranquil, without beginning or end, inactive, of the nature of endless bliss. (237)

> That supreme *brahman* which transcends all speech is accessible to the eye of pure enlightenment. It is pure Awareness, the beginningless Reality. You are that *brahman!* Contemplate it yourself. (255)

The mystical experience of the singular Being, called *brahman* or *ātman*, is so overpowering that the adepts are absolutely convinced that they have encountered something that is infinitely more real than anything related by the senses. They do not deny the myriad of forms in the universe. Their argument is rather that the senses do not give us a true picture of what there is. They firmly maintain that the mind of the unenlightened individual definitely distorts reality by splitting it up into so many compartments. These compartments are the multiple entities located in the space-time world as we encounter it. In contrast, the single Being is an uninterrupted continuum where time stands still and the concept "space" is meaningless.

Since the world of multiplicity is the result of imperfect knowledge or spiritual blindness (*avidyā*) that blocks out the knowledge of the single Being, it logically follows that this ultimate Real must also be our true nature. It is the underlying purpose of any form of Yoga to eliminate all false identities that a person assumes in the course of a lifetime, and to bring the spiritual aspirant to his or her authentic identity, which is none other than the transcendental Ground or Self. When looked upon as the ultimate foundation of the manifold universe, this singular Reality is called *brahman*, whilst from a psychological viewpoint as the inmost essence of the person it is designated as *ātman*. *Brahman* and *ātman* signify one and the same all-pervasive Being.

The recovery of our true nature takes place in the act of enlightenment (*bodhi*) through the agency of Yoga. The process leading up to this supreme illumination is always the same: The mind is withdrawn from all external things and centered inward either with or without the help of a "prop," such as a potent sound (*mantra*) or a potent mental image (*yantra*), and so on.

In Tāraka-Yoga, the switch by which the ordinary consciousness is converted into the continuous Awareness (*cit*) of the single Being is a series of exercises in which light phenomena play a decisive role. That inner light is produced by a technique known as *shāmbhavī-mudrā* in Tantra and Hatha-Yoga. Seated comfortably in the *siddha-āsana* or any other posture, the *yogins* fix their sight on the "cavern in the middle of the space between the eyebrows" (i.e., in the middle of the head). The eyes can either be open or closed; the eyebrows may be slightly raised.

Whichever way this practice is executed, it always involves a new kind of looking by means of which the area of the forehead is brought into focus and somehow "energized." In terms of the esoteric physiology of Hatha-Yoga, this implies the activation of the sixth center, the so-called *ājnā-cakra*.

The light phenomena experienced in Tāraka-Yoga do not derive from any external source such as the Sun or other luminous objects. These lights are of a very special nature and are absolutely private occurrences. It is difficult to say precisely what they are. Neurophysiology and the psychology of altered states of consciousness are still in their infancy and do not have much to offer in the line of a sound explanation. At any rate, it would be totally misleading to regard these experiences as due merely to the excitation of the optical nerves. They differ qualitatively from the kind of light flashes produced by, say, manual stimulation of the optical nerves.

Nor must these photisms be confused with hypnagogic images as experienced before sleep. The *tāraka* lights are extremely vivid and have a stunning quality of authenticity and reality. Whatever they may be in physiological terms, to the practitioners of Yoga they represent signs of progress on the inward path. As practitioners succeed in emptying their mind of the sensory input and the images or word fragments bubbling up from the subconscious, their experience of radiant light becomes increasingly more intense and real.

According to the *Advaya-Tāraka-Upanishad*, there are three clearly discernible stages of achievement on this path of Yoga. These are referred to as the "three signs" (*tri-lakshya*). The first is known as the "inner sign" (*antar-lakshya*), the second as the "external sign" (*bahir-lakshya*), and the third as the "intermediate sign" (*madhya-lakshya*). These can be said to constitute different phases of *shāmbhavī-mudrā*, the "gesture" or "seal" of Shāmbhu, Lord Shiva.

In keeping with Tantric imagery and its detailed esoteric "geography" of the human body, the *Advaya-Tāraka-Upanishad* provides a concise description of the subtle energy centers (*cakra*) and channels (*nādī*). According to this text, the axis of the body extending from the perineum to the crown of the head is a luminous channel in which is seated the mysterious force called *kundalinī-shakti*.

This "serpent power" is described as being radiant like myriads of lightning flashes. Even though resting dormant at the bottom of the central duct, the *kundalinī* illuminates the entire channel known as the *sushumnā-nādī*. This indescribable luminosity can be seen by *yogins* when they focus their inward eye on the "mental window" situated at the forehead. This locus is technically referred to as *lalāta-mandala* ("forehead circle").

Blocking the ears with their forefingers, the *yogins* can hear the sound *phu* inwardly, and their consciousness space begins to be filled with a phosphorescent bluish light. At the same time a feeling of great bliss suffuses their entire being. This is the first stage of *shāmbhavī-mudrā*, and is known as the "perception of the inner sign" (*antar-lakshya-lakshana*). It is also called *tejo-dhyāna* or "fire meditation" in the *Gheranda-Samhitā*. The experience is quite transient and needs to be repeated to become stable, so that it can be used as a stepping-stone for further efforts on the spiritual path.

The second phase of *shāmbhavī-mudrā* is the "perception of the external sign" (*bahir-lakshya-lakshana*). It is described as the visual experience of an external field of different colors appearing at a distance of between two and six inches from the forehead. It must be understood as a highly dynamic field with waves of blue, red, orange, and similar colors, and with shafts of gold at the fringes. This is experienced with open eyes, and the colorful field is apparently superimposed on the ordinary perceptual image. Thus in the second phase, the internal vision of light is gradually externalized. This technique is said to be perfected when the luminous ether or field is steadily perceived about six inches above the head.

In the third stage of the experiment, the "perception of the intermediate sign" (*madhya-lakshya-lakshana*), everything happens in a greatly intensified manner, and consciousness becomes so absorbed in the experience that one can no longer properly speak of it as a vision or perception. This is *samādhi*, the merging of subject and object. The practitioner *becomes* his or her experiences. The "eternal field" that he or she perceives or, more precisely lives, is both internal and external, and it can assume any of these five forms: (1) *guna-rahita-ākāsha*: the ether-space devoid of quality, (2) *parama-ākāsha*: the supreme ether-space, (3) *mahā-ākāsha*: the great ether-space, (4) *tattva-ākāsha*: the ether-space of verity, and (5) *sūrya-ākāsha*: the solar ether-space.

These represent distinct experiences associated with specific colors and intensities. Ideally the progression is from the first up to the fifth. This last luminous field is compared to the joint radiance of a hundred thousand suns. On this level the *yogin's* identification with the "delivering" or *tāraka* sign is fully accomplished.

Only one more step remains to be taken, namely the realization of the transmental (*amanaska*) Reality, which is also known as *tāraka*. Thus the word *tāraka* is used in a double sense. On one hand it refers to the "signs" or visionary experiences induced by *shāmbhavī-mudrā*, and on the other hand it signifies the singular Being itself. This double usage may be misleading for the layman, but to the initiate who has come to understand the nondual basis of existence it is extremely meaningful: The many signs of the unitary Being are not really external to the supreme *tāraka* but are merely so many manifestations of it conjured up by the unenlightened mind, which is unable to perceive the highest truth directly.

The transmental *tāraka* is synonymous with *nirvikalpa-samādhi*. In this state, the spiritual practitioner is the single Being apprehending itself by itself. Here the *yogin's* inward odyssey finds its fulfillment. Not only is the practitioner's consciousness transmuted into pure Awareness, there seem to be also marked changes in body chemistry. He or she is said to need almost no food, to have conquered sleep, and yet to be strong in body and sound in mind.

The photistic path of Tāraka-Yoga utilizes phenomena that were undoubtedly known even in archaic times. We know, for instance, that light phenomena play an important role in Shamanism, which has ancient roots that clearly antedate Yoga. Moreover, the ultimate Reality itself is often called "light" (*jyotis*) in the earliest Vedānta scriptures.

Surprisingly enough, we do not find this usage in the extant works on Tāraka-Yoga. Nowhere do they speak of the absolute Reality as being luminous. Instead, it is said to be transmental, that is, transcending the categories of the mind. Thus, it presumably also transcends anything that the mind might experience or conceptualize as "light." In Tāraka-Yoga, experiences of light precede the ultimate realization. Liberation thus implies a leap beyond photisms, indeed beyond any other experiences generated along the yogic path. The transmental (*unmanī*) condition reveals the eternal bliss (*ānanda*) of the Absolute. However, this bliss is not a content of experience but the very being of the liberated person. As the *Mandala-Brāhmana-Upanishad* (11.5.3–4) puts it:

The *yogins* become that ocean of bliss.

Compared with that [absolute bliss], Indra and the other [deities] are only moderately blissful. Thus he who has attained [ultimate] bliss is a supreme *yogin*.

68

Yantra-Yoga
Divine Geometry

IN THEIR ENDEAVOR to intensify consciousness and transcend its ordinary limitations, *yogins* have taken advantage of the entire gamut of human expression and potential. Thus, for example, we find that they utilized our readiness for action in Karma-Yoga, our innate devotional ability in Bhakti-Yoga, our ability to produce complex sound patterns in Mantra-Yoga, our capacity for concentration in Rāja-Yoga, and our faculty of discrimination in Jnāna-Yoga. The *yogins* naturally also made use of the most powerful among the senses—the visual sense—in conjunction with our capacity for visualization.

Yogic discipline is essentially a matter of inner focusing, centeredness, or mindfulness. In some schools, this focusing involves actual visualization, or imaging, in which a definite object is held mentally for a prolonged period of time to produce a shift in awareness. Tantra, for instance, employs geometric designs known as *yantras*, which are considered highly efficient tools for concentrating the wandering mind.

According to Tantric philosophy, the many forms in the universe have not only their own distinctive shape perceptible to the physical eye but also their individual "cosmography." That is to say, everything—whether animate or inanimate—carries within itself a faithful "memory tape" of its genesis. Moreover, the story of the cosmos as a whole is also inscribed in it. This is so because even the smallest particles in the cosmos mirror the total structure of the universe. In this sense, every perceptible form can be said to be a *yantra*.

This way of looking at existence is typical of all traditional societies, which regard the world as a sacred event. Traditionally, religion has been a way of acknowledging the fact that there is a link between Heaven and Earth. The temples and pyramids of the ancient world were erected to emphasize that connection. It is only in recent centuries that this worldview has been progressively undermined by the ideology of scientism, which seeks to "demythologize" our existence, forgetting that we cannot live by intellect alone.

In their quest for simplicity of understanding and reconnection with the sacred, the metaphysicians of Tantra arrived at the conclusion that every form in the cosmos can be reduced to a definite number of primary geometrical figures, such as the point, line, triangle, square, and circle. These are thought to have a fixed symbolic value. In combination, they are considered to be expressive of particular qualities as embodied in certain aspects of creation.

In the narrow technical sense, a *yantra* is a complex geometrical pattern specifically employed in Tantra as an "instrument"—which is the literal meaning of the word *yantra*—for internalizing consciousness and transcending the ordinary mind. The *Tantra-Tattva* (folio 519), a late Tantric scripture, states that a *yantra* is so called because it controls (*niyantrana*) the passions and hence also suffering.

A *yantra* is deemed to be a vessel or seat for certain deities representing major creative forces in the universe—such as Lakshmī (bringer of good fortune), Vishnu (the all-pervader), or the elephant-headed Ganapati or Ganesha (remover of obstacles).

During a typical Tantric ceremony, these deities are invoked through the recitation of potent sounds (*mantra*), sacred hand gestures (*mudrā*), breath control (*prānāyāma*), and a great variety of other ritual techniques. One of the principal practices is to create the respective *yantra* of the deity to be worshiped. This is done by drawing the geometric design on paper or wood or into sand, or by engraving it on metal, or sometimes by modeling it in three dimensions.

But drawing or modeling the *yantra* externally is not enough. Gradually the Tantric practitioner must establish the *yantra* within himself, through intense concentration and visualization. He has to build up a vivid three-dimensional model of the *yantra* within his own mind. Or rather, he must come to realize experientially that his body is in truth identical in form with that *yantra*.

This is a very difficult and lengthy process. For us moderns it might even seem to be an impossible task, because we no longer enjoy our ancestors' excellent memory. Traditional societies transmitted their knowledge orally rather than in written form. For instance, the hymns of the *Vedas* and the verses and prose passages of the *Upanishads* were originally all memorized, and with astonishing accuracy. However, with the increasing use of books, this wonderful mnemonic facility has been largely lost. But memory is crucial to the kind of visualization called for in Yoga, especially Tantra-Yoga.

The mentally constructed *yantra* must become so vivid that it feels alive. When the practitioner is successful at this inner work, the *yantra* turns into a vibrating force field that completely absorbs her attention. In due course, she can no longer tell whether the *yantra* is within herself or she is within the *yantra*. Her consciousness is progressively carried into a deep absorption, where she becomes completely oblivious to her surroundings. Her senses no longer register external stimuli, and she lives entirely in their inner world. Finally, she becomes aware of the deity (i.e., the personalized creative force) of the *yantra* itself.

Meditative absorption (*dhyāna*) is characterized by a gradual abolition of the subject-object barrier that is fundamental to the ordinary waking consciousness. At the end of the process lies the complete unification of subject and object, the merging of the knower, the known, and the act of knowing. At this point all duality is transcended. This state is called *samādhi*, or "ecstasy."

There are two fundamental types of *samādhi*, a "lower" and a "higher." The former has as its base a "form" (*rūpa*), or focal point, with which the experiencing subject is merging. In the latter type of *samādhi*, there is a total absence of contents in consciousness. Consciousness, or rather awareness (*cit*), abides in itself. The empirical consciousness is temporarily abolished, making room for the transcendental "witness" (*sākshin*). This is the condition referred to as Self-realization or liberation.

The meditative experience of the deity of a particular *yantra* belongs to the "lower" mode of *samādhi*. It is considered an invaluable preparation for the ultimate realization of the universal Self.

At the outset of one's practice the *yantra* should, paradoxically, be more complex. Once a certain measure of success in concentration and visualization has been achieved through regular exercise, the *yantra* can be very much simplified. The *yantra* can be internally or externally constructed in two ways. It can be imaged from the innermost point (the *bindu*) going outward, in accordance with the process of cosmic evolution. Or it can be visualized from the outermost circumference going toward the center, in alignment with the process of meditative absorption (or involution). The symbolism of the constituent elements of a *yantra* is comparatively simple. But the inner meaning of a *yantra*, embodied in its deity, can only be fully grasped when it is experienced inwardly.

The principal element of any *yantra*, though not always articulated, is the point or *bindu* (drop). It represents that point in space and time where any object comes into manifestation. The *bindu* stands between manifestation and the unmanifest, between actuality and potentiality. It is the creative matrix, the primary structure, from which issues the whole cosmos in its multiformity. This is true both of the physical world and the psychological universe, macrocosm and microcosm.

Manifestation can only occur with movement. Geometrically, this is expressed by a line or a combination of lines. The ascending movement is depicted by an upward pointing triangle, symbolizing the male principle in the universe, or *shiva*. By way of analogy, it is connected with the element of fire and mental activity in general. Its numerical value is 3. The triangle that points downward stands for the female creative principle, or *shakti*, embodying the activity of *shiva*. It is linked with the element of water, and its numerical value is 2.

The dodecagon, one of the more common elements in *yantras*, is composed of an upward- and a downward-pointing triangle. It symbolizes the state of balance of the manifested world. The existence of the cosmos is made possible by a perfect dynamic equilibrium between opposing forces.

The state of chaos or negation is depicted in the form of two vertically arranged triangles meeting at their tips, thus forming the "drum of Shiva." God Shiva here represents the principle of destruction and thus also of renewal.

The square represents the element of earth *(bhū)*; its numerical value is 4. This symbolism is almost universal.

The circle is the symbol of periodicity and rhythm. It can also signify the latent "coiled" energy inherent in matter. It is connected with the fifth element, ether *(ākāsha)*. Its numerical value is 1 or 10, respectively.

The hexagon, as the symbol of the element of air *(vāyu)*, represents dispersed movement.

The lotuses in various *yantras* signify particular entities or personified energies, which are identifiable by the number of petals. The eight-petaled lotus, for example, is indicative of God Vishnu the preserver.

The Tantric scriptures mention and describe a great number of *yantras*. Most of them are put to spiritual use. But there are some that are employed specifically in order to cure illnesses or to obtain material benefits. The most celebrated *yantra* is unquestionably the *shrī-yantra*, also called the *shrī-cakra* (auspicious wheel). It is a symbolical archetype of the cosmos and, by way of analogy, of the human body. It is the great symbol of the Goddess *(devī)*, or Shakti, both in her transcendental and immanent form.

Devī stands for the female principle in the universe, the power or energy that is responsible for all creation.

According to Tantric philosophy, Goddess and God are really one. Both together constitute the primordial Unity, the singular Reality beyond all phenomena. Their separation, as experienced on the empirical level, is the reason for all human suffering. Self-realization consists in the discovery that, on the ultimate level of existence, God and Goddess are forever embracing one another, and the Self-realized adept participates in the delight of their eternal union.

The *shrī-yantra*, as employed in Tantric liturgy, serves to remind the *yogin* or *yoginī* of the ultimate nondistinction, or unity, between subject and object. This *yantra* is composed of nine juxtaposed triangles, which are arranged in such a way that they produce a total of forty-three small triangles. Four of the nine primary triangles point upward, representing the male cosmic energy; five of them point downward, symbolizing the female cosmic power.

These triangles are surrounded by an eight-petaled lotus symbolizing Vishnu, the all-pervading ascending tendency in the macrocosm and microcosm. The next lotus, with sixteen petals, represents the attainment of the object of desire, particularly the power over the mind and sense-organs. Enclosing this lotus are four concentric lines that are symbolically connected with the two lotuses and the triangles. The triple-line surround is called "Earth city" (*bhū-pura*); it symbolizes the three spheres of the world, and microcosmically speaking, the human body.

In Southern India, the *shrī-yantra* is considered an object of worship. Some of the medieval and later Hindu temples contain shrines in which a smaller altar is to be found. Tradition has it that these altars enshrine engravings of the *shrī-yantra*. For reasons of health and, sadly, also for purposes of black magic, the *shrī-yantra* is engraved on a thin gold, silver, or copper foil that is rolled into a cylinder and placed in a metallic case to be worn as a kind of amulet.

A much more detailed pictorial version of the *yantra* is the *mandala*, as used in Tibetan (Vajrayāna) Buddhism. Instead of a point, imaginary or actually indicated, the *mandala* has as its center the Primordial Buddha (Ādi-Buddha) from whom proceed in all four directions the "Four Paradises" supervised by various Buddhas, or enlightened beings. Outside the inner "walls" of these paradisiacal fields are typically the Four Human Buddhas and the Four Guardians.

Yantra-Yoga is a form of "inner worship" (*antar-pūjā*), usually of the Goddess. After the Goddess is invoked through *mantra*, or potent sound, she must be invited into, and properly installed in, the *yantra*, which is her body. Since the internally visualized *yantra* is none other than the practitioner's own body-mind, the installation of the Goddess means that he or she is now one with the deity.

Now begins the still more difficult task of progressively dissolving the *yantra*—proceeding from its outermost to its innermost elements. Since the *yantra* is experienced as one's own body-mind, this dissolution implies the dismantling of one's inner world. When consciousness has been reduced to the absolute zero of the *bindu*, a radical switch occurs. The *yogin* or *yoginī* becomes identical with the ultimate Reality, which is superconscious, omnipresent, and eternal. Thus, the *yantra* merely serves as a means of gradually reducing the complexities of the mind until the simplicity of the transcendental Self, or Reality, is recovered. This recovery is enlightenment.

❧ 69 ❧
What Is Tantra?

IN RECENT YEARS, Tantra has become increasingly popular. Unfortunately, this trend has not led to a better understanding of this ancient spiritual tradition. If anything, Tantra's popularity in the West—and the accompanying "popularization"—has caused more misunderstanding and confusion. If we were to pick up any New Age magazine, we would see advertisements for Tantric workshops promising both spiritual knowledge and fun. What is commonly marketed as Tantra, however, is at best sexual sensitivity training and at worst sex with a patina of Asian mystique. Not surprisingly, many Yoga students equate Tantra with sexual practices and "fun." Nothing could be further from the truth.

Authentic Tantra is essentially a liberation teaching (*moksha-shāstra*), with the explicit purpose of leading practitioners to enlightenment. Ritual sex (*maithunā*), which is the focus of Western "Neo-Tantrism," is practiced only in left-hand schools of Tantra. Mainstream (*samaya*) Tantra has always frowned on extremist practices and favored an approach that permits householder *yogins* and *yoginīs* balanced sexual activity and sexual abstinence for ascetics.

Significantly, even those schools that include ritual sex in their repertoire typically emphasize ritual over sex, which is not to say that there have not been *tāntrikas* who failed to live up to the great ideals of this extraordinary tradition. Indeed, the orgiastic excesses of some Tantric schools were responsible for Tantra's eventual ill repute in India. Another reason for the decline of Tantra was its frequent association with black magic. But the failure of some practitioners must not blind us to the great insights and achievements of Tantra as a whole.

Perhaps the modern preoccupation with ritual "Tantric" sex is simply the result of our society's moral confusion and uneasiness about sexuality (the so-called sexual revolution notwithstanding). Be that as it may, students of Yoga should know that Tantra is a legitimate yogic orientation. It represents a grand cultural-philosophical synthesis, which came to the fore in the early centuries of the Common Era and peaked around 1200 C.E. Originally, the Tantric teachings were transmitted orally, and even the oldest available Tantric scriptures—also called *Tantras*—represent a more mature stage of development. But these texts, written mostly in Sanskrit (but, as far as Buddhist Tantra is concerned, preserved mostly in Tibetan), give us a good idea of the nature of the Tantric teachings from c. 500 C.E. onward.

From the outset, Tantra understood itself as a "new age" teaching intended for the *kali-yuga*, the Dark Age of moral and spiritual decline, which is still in full swing today. The Tantric adepts felt that the *Vedas* (in the case of Hindus) and the Pali *Suttas* (in the case of Buddhists) had lost their efficacy and a new approach was needed. In particular, Tantra offered new rituals, but it also put forward new philosophical ideas or, rather, gave old ideas a new look and feel. This process went hand in hand with the development of a new technical language and symbolism, which makes the *Tantras* challenging reading.

Tantra embraces both the path of direct realization (in which one recognizes one's true nature through the agency of one's past good karma and/or the grace of the guru or the ultimate Reality itself) and the graduated path (which employs a variety of disciplines and techniques, notably rituals of various kinds, that enable one to progressively purify oneself until true knowledge shines forth).

In terms of the spiritual path, Tantra understands the body and the world at large not as obstacles to enlightenment, but as the very foundation of yogic discipline. Body and world are not illusory, as taught in some schools of Vedānta (or Jnāna-Yoga), but are manifestations of the ultimate Reality. Therefore they must never be ignored, neglected, or denounced but, instead, viewed in their proper context and duly respected. The body, according to Tantra, holds all the secrets of the universe. It is a miniature replica of the macrocosm. The Tantric adepts also understood the body as a temple of the Divine—an idea present already in ancient Upanishadic times but not followed through.

These notions led, around 1000 C.E., to the creation of Hatha-Yoga, which is in fact a form of Tantric Yoga. The purpose of traditional Hatha-Yoga is to awaken the body's dormant spiritual potency, the "serpent power" or *kundalinī-shakti*. This is also at the heart of Tantra. The serpent power is none other than the power of the transcendental Reality manifesting in the finite human body.

The ultimate spiritual goal of enlightenment, or liberation, is achieved when the awakened serpent power has completely transformed the ordinary material body into a body of light, or what the Buddhist *tāntrikas* know as the "rainbow body" and the Christians as the "body of glory." That body is immortal, infinitely plastic (i.e., capable of assuming any shape), and endowed with all kinds of exceptional capacities (*siddhi*). The *Yoga-Shikhā-Upanishad* (1.25–26) states:

> Embodied beings are said to be twofold: ripe and unripe.

> Unripe embodied beings lack Yoga; the ripe ones are with Yoga. Through the fire of Yoga, the entire body is rendered sentient and free from grief.

> The unripe body, however, should be understood to be insentient, earthen, and bestowing suffering.

For the Tantric adepts, liberation is not a matter of entering some alternate dimension apart from the sensory world but of transmuting the body-mind in the "light" of the Ultimate. Surely this noble goal is worthy of our consideration.

❧ 70 ❧

Sex, Asceticism, and Mythology

FRIEDRICH NIETZSCHE, the nineteenth-century German philosopher who declared the death of God, observed that the human being is a rope stretched between animal and deity. He could as easily have likened us to the tension between sex hormones and higher cerebral impulses. The metaphor, like most metaphors, is only partly accurate, because we also *are* our genitals just as we *are* our brain and all the other aspects of our bodily being. Of course, we also are a great deal more than the body or its various parts, as serious practitioners of different spiritual disciplines throughout the ages have discovered for themselves.

Nevertheless, the dynamic between biological needs, specifically genital urges, and higher evolutionary or transpersonal aspirations is a crucial part of all moral, religious, and spiritual traditions of the world. Typically, we experience these two sets of wants or needs as being at war with each other: Don't let the cerebrum know what the genitals are doing. Suppress your desires. Curb your sexual curiosity. Feel ashamed about having genitals.

This body- and sex-negative orientation is epitomized in the religious doctrine according to which the "flesh" is the enemy of the "Spirit." For love to be "pure," it must be devoid of sexual connotations. At best sex is regarded as a necessary evil. As the British mathematician-philosopher Bertrand Russell pointed out, this view has caused millions of people great misery.[1] For, they had to suppress their sexual instincts in the hope of a better life in the hereafter, where, as sexless (possibly even disembodied) angelic beings, they could participate in the joys of heaven beyond all genitality and sexual complications.

This dualistic idea, which splits the human being into genital or sensual and spiritual or ascetical compartments, is at home in the Judeo-Christian tradition and Islam as much as it is in certain schools of Hinduism and Buddhism. For instance, the ancient *Rig-Veda* (1.179), the Old Testament of Hinduism, records a domestic quarrel between Sage Agastya and his wife Lopamudrā. The cause of their quarrel was—of course—sex. Agastya, who was a renowned ascetic and a paragon of the virtue of chastity (*brahmacarya*) was, frankly, neglecting his wife. In other words, he preferred to meditate in solitude over making love to her. Understandably, she was beginning to feel frustrated, and so she started to complain and make demands. At first, the sage valiantly defended his position. No doubt, she would have expected no less of him. Lopamudrā, who knew her husband well, was not inexperienced in the art of seduction and bit by bit Agastya succumbed to her womanly wiles. No sooner had he broken his vow of sexual abstinence than he felt great compunction. To "purify" himself again, he made all kinds of sacrificial offerings to the gods. Probably a now contented Lopamudrā was aiding him in his rituals.

We may speculate that the intimate conversation between the couple found its way into the most venerated part of the sacred literature of the Hindus because it described a common situation in ancient times: a householder-ascetic struggling with his own and his wife's sexuality in the midst of a demanding spiritual life. This struggle, which has brought many would-be ascetics to their knees, has been fought by men and women ever since religions began to preach the idea that in order to fulfill spiritual life one must completely curb the passions of the flesh. Whole traditions arose that were based on this mistaken idea, namely that communion with the Divine, or liberation, depends on repressing, confining, or somehow "sublimating" the sexual urge.

Certainly, utter renunciation of sex was the grand ideal to which countless ascetics in ancient India aspired. Many of them came to be remembered in the popular and sacred literature. A good many, however, are remembered for failing to uphold this supreme ideal. Thus, the *Mahābhārata* epic and the *Purānas* tell many tales of fallen ascetics. A favorite story-telling motif is that of a particularly zealous penitent being sorely tempted by an unearthly damsel, sent by one of the deities to test the ascetic's determination and patience.

In the *Rāmāyana* epic (1.62), we hear of the illustrious sage Vishvamitra whose passion was inflamed when he saw beautiful Menakā bathing naked in a stream near his hermitage. His love affair with her lasted for a full ten years, at which point he "came to his senses" and resumed, with doubly fierce resolution, his ascetic mode of life. Sharadvant, a mighty *yogin* and skilled archer, was tested in a similar fashion. When he spotted a scantily clad maiden he temporarily lost control over his mind, stood agape, and involuntarily dropped his bow and arrows, as well as his semen. The famous sages Vyāsa, Kashyapa, Bharadvāja, Mankanaka, and Dahica experienced similar mishaps.

For the ascetic, lust is the ally of death. The reason for this is that the loss of semen (*bindu*) signals to him the loss of power, energy, and hard-earned karmic merit. The ascetic needs good merit to cheat the iron law of *karma*, and he requires the body's energy to accomplish the magnificent work of self-transformation that is the goal of all austerities. The ascetic is a hoarder of psychosomatic energy. He guards all bodily openings, especially the genitals. Semen is, for him, not merely semen but a substance of power that must be accumulated, not squandered. The typical ascetic is always worrying about the involuntary loss of semen, or becoming sexually aroused to the point where he loses control over his thoughts. That chastity (*brahmacarya*) must not be confused with self-emasculation is a point made in many of the stories:

Whenever a *yogin* has been distracted from his single-minded discipline, he proves to be a most virile and vigorous lover. In India, it is well known that *yogins* acquire great sexual attractiveness, and that this is one of the dangers lurking on the spiritual path. This is also one of the reasons why not a few Western ladies swoon over their favorite swami, often without understanding that the secret of his sexual attractiveness lies in his prolonged sexual abstinence. Little wonder that *yogins* have been warned from time immemorial to steer clear of the female gender. But this traditional warning merely plays into the body-negative inclinations of many ascetics, and it encourages "spiritual narcissism" rather than the enlightened attitude of love and compassion.

That ascetics are not eunuchs is best exemplified in the person of Shiva, the destroyer aspect of the Hindu trinity. He is both ascetic and sex fiend par excellence. Shiva's dual nature is brought out beautifully in the *Purānas*, India's traditional encyclopedia-like compilations in Sanskrit, which contain numerous myths, legends, and philosophical as well as theological accounts. The following is a story from the *Skanda-Purāna* (1.1.34), which portrays the divine Shiva sporting a range of very human character traits.

Shiva played dice with his celestial spouse, Pārvatī, who beat him by cheating. Angry at having lost, Shiva started a noisy quarrel. To cool his temper, which threatened to upset whole worlds, he took to the forest. In the manner of a true ascetic, he stripped off all his clothes and enjoyed the solitude. Pārvatī, however, felt twinges of guilt about her cheating and also was filled with longing for her husband. Taking a friend's good advice, she decided to ask for forgiveness. She assumed the form of a most beautiful maiden, magically transported herself into the forest, and appeared before Shiva.

The great lord of *yogins* was stirred from his meditation. When he saw the voluptuous damsel, he was instantly filled with desire. He reached out for her, but she promptly vanished into thin air. Tormented by his lust for that mysterious beauty, Shiva took to wandering. Then one day he encountered her again. This time he was careful to approach her with less impetuousness. The maiden told him that she was in search of a husband who is all-knowing and in control of his emotions. Without batting an eyelid, Shiva volunteered himself immediately. However, the beauty told him that he could not possibly be qualified to be her husband, since he had abandoned his wife, Pārvatī, whose love he had won by his excessive austerities. Shiva denied this charge.

Then, changing her tactics, the maiden hailed him as the lord of ascetics and the master of Kāma, the deity of passion. Shiva's response to this was to attempt to take the girl by force. She demanded to be released at once, and firmly instructed him to ask her father for permission first. Shiva consented. The maiden's father failed to understand how the lord of the universe could possibly be so captivated by, and deluded about, any woman, however lovely. This provoked the sage Nārada to poke fun at Shiva, observing that contact with women always makes men ridiculous. Nārada's words made their point.

Shiva suddenly realized his wife's charade. He roared with laughter. But then he set out to perform fierce austerities that would make all beings tremble in fear. Pārvatī promptly assumed her real form and prostrating herself before the mighty god, asked him for forgiveness. Shiva was appeased by this gesture and returned to his celestial abode with her—no doubt to resume his eternal play as well as intermittent domestic quarrels with Pārvatī.

This story, like so many others, depicts Shiva as a figure full of contradictions. He is the supreme deity, and yet he commits the all-too-human folly of lusting after a girl whose beauty is by all appearances as ephemeral as any mortal being's. He is capable of the most intense ascetic fervor and at the same time falls prey to the very desire that he once conquered in the form of Kāma, the deity of desire. He takes himself very seriously, and then again he can break into cosmic laughter over his seeming lapse of divine stature. He assumes the role of a fool who can be tricked at dice, but he is the omniscient, all-powerful lord of creation who, by a single intention, can plunge the universe into nothingness.

Judged by mortal standards, Shiva is an impossibility. But, then, Shiva is not subject to mortality or human-made standards. He is *all* possibilities of life at once. He *is* life. As such Shiva is an instructive symbol for the spiritual practitioner who senses that one can embrace a discipline of self-transcendence without having to turn one's back on life.

Shiva's eroticism is a slap in the face for all those ascetics who associate their personal salvation with sexual sublimation or, worse, with rigid control of the natural appetites. Shiva's life-affirming character embodies wisdom that goes beyond the conventional religious view of things. It is the kind of wisdom that is the foundation of the schools of Indian and Tibetan Tantra and that also informs the "sexual alchemy" of the later Taoist masters in China.

Both the Tantric masters and the Taoist adepts knew that sexuality in itself is not a hindrance to spiritual maturation. They promoted, on the contrary, the idea that an impotent eunuch (*klaibya*) stands a slim chance of realizing the supreme potential of spiritual evolution—enlightenment, or liberation. Instead of recommending the anxious suppression of the libido lest it should interfere with the sacred task of spiritual transformation, they favored a sex-positive philosophy. They even designed special practices to utilize this most powerful impulse in us for the process of psychospiritual transmutation. Of course, they did not condone the kind of "sexploitation" that is the liability of the ordinary individual, particularly in our post-sexual-revolution days. Rather, they were interested in the right use of the sexual energy.

In Taoism, the accent lies on a balanced healthy life through the well-regulated employment of sexuality, by which a person may become sensitive to the spiritual dimension. In Tantra, the sexual disciplines primarily serve the purpose of self-transcendence to the point of utter bliss. In the former tradition, the "sexual arts" are closely connected with medicine; in the latter tradition they form part of the liberation technology better known as "Yoga." Whereas in Taoism sexual intercourse without male orgasm is used to manipulate the hormonal system of the body for better health, in Tantra the focus is principally on the energy exchange between the sex partners. In the Tantric tradition, the male bias is more overt than in the schools of Taoism, though in the latter tradition it is implicit in the prescription to preserve the semen at all costs.

In Hindu Tantra, where intercourse is connected with the notion of sacrifice (*yajna*), the ritual rule against seminal emission is not as strict as in Buddhist Tantra. But for both traditions the crux of this sexual ritualism is the same: to restore the body-mind to perfect equilibrium, which coincides with the absolute bliss of enlightenment. The general idea behind these schools of thought is that we are, from birth on, in a state of disequilibrium because of the differentiation of our physical bodies into male and female. This differentiation, known as dimorphism in Western physiology, sets up a tension in us, which we then seek to release by trying to merge with the opposite sex, either sexually or emotionally, or both.

Orgasm is the closest simulation of the absolute bliss (*ānanda*) for which we all are unconsciously striving. But orgasmic pleasure is only a trickle in comparison to that bliss, and it is of course disappointingly ephemeral. The nervous discharge that accompanies orgasm creates a momentary state of balance, but that balance is on a very reduced level of energy.

The Tantric practitioners recognize the error in this popular approach, which seeks self-completion by external means, namely sexual union. They are more interested in heightening the level of psychosomatic energy and in intensifying awareness, until there is the breakthrough into the transcendental dimension of bliss. They engage sexual intercourse as a spiritual discipline rather than for hedonistic reasons. This entails the insight that every individual is, psychologically speaking, both male and female, and that therefore the desired unitive or balanced state does not occur externally but internally, in consciousness. Thus, for the Tantric practitioner, the outward sexual act is essentially a symbolic ritual of the real work, which is performed in consciousness. Indeed, the right-hand schools of Tantra do not even condone actual sexual congress.

However, the left-hand approach, which involves sexual intercourse (*maithunā*) with a suitable partner, has the advantage of increasing the level of psychosomatic energy and thus of including the physical dimension in the process of psychospiritual transformation. Actual sexual intercourse involves an energy exchange between the partners in the Tantric ritual, which enhances the unification process that is strived for on the level of consciousness.

At the point of enlightenment, the Tantric practitioner realizes the transcendental unity of Male and Female, Shiva and Shakti. This condition is known as "great delight" or *mahā-sukha*, since it cannot be diminished by anything, not even by the act of ejaculation, which typically concludes the male partner's experience of sexual pleasure in ordinary circumstances.

Tantra is the technology of joy on many levels—from sexual pleasure to transcendental bliss, but always from the perspective of spiritual growth. It is a yogic art that explores the hidden dimensions of the unity of the body and the mind, which modern science is only now beginning to acknowledge. It reminds us that our guilt about sex is only an added complication that we superimpose on our false relationship to sexual pleasure. Instead of viewing sex as a means of higher human growth, we tend to use it as a fleeting consolation or a way of asserting power and dominance over another. Perhaps our guilt feelings are not so much about engaging our "lower" functions as about not finding the bliss of transcendental consciousness.

Tantra challenges us to a radically different view about ourselves and sexuality: to view sex as a lawful, if limited expression of our innate bliss, and at the same time as a means of getting in touch with that unalloyed delight that is the very essence of reality. According to Tantra, the body is the temple of the divine or transcendental Reality. But for this to be functionally true of us, and not merely in principle true, we must discover and live from the point of view of that great delight. Then everything, including our sexuality, will be transformed. Our lives become creative play (*līlā*).

PART FIVE

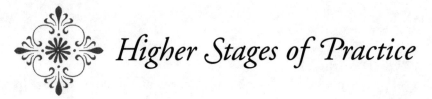 *Higher Stages of Practice*

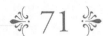

71

Pathways to Relaxation and Meditation

RELAXATION AS AN ATTITUDE

Two thousand years ago, the great Yoga master Patanjali stated in his *Yoga-Sūtra* (2.47) that the yogic postures are to be accomplished by relaxing all stressful effort. This prescription captures the very spirit of Yoga and applies to all yogic practices.

Stressful effort—"trying too hard"—is always a sign that our ego is in the way: We are not in the flow of things and are trying to make something happen, perhaps even by sheer force. However, this attitude predictably creates tensions in us that sooner or later have their negative side effects in our emotions and our body. Stressful struggle is ultimately a self-defeating strategy. Are we, then, to do away with all effort? The short answer is: this would be impossible. Even an enlightened being, who is perfectly harmonized with the flow of life, must make some effort to eat, drink, walk, or talk. From the inside, these activities all appear to happen of their own accord, but so long as we are embodied, we have to perform actions. All actions have an element of effort, that is, an investment of energy. The difference between the effort of an enlightened being and of an ordinary person is that the former does not subjectively experience stress from the effort.

What if an enlightened being were to climb Mount Everest or K2? Surely, he or she would experience the same physical hardship as any other climber. To give a more passive example: What if an enlightened being were exposed to blaring disco music for hours on end? His or her body would undoubtedly feel the onslaught of the sound waves, but this would not change the inner bliss one iota. What if an enlightened being had to endure an hour's worth of root canals without Novocain? There would most likely be pain, but it would be experienced through buffering layers of indifference, as if the pain occurred at a distance. Some *yogins* acquire this ability long before they are enlightened. Certainly the enlightened being would not add fretful anticipation of pain to the actual pain.

Enlightenment does away with the illusion of the ego, of being an encapsulated self separate from all others. No ego, no stress. No stress, no suffering. Perhaps that is why so many advanced adepts have uncreased foreheads and soft childlike bodies. Also, when we look at their pictures more closely, we find that their pupils tend to be dilated. Dilation normally is a sign of fear or surprise. Since all adepts claim to have transcended fear, we could conclude that they are in a perpetual state of surprise. In fact, one school of Yoga — Kashmiri Shaivism — speaks of ecstasy as a condition of astonishment (camatkāra).

Relaxation is first and foremost the release of the ego illusion. So long as we identify with our name, our body, our belongings, our relationships, and our reputation, we leave the door wide open for suffering (duhkha). In the course of our life, we are likely to experience physical discomfort and loss of a relative or dear friend. We may have our wallet or car stolen or become the target of envy or unfriendly gossip. If we are identified with the ego-personality and all it stands for, these eventualities will inevitably cause us disappointment, frustration, anger, sorrow, grief, envy, jealousy, and all the many other negative emotions that seem to make up much of ordinary life. However, as we relax the ego's grip, these emotions will affect us less and less, and in the truly accomplished yogin they are virtually absent.

The entire moral code of Yoga may be understood as a means of letting go of the "fist" of the ego. Thus the five yamas or "disciplines" — nonharming, truthfulness, nonstealing, chastity, and greedlessness — represent a comprehensive orientation of relaxation. Likewise the five niyamas or "restraints" — purity, contentment, asceticism, study, and dedication to a higher principle — include this element of relaxation. Thus through the practice of purity, we release all concern for the lower or material nature. Through contentment, we let go of grasping for "stuff." Through asceticism, we relax the habit of convenience and self-pleasuring. Through study, we let go of the habit of jumping from one thing to the next and instead cultivate mental discipline. Through dedication to a higher principle — usually understood as devotion to the Lord (īshvara) — we relax the stressful effort of holding on tightly to our ego-personality.

Another term for this orientation is "equanimity" or its cognate "evenness" (samatva). This kind of balanced attitude lies at the base of the other limbs of Yoga as well. Thus the practice of postures, breath control, sensory inhibition, concentration, meditation, and ecstatic unification cannot succeed without deconditioning ourselves from the habit of stressful effort. In the case of the postures, "trying too hard" can cause painful tearing of tendons and ligaments. Overdoing breath control can lead to still more serious injuries, including damage of the heart muscle.

When we effortfully push the practice of sensory inhibition, we may experience the shock of encountering our inner world in a state of disarray. This is one of the problems of using artificial means (such as psychedelics) to access the deeper reaches of consciousness by force. Concentration without relaxation will merely give one a headache. Similarly, forced meditation only produces increased nervousness. Ecstasy (*samādhi*), which is a total switch in consciousness, will not even come about naturally in the absence of relaxation. If we prematurely force our way into the ecstatic experience through drugs or other artificial means, we are likely to invite confusion, delusion, or possibly even a psychotic breakdown. The experience itself may not be genuine either but merely a simulation and therefore may not be capable of yielding any positive spiritual results.

THE RELAXATION RESPONSE

The path of Yoga—from beginning to end—can be understood as a progressive relaxation of body and mind. This attitude of relaxation can be fostered through specific exercises in somatic relaxation. Hatha-Yoga provides a number of such exercises, and a good introduction and interpretation is Judith Lasater's *Relax and Renew*.[1]

In the Western world, the need for conscious relaxation was first discussed by the American physician Edmund Jacobson (1885–1976), inventor of progressive muscle relaxation. He used his exercises to treat hypertension, insomnia, indigestion, colitis, and "nervousness." His book *You Must Relax* was published in 1934, the same year that a raging storm in the "Dust Bowl" carried off an estimated 650 million tons of top soil, Mao Tse Tung and about 100,000 communists began their 10,000-mile march to evade the Chinese government under the leadership of Chiang Kai-Shek, and in Germany Adolf Hitler was fatefully declared "Führer."

Jacobson's pioneering work stimulated further research on relaxation, and in the 1970s, Herbert Benson, a professor of medicine at Harvard University, brought relaxation to the attention of millions of Americans through his articles in *Good Housekeeping* and *Family Circle*, and subsequently his books *The Relaxation Response* (1975) and *Beyond the Relaxation Response* (1984). Benson explains the relaxation response as follows:

When the fight-or-flight response is evoked, it brings into play the sympathetic nervous system, which is part of the autonomic, or involuntary nervous system. The sympathetic nervous system acts by secreting specific hormones: adrenalin or epinephrine or noradrenalin or norepinephrine. These hormones, epinephrine and its related substances, bring about the physiologic changes of increased blood pressure, heart rate, and body metabolism. . . . While the fight-or-flight response is associated with the overactivity of the sympathetic nervous system, there is another response that leads to a quieting of the same nervous system. Indeed, there is evidence that hypertensive subjects can lower their blood pressure by regularly eliciting this other response. This is the Relaxation Response . . .[2]

Benson called hypertension a "hidden epidemic," which he related directly to stress leading to the fight-or-flight syndrome. Contrary to popular opinion, stressful living is nothing new. Four thousand six hundred years ago, as Benson pointed out, a Chinese chronicler lamented the temper of his own era, which was marked by calamity, disobedience, rebellion, grief, and inner bitterness. We find similar laments on Sumerian tablets engraved nearly five thousand years ago. We know from history that a comparable situation has prevailed throughout the ages in many cultures. It is true, though, that in our own time the fast pace of life is causing an unprecedented degree of stress to an unparalleled number of people around the world.

Conscious relaxation has proven to be an effective means of combating stress and its harmful physiological effects. Benson developed his own technique for achieving the relaxation response but is well acquainted with traditional yogic methods. In the late 1960s, at Harvard's Thorndike Memorial Laboratory of the Boston City Hospital, he did in fact conduct research on Transcendental Meditation, the popular method promoted by Maharishi Mahesh Yogi. This method is simple Mantra-Yoga, in which initiates are given a mantra to recite. But *mantra-japa* is just one of many ways that Yoga masters recommend for relaxing the body and mind. In Hatha-Yoga, for instance, relaxation is tackled directly at the level of the body.

YOGIC RELAXATION

The most common Sanskrit name for the relaxation posture is *shavāsana*, composed of *shava* ("corpse") and *āsana* ("posture"). Most Western writers translate this as "dead pose," which more accurately conveys the Sanskrit synonym *mrita-āsana*. This is a curious designation. As Swami Gitananda of South India observed, the Yoga masters have generally been very astute in naming the yogic postures but in this case may have created a misnomer.[3] As he pointed out, the practitioner resting in *shava-āsana* is far from dead. However, the venerable Swami conceded that this graphic expression was intended to suggest a motionless state lacking all tension, reminiscent of a corpse.

Because the word "corpse" in this context offends both Western and Eastern sensibilities, even many Indian Yoga teachers have renamed this practice, calling it *shānta-āsana* ("tranquil posture"), *prashānta-āsana* ("quiet posture"), *nishcala-āsana* ("immobile posture"), or *acala-kriyā* ("unmoving practice"). Swami Gitananda proposed *prashrita-āsana* ("lying down posture").[4] Why not call it *shaithilya-āsana* ("relaxation posture"), since the prone position is the most frequently used way of relaxing the body? *Shaithilya*, by the way, is a term used already in the *Yoga-Sūtra* (2.47) in connection with the relaxation of effort (*prayatna*) in the execution of yogic postures. *Shava-āsana* makes relaxation itself the focal point. Here is a succinct description of this technique:

1. Lie flat on your back, with the feet slightly apart and the hands—palms up—about a foot away from the body.

2. Close your eyes and mouth, breathing naturally through the nose.

3. Scan your body and let go of all tension, paying special attention to the shoulders, facial muscles, chest muscles, and abdominal muscles.

4. Remain aware of the whole body, while allowing the breath to flow naturally.

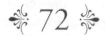

72

What Is Meditation?

WHEN WE EXAMINE the quite extensive literature on meditation, we find that meditation has been explained in many different ways. Here are some of the explanations I encountered while writing this essay:

> Meditation is a method by which a person concentrates more and more upon less and less. The aim is to empty the mind while, paradoxically, remaining alert.[1]

> The concept "meditation" refers to a set of techniques that are the production of another type of psychology, one that aims at personal rather than intellectual knowledge. As such, the exercises are designed to produce an alteration in consciousness—a shift away from the active, outward-oriented, linear mode and toward the receptive and quiescent mode, and usually a shift from an external focus of attention to an internal one.[2]

> Meditation is a procedure that allows one to investigate the process of one's own consciousness and experiencing, and to discover the more basic, underlying qualities of one's existence as an intimate reality.[3]

> Meditation . . . is a deliberate switching-off of these external stimuli that prepare the nervous system for fight or flight, and a courting of the heretofore unconscious stimuli which have hitherto been reduced to a minimum by the process of individual selective awareness.[4]

> Basically, meditation can be described as any discipline that aims at enhancing awareness through the conscious directing of attention.[5]

It is evident from the above explanations that meditation is a complex phenomenon that can be viewed from many different angles. Each explanation both reveals and obscures. In the final analysis, it proves to be an elusive, even mysterious process.

While we can meaningfully talk about meditation, just as we can talk about love or life itself, we have to meditate, live, and love in order to truly understand what these things mean. Here I will talk about meditation, basing myself principally on the sacred literature of Hinduism and, secondarily, on my own experience as a meditator. Specifically, I will make use of the *Rig-Veda*, some of the *Upanishads*, the *Bhagavad-Gītā*, the *Yoga-Sūtra*, and some of the scriptures on Hatha-Yoga.

Beginning with the meditation practices described in the ancient *Vedas* well over three thousand years ago: As the British Vedicist Jeanine Miller has shown, the bards (*rishi*) who composed the Vedic hymns were not merely inspired poets but *seers*; they claimed to have *seen* the hymns.[6] Then they *sang* what had been revealed to them in their visions. Thus, the Vedic hymns are, by and large, songs of praise used during various ritual occasions.

The visions of these seer-bards are called *dhī*. This word is derived from the same root that also yielded the word *dhyāna*, which is the most common designation for "meditation" in the Sanskrit language.

The *rishis* gave their meditative activity the technical designation *brahman*, a word they derived from the verbal root *brih*, meaning "to grow, expand." *Brahman*, in the ancient Vedic sense, is the magical act of "drawing forth" sacred power from the psyche. It is, as Miller explained, a recapitulation of the cosmogonic process itself. The seer's *brahman* duplicates, psychologically, the genesis of the universe itself, which emerged from the transcendental Reality, which is neither being nor nonbeing.

In this meditative state, illumined vision (*dhī*) occurs. Through *brahman*, which is always "god-given" (*deva-datta*), the "Sun" is made manifest. That is to say, meditation manifests splendorous light of the transcendental Reality, the luminous Superconsciousness, which was later called *cit*. The Vedic seers knew that the effulgence of stars and the radiance to be discovered in the heart are aspects of the same principle. Miller distinguished three types of *brahman* meditation: (1) *mantric meditation*, or the absorption of attention in and through sound (mantra), (2) *visual meditation*, or the generation of illumined thought (*dhī*) during which a particular deity is invoked, and (3) *absorption in mind and heart*, or the deepening of meditation by pondering the illumined insight (*dhī* or *manīshā*) further.

The Vedic seers themselves also knew of a "fourth *brahman*," which Miller identified as the ecstatic state beyond meditation. It is in this fourth *brahman* that the seers experienced great joy and freedom from fear, as well as immortality (*amrita*).

The Vedic notion of meditation is associated with a number of other key concepts, notably *hrid* ("heart"), *tapas* ("flame-power"), *kratu* ("creative will"), and *rita* ("truth" or "cosmic order"). The heart stands for inwardness, our inner life, as concentrated in the faculty of higher feeling, which has anciently been connected with the physical heart. The heart is the "cave" in which the hidden treasure may be found—an almost universal idea in the religious traditions of the world.

Tapas, again, is generally rendered as "asceticism" but has far deeper connotations. It is first and foremost the inner glow and power achieved through utmost self-discipline, and it corresponds to the self-confinement exercised by the primordial Being in producing the multifarious universe. The ascetic's *tapas,* in other words, is an exact symbolic duplication of the Creator's original act of self-sacrifice, which brought forth the cosmos.

Self-discipline is not so much a matter of negation as the creative channeling of primal energies. This idea is captured in the word *kratu,* often translated as "will." *Kratu* is the psychological power behind the incredible work of *tapas.* It is the will to bring what is originally invisible into the visible realm, so that it can be understood. The visions of the Vedic *rishis* are the product of their inner determination to create.

Such creation always follows universal laws, and the resultant visions are expressions of the cosmic order (*rita*). Conforming to the invisible order of the universe, they render the divine truth tangible. The *rishis* are, therefore, conveyors of the truth, the primordial harmony underlying all appearances. We can appreciate the immense richness of the Vedic seers' spiritual understanding of life.

The considerable wealth of their religious and mystical ideas was increased in subsequent times. From the second millennium B.C.E. onward, the Hindu sages composed the *Upanishads.* These are esoteric explanations and expositions of the Vedic lore, but in many ways they represent a new orientation. In keeping with this change, meditation was henceforth called *dhyāna.* We also find in the *Upanishads* the earliest references to the tradition of Yoga, which gradually evolved into the "six-limbed" (*shad-anga*) and then the eight-limbed" (*ashta-anga*) path.

Moreover, the Vedic key word *brahman* now acquired a new meaning. From then on it referred no longer to the state of meditation but to the Divine or ultimate Reality itself, signifying the great powerful expanse of the sacred. As the core of the psyche or mind, that same Reality came to be known as the "Self" (*ātman*).

In the *Chāndogya-Upanishad* (7.6.1), one of oldest of these scriptures, we find a most interesting passage, which provides an important clue about meditation. It reads:

> Meditation (*dhyāna*), assuredly, is more than thought. The Earth meditates, as it were (*iva*). The atmosphere meditates, as it were. Heaven meditates, as it were. The waters meditate, as it were. Mountains meditate, as it were. Gods and men meditate, as it were. Hence those among men here who attain greatness—they are, as it were, a part of the estate of meditation. Now, those who are small are quarrelers, maligners, slanderers. But those who are superior are, as it were, a part of the estate of meditation. [Therefore] appreciate meditation.

What does all this mean? First of all, we are told that meditation is more than thought. The Sanskrit text uses the word *citta*, which, we are told in the preceding passage, is more than intention (*samkalpa*), which, in turn, is more than intellection (*manas*). Here *citta* probably signifies ordinary consciousness. Thus, meditation is "more than" the average consciousness. In fact, it is a higher form of awareness.

But why does the anonymous author state that "the Earth meditates as it were"? Or that "mountains meditate as it were"? The phrase "as it were" (*iva*) makes it clear that he did not want us to think that the mountains were engaged in a deliberate exercise. Nevertheless, he insisted, they were engaged in something resembling meditation. If we take a leisurely hike in the countryside with no worries on our mind, simply experiencing the hills, trees, and brooks, we will no doubt be struck by their stillness, their utmost simplicity. They simply abide without any concerns or problems. This is exactly the condition of meditation. Meditation is simply being present in the way hills, trees, and brooks are present.

Meditation is abiding. The old word "abide" comes from the Anglo-Saxon *bidan* meaning "to wait." Meditation is indeed a kind of waiting, though not the semiconscious, nervous waiting that typically happens when we stand at a bus stop or sit in the reception area of a dentist's office. Meditative waiting is resting in the present, without the usual flight into thought. It is "just sitting," as the Zen Buddhists put it. Meditation is thus a form of centering, which involves our disengagement from the machine of the mind and our resting in the heart.

The Upanishadic sages preserved many of the Vedic spiritual motifs. Thus they placed the Self in the heart. One of the Sanskrit words for "heart" is *hridaya*. In the *Chāndogya-Upanishad* (8.3.3), the word is fancifully explained as "that which is in the heart" (*hridy ayam*), meaning the Self.

By practicing the "friction" of meditation, one may see the "resplendent deity" (*deva*) who is hidden within the heart, declares the *Shvetāsh-vatara-Upanishad* (1.14). This practice is done by using the body as the lower friction-stick and the syllable *om* as the upper friction-stick. Through the combined action of the two sticks the spiritual fire is kindled. This notion takes us back to the Vedic *tapas*, which includes an element of tension or friction as well. Through "glow" or *tapas*, the ascetic supercharges his or her body with transformative energy, which, in the end, yields the desired meditative vision of the Divine.

Some time during the fifth or fourth century B.C.E. the *Bhagavad-Gītā* was composed. This wonderful scripture is deemed an honorary *Upanishad*. The word *dhyāna* occurs many times in this work, as does the term *yoga*. In fact, the sixth chapter bears the title *dhyāna-yoga*, and verses 10 to 15 offer a summary of the meditative approach taught by the God-man Krishna.

In verse 12.12, again, *dhyāna* is said to be better than wisdom (*jnāna*), because it gives rise to the renunciation of action's fruit and to peace.

In the *Gītā*, the God-man Krishna asks his disciple Arjuna to yoke his higher mind (*buddhi*) by fastening it on him. In this way the entire body-mind becomes focused as well. Krishna speaks of those who have renounced all actions in him and who are intent on him alone, worshiping him by contemplating him through the practice of Yoga. This is an early statement of the practice of *guru-yoga*, where the adept-teacher serves as a focal point for the disciple's meditative and devotional life. The underlying idea is that the Self-realized master is a doorway to the Divine.

In the *Maitrāyanīya-Upanishad* (6.18), which dates back to the second or third century B.C.E., we find the first formulation of the yogic path as a process of clearly demarcated stages called "limbs" (*anga*). This scripture enumerates them as follows: breath control (*prānāyāma*), sensory inhibition (*pratyāhāra*), meditation (*dhyāna*), concentration (*dhāranā*), appraisal (*tarka*), and ecstasy (*samādhi*), in this order. Thus meditation appears as the third of six "limbs." It is uncertain why concentration succeeds rather than precedes meditation, though perhaps this is a hint at the fact that concentration and meditation are closely linked inner processes.

The practice of *tarka*, here translated as "appraisal," is not explained in the *Maitrāyanīya-Upanishad*. However, it likely refers to the exercise of careful examination of the quality and effects of one's meditation. Without self-criticism, the moods and visions engendered by meditation can become obstacles to the spiritual process. The Yoga practitioners must apply discrimination to their life as a whole, but especially to the manifestations of their own psyche. As the contemporary philosopher-sage Paul Brunton put it:

> Meditation must be accompanied by constant effort in the direction of honest self-examination. All thoughts and feelings which act as a barrier between the individual and his Ultimate Goal must be overcome. This requires acute self-observation and inner purification. . . . He must be on his guard against the falsifications, the rationalizations, and the deceptions unconsciously practiced by his ego when the self-analysis exercises become uncomfortable, humiliating, or painful. Nor should he allow himself to fall into the pit of self-pity.[7]

Formulations like those of the *Maitrāyanīya-Upanishad* prepared the way for the classical eightfold path of Patanjali, who probably lived in the second century C.E. In Patanjali's school, meditation figures as the seventh "limb." It is immediately preceded by the practice of concentration and succeeded by ecstasy. The fact that there are these stages reminds us that meditation is not an end in itself. It is simply a means to Self-realization through the mediating practice of ecstatic self-transcendence.

It is very important to realize that meditation is an integral part of the spiritual path. This means it cannot be practiced successfully apart from the other "limbs." Moreover, *dhyāna* is not a self-contained state, but its thrust is toward its own transcendence, that is, toward ecstasy, or *samādhi*. *Dhyāna* makes no sense outside the context of enlightenment, or spiritual liberation.

How did Patanjali explain *dhyāna*? In aphorism 3.2, he tells us that "meditation is the one-directional-flow (*eka-tānatā*) of ideas with regard to the [object of meditation]." We cannot understand this rather technical aphorism in isolation. It refers back to concentration. In fact, we cannot understand the meditative process according to Patanjali without going still further back, namely to the practice of posture (*āsana*). Meditation really starts there. For, posture involves a high degree of relaxation and, as Patanjali puts it in aphorism 2.47, one's "coinciding with the infinite [space of consciousness]."

This practice induces a measure of insensitivity to external stimuli, thus naturally leading over into the practice of sensory withdrawal (*pratyāhāra*) followed by concentration and meditation.

In aphorism 2.11, which is often glossed over by readers of the *Yoga-Sūtra*, Patanjali tells us another very important fact about meditation. He states that "the fluctuations of these [causes of suffering, or *kleshas*] are to be overcome by meditation." In other words, meditation rather than ecstasy is the means of transcending the mind's perpetual fluctuations (*vritti*). The fluctuations, again, are merely one of the manifestations of the causes of suffering (*klesha*), namely spiritual ignorance, the sense of individuality, passionate attachment to beings and things, the emotion of aversion, and the thirst for life. Another, subtler, aspect of the causes of suffering comprises the special mental acts (called *prajnā*) associated with the lower stages of ecstasy, which are distinct from ordinary thoughts. At any rate, the ecstatic state cannot even occur until the *vrittis* have been brought under control in meditation!

The specific task of the different forms of conscious ecstasy (*samprajnāta-samādhi*), composing the lower level of ecstasy, is to get the presented ideas (*pratyaya*) under control. These are spontaneous thought forms, higher types of insight (*prajnā*) arising in the ecstatic state. They need to be transcended so that the condition of supraconscious ecstasy (*asamprajnāta-samādhi*) can come about, which is the threshold to liberation.

We may note here that, for Patanjali, any locus (*desha*) is as good as any other for focusing the mind and achieving the meditative state. His broad-minded attitude permitted the elaboration of meditation techniques in subsequent times. One of these later developments represents the typical meditation practice in Hatha-Yoga, which is a complex *visualization* technique. Just how complex this meditation can be is best illustrated by the following passage from the seventeenth-century *Gheranda-Samhitā* (6.2–8):

> [Let the *yogin*] visualize that there is a great sea of nectar in his own heart; that in the middle of that [sea] there is an island of precious stones, the sand of which [consists of] pulverized gems; that on all sides of it are *nīpa* trees laden with sweet blossoms; that next to these trees, like a rampart, there is a row of flowering trees such as *mālatī, mallikā, jātī, kesarā, campakā, parijātā,* and *padma,* and that the fragrance of their blossoms is spreading all round in every direction. In the middle of this garden, let the *yogin* visualize that there is a beautiful *kalpa* tree with four branches, representing the four *Vedas*, and that it is laden with blossoms and fruits. Beetles are humming there and cuckoos are singing. Beneath that [tree] let him visualize a great platform of precious gems. Let the *yogin* [further]

visualize that in its center there is a beautiful throne inlaid with jewels. On that [throne] let the *yogin* visualize his particular deity (*devatā*), as taught by the teacher [who will instruct him about] the appropriate form, adornment, and vehicle of that deity. Know the constant meditation of such a form to be "coarse meditation" (*sthūla-dhyāna*).

Meditation, often of the visualizing variety, has also been a part of the Western religious and esoteric traditions. Often this practice took the form of prayer and visualization combined, as in the case of the "heart prayer" of the Eastern Church. Christian monastics also used mantras like "Hail Mary" in their practice (*exercitium*). But these efforts never produced a system of meditation as intricate as the systems we encounter in Hinduism and Buddhism. Nevertheless, practitioners of Eastern meditation techniques can certainly benefit from studying Christian approaches. Conversely, spiritual seekers adopting Christian forms of prayer and meditation are clearly able to enrich their practice by a close study of Eastern methods.

Today the West is pioneering the scientific exploration of meditation. This interest was chiefly initiated by practitioners of Transcendental Meditation (TM), the system promulgated in the West by Maharishi Mahesh Yogi.[8] It seems fitting, therefore, to comment briefly on this particular approach. Despite all the secrecy surrounding it, TM is really a form of Mantra-Yoga, supposedly the simplest type of Yoga. Initiates are given, usually for a substantial fee and with a solemn promise of secrecy, their own specific mantra taken from a limited pool of such "words of power" as *om*, *ram*, or *bam*. They are then asked to focus their attention on and through that sacred sound during each meditative session.

Many claims have been made about TM, ranging from simple physiological effects to extraordinary parapsychological phenomena. One of the more interesting, if controversial, claims concerns the "field effect" of meditation. It is said that TM is an effective means of improving the psychic environment of the world, capable of preventing war and other similar disasters. As any meditator can confirm, the meditative state not only has a benign effect on his or her own inner environment but *can* also extend to other beings who are directly exposed to the meditator's peaceful presence. How far-reaching this effect is and how it functions remains to be fully investigated.

Psychologists have succeeded in giving us a fairly good picture of what happens physiologically and psychologically in meditation. They have shown that meditation is an unusual but largely beneficial condition. They also have furnished us all kinds of operational facts about it, such as the correlation that exists between certain levels of meditative experiencing and brain waves. In fact, this discovery has led to a whole new technology, known as "biofeedback," which has the purpose of facilitating the induction of brain waves characteristic of relaxation and meditation.

Whatever the usefulness of this technology may be, we must realize that it can never be a substitute for spiritual maturation. While we may trick our nervous system into functioning in certain ways by wiring ourselves to sophisticated gadgetry, there is no real shortcut on the path to enlightenment. The same argument applies to the ingestion of "mind-altering" drugs. In the final analysis, for meditation to truly serve our quest for personal wholeness, it must be integrated with a sound spiritual orientation and sustained overall discipline. Genuine meditation practice always unfolds in the context of our encounter with the sacred dimension, and this necessarily involves the transcendence of the ego or, in old-fashioned terms, self-surrender.

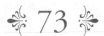

73

Prayer in Yoga

TRADITIONAL YOGA practitioners have long considered prayer (*prārthanā*) beneficial, and prayer is in fact a widespread and important yogic practice. Does that make Yoga a religious activity? It all depends on how one defines religion. It is necessary to distinguish between religion and spirituality. The former emphasizes external authority (a paternalistic deity and priesthood) and the need for mediation between oneself and the ultimate Reality, as well as conformation to a prescribed set of moral behavior under the threat of incurring sin. The latter relies primarily on intrinsic authority ("Self" or "Inner Ruler") and voluntary self-discipline based on self-understanding. If, in the case of a spiritual tradition, external authority (e.g., a guru) is involved, it is understood that he or she is merely a manifestation of the same Self or Reality that is one's own true nature.

Thus prayer can be either *religious* or *spiritual* — or also plain neurotic — depending on how we approach it. Some forms of Yoga are more religious than others, but all Yoga is spiritually based, because its essential goal is to lead practitioners beyond all external authority and mental projections into a state of transconceptual realization called *moksha, mukti, kaivalya, bodhi,* or *nirvāna* — all signifying liberation, freedom, or enlightenment. Even those schools of Yoga that conceptualize the ultimate Reality as a Divine Person (*uttama-purusha*), who infinitely surpasses the human being, teach that enlightenment transcends the body and the mind.

If prayer is engaged as a deeply self-transcending, self-transformative practice, it becomes a *spiritual* discipline. Who, then, are we praying to? That depends on our personal orientation and the tradition to which we belong, if we belong to one. Thus, if we are practitioners of Hindu Yoga, the focus of our prayerful attention could be Shiva, Devī (in her many forms), Krishna, Ganesha, Hanumat, or our own guru or some other great master (who serves as a "signal of transcendence"). In Buddhist Yoga, the object of prayer can be the Buddha, Avalokiteshvara, Tārā, or any of the other numerous focal points of devotion.

Through prayer we make a connection with the higher Reality in whatever form we might conceptualize or visualize it. The Yoga tradition most commonly explains this connection as being not merely symbolic or intrapsychic but objectively real. However we might think about it, it works! Medical professionals have demonstrated the effectiveness of prayer in health and healing in several independent studies. American physician Larry Dossey states in his widely read book *Healing Words*:

> Experiments . . . showed that prayer positively affected high blood pressure, wounds, heart attacks, headaches, and anxiety. . . . Over time I decided that *not* to employ prayer with my patients was the equivalent of deliberately withholding a potent drug or surgical procedure."[1]

Modern medicine is merely rediscovering what the *yogins* and *yoginīs* knew long ago. Rediscover this power of prayer for yourself and others.

❧ 74 ❧

The Ecstatic State

THE LAST "LIMB" (*anga*) of Patanjali's eightfold path, as mapped out in the *Yoga-Sūtra*, is ecstasy or *samādhi*. Importantly, however, it is not as often thought, even in India, the final goal of Yoga. The ultimate destination of the yogic journey is not any altered state of consciousness but pure Consciousness or Awareness itself, which is the same as liberation or enlightenment.

Just as "one-pointedness" (*eka-agratā*) is the essence of concentration and "one-flowness" (*eka-tānatā*) that of meditation, so "coinciding" or literally "falling together" (*samāpatti*) is the essence of ecstasy. Our ordinary state of consciousness is based on the clear-cut distinction between subject and object. In the processes of concentration and meditation, this differentiation becomes gradually blurred, and in the ecstatic state, it is altogether transcended. *Samādhi*, which can stand for both the technique and state of ecstasy, can be understood as the temporary identification of the contemplating subject with the contemplated object. As meditation proceeds, the object of meditation looms ever more large in the meditator's consciousness. In *samādhi*, the object alone survives—or nearly so, because in the lower forms of ecstasy there still is cognitive activity happening.

Already the Upanishadic sages over three millennia ago taught the profound esoteric truth that we become what we contemplate. Without a doubt, they derived this insight from their ecstatic experiences. Through the practice of concentration, the *yogin* selects and focuses upon a specific object. Then through meditation, he increasingly penetrates that object with his single-pointed attention. Finally, in the ecstatic state, he *becomes* the contemplated object in consciousness. The Latin tradition knows this condition as *coincidentia oppositorum*, the coinciding of opposites, which describes accurately the nature of the *samādhi* state. Ordinarily, subject and object are opposed to each other. The latter is thought to exist outside and apart from the cognizing subject. This barrier is lifted in the ecstatic condition.

Some talk about this condition as if it were all of a piece, which is definitely not the case. Rather Yoga, like many other spiritual traditions, recognizes the existence of a ladder of ecstatic unification comprising many rungs or stages. In Hinduism, Patanjali's model of ecstatic states is perhaps the most detailed. He distinguishes between two fundamental types of ecstasy: (1) *samprajnāta-samādhi*, or ecstasy connected with higher insights (*prajnā*), and (2) *asampra-jnāta-samādhi*, or ecstasy unaccompanied by higher insights.

In Vedānta, these two types are respectively known as *savikalpa-samādhi* and *nirvikalpa-samādhi*. Here *vikalpa* ("ideation," "concept," "form") takes the place of *prajnā* ("wisdom," "knowledge," "insight"). In some schools, the synonyms *sabīja-samādhi* ("ecstasy with seed") and *nirbīja-samādhi* ("ecstasy without seed") are used. Here the term "seed" stands for mental activity, which creates subconscious activators (*samskāra*), or karmic deposit, leading to more mental activity in the future. According to Patanjali, *nirbīja-samādhi* constitutes the final phase of *asamprajnāta-samādhi*, when all subconscious karmic factors have been eliminated, and the *yogin* enters into the state of liberation itself.

Only in the *asamprajnāta/nirvikalpa/nirbīja* type of *samādhi*, which is considered higher or superior to the other, does the transcendental Awareness—the ultimate or true Subject—shine forth without intrusion of mental activity. In other words, it has no mental contents. Both body and mind are truly transcended, at least temporarily. All other forms of ecstasy remain within the purview of empirical reality, the world of change (*samsāra*). Whereas *asamprajnāta-samādhi* has no subdivisions, because it has no object with which the *yogin* identifies, *samprajnāta-samādhi* comprises various grades, which Patanjali categorized as follows:

- *savitarka-samādhi*, or simply *vitarka-samādhi* — ecstatic identification with the external or "coarse" (*sthūla*) aspect of the contemplated object and connected with conscious content (*pratyaya*) of the type known as *prajnā* (higher insight); because these higher insights relate to the coarse level of an object, they are called *vitarka* ("cogitation," "reflection," "consideration," "deliberation," etc.);
- *nirvitarka-samādhi* — ecstatic identification with the external or coarse aspect of the contemplated object but without the arising of higher insights; the conscious content is the contemplated object itself;
- *savicāra-samādhi* or simply *vicāra-samādhi* — ecstatic identification with the inner or "subtle" (*sūkshma*) aspect of the contemplated object and connected with conscious content of the type known as *prajnā*; because these higher insights relate to the subtle level of an object, they are called *vicāra* ("cogitation," "reflection," "investigation," "examination," etc.);

- *nirvicāra-samādhi* — ecstatic identification with the inner or subtle aspect of the contemplated object but without the arising of higher insights; the conscious content is the contemplated object itself.

The mental activity (*pratyaya*) in these four lower forms of ecstasy must not be confused with our familiar meandering thought processes (*vritti*). As the *Yoga-Sūtra* (2.11) makes clear, these must be thoroughly controlled through concentration and meditation before the switch from the empirical to the ecstatic consciousness can occur. These recurring noetic acts in the *samprajnāta* ecstasy have a palpable immediacy that distinguishes them from the usual vague ramblings of the mind confronting an object. They are pure thought, instant recognitions, or certainties of understanding. They are suprawakeful knowing, a form of thinking that is not identical with the sense-based semiconscious, automatic activity of the ordinary mind. They are spontaneous and transparent flashes of awareness and understanding, born of the unmediated experience of the object of contemplation.

In yogic terminology, these ecstatic supercognitions are direct or unmediated apprehension (*sakshātkāra*), which is not confined to the present structure of the object of contemplation. As Vijnāna Bhikshu explained in his *Yoga-Sāra-Samgraha* (chapter 1), this ecstatic knowing extends also to the contemplated object's past and future forms and, in *vicāra-samādhi* also to its subtle energetic essence. What this means can only be understood within the framework of the ontology of Yoga and Sāmkhya: Cosmic reality, called *prakriti*, is not only the familiar visible world; it also includes an inner or subtle dimension that is hierarchically stratified.

This invisible realm of cosmic existence ranges from a pure transcendental matrix of potentiality (called *pradhāna*) to the plane of the *logos* or higher mind (*buddhi*) and, further still, to the level of the "I-maker" (*ahamkāra* or, as Patanjali has it, *asmitā*), the sense-bound lower mind (*manas*), the senses (*indriya*), and the energetic templates (*tanmātra*) underlying the coarse elements (*bhūta*) that compose the visible universe. This ancient model, which was originally the product of much meditative and ecstatic introspection, seeks to explain the evolution from the One to the Many.

The culmination of *samprajnāta-samādhi*, which is connected with an objective prop, is reached when the personality core (*sattva = buddhi*) shines forth with a degree of translucency comparable to that of the transcendental Self (*purusha*). Here is the threshold that leads to the nonobjective, supraconscious ecstasy, which consists in pure Awareness, or the Self/Spirit itself.

The avenue for rediscovering the innate freedom of the transcendental Self, the eternal Witness, is the elimination of all the karmic traces that our experiences, life after life, have left behind as imprints in the depth of the mind. This is accomplished in *asamprajnāta-samādhi*, the state of supra-conscious ecstasy. This elusive state progressively burns out all subliminal residua responsible for the formation of empirical consciousness and thus of the experience of duality and alienation from the transcendental Self. Thus this ecstatic state is responsible for a total remolding of the human being whereby we remember our true nature as transcendental Being-Awareness.

When all karmic seeds have been burned in the seedless ecstasy (*nirbīja-samādhi*), enlightenment or liberation ensues, which Patanjali calls *kaivalya* or "aloneness," since the transcendental Reality, or the Self, stands in its own glory without interference from any mental obscurations.

Patanjali refers to this ultimate phase of the supraconscious ecstasy also as *dharma-megha-samādhi*, or "ecstasy of the cloud of *dharma*." It is not clear in what sense the word *dharma* is used in this context. The classical exegetes have interpreted it as "virtue," and this explanation seems to have satisfied most scholars. However, in view of the fact that the liberated being is said to have transcended good and evil, this interpretation does not ring quite true. In my monograph *The Philosophy of Classical Yoga*, I have therefore proposed that *dharma* here refers to the primary constituents (*guna*) of the world ground, which are finally being transcended. The "cloud" of the primary constituents is the final veil in the process of dissolving: the *gunas* themselves resolve back into the transcendental ground of the cosmos.

Thus the process of yogic involution takes place in distinct stages, which can be understood in terms of levels of achievement or accomplishment. In his tenth-century *Tattva-Vaishāradī* (1.17), Vācaspati Mishra compares the *yogin* practicing ecstasy to an archer who shoots at increasingly smaller and more distant targets. Such scales of ecstatic involution, however, are intended to serve as a general map only and are seldom strictly adhered to in practice. Fully accomplished adepts (*siddha*), like the nineteenth-century spiritual virtuoso Ramakrishna, are able to enter any ecstatic state at will.

Most importantly, none of the above-mentioned states of *samādhi* amount to ultimate liberation or enlightenment. Although *asamprajnāta-* or *nirvikalpa-samādhi* does in fact disclose the transcendental Self, it is an incomplete realization, as it depends on a radical introversion of consciousness and is temporary and exclusive of bodily awareness. Full enlightenment, by contrast, does not depend on the extraversion or introversion of attention and it also is permanent. Some schools of Yoga call this ultimate realization *sahaja-samādhi* or "spontaneous ecstasy." The term *sahaja* literally means "together born," suggesting that in this realization, the normally operative distinction between the empirical reality and the transcendental Reality no longer applies.

This unsurpassable realization is the goal of all authentic Yoga.

The Serpent Power and Spiritual Life

THE KUNDALINI CONCEPT, which belongs to the heritage of Tantra-Yoga, is one of the more obscure notions of India's spiritual heritage; yet it also happens to be one of the most important and fascinating ones. The word means "she who is coiled" and refers to the divine potential locked away in the human body. Often called the "serpent power," the *kundalinī* is the Energy of Consciousness (*cit-shakti*), or Goddess Power (*devī-shakti*).

According to Tantric metaphysics, the ultimate or divine Reality is far from impotent and possesses all conceivable (and inconceivable) powers. On the one hand, it is pure Consciousness; on the other, pure Energy. The Tantric branch of Kashmiri Shaivism speaks of the ultimate Reality as a supervibration (*spandana*). Everything else is but a stepped-down version of that incomprehensible vastness of Energy. The energies of the manifest physical cosmos are a mere trickle by comparison. It is the life energy (*prāna*) that animates and sustains the human body; but it is the *kundalinī* that, when awakened from its dormant state, transforms the body from a sentient biological organism into a field of light transcending the laws of Nature and fully responsive to the enlightened will of the Yoga adept. The goal of all schools of Tantra-Yoga, as with any form of Yoga, is enlightenment or liberation. But many Tantric schools seek the kind of enlightenment that includes the body and the world. Thus the Tantric adepts speak of a *vajra-deha* ("adamantine body") or *divya-deha* ("divine body").

The *kundalinī* is instrumental in the creation of this extraordinary vehicle of the enlightened adept. According to Tantra, it underlies all spiritual evolution. Not all branches or schools of Yoga, however, avail themselves of this concept. In fact, this concept did not come into vogue until the emergence of Tantra around 500 C.E. Thus it is not mentioned in the *Vedas*, the early *Upanishads*, the *Bhagavad-Gītā*, or the *Yoga-Sūtra* (c. 200 C.E.). But later texts, like the *Bhakti-Sūtras* ascribed to Nārada and Shāndilya respectively, make no reference to it. There is some discussion about whether the Tantric claim to the universality of the *kundalinī* is in fact correct, or whether enlightenment is possible without the involvement of the *kunda-lini* process.

Since there have been adepts who claimed to be enlightened but did not experience the typical symptoms of a *kundalini* awakening, we may assume that enlightenment is possible without manifestation of the typical symptoms, such as the experience of explosive luminosity, inner sounds, sensations of heat, dizziness, drowsiness, inability to sleep, and so on. In his book *The Kundalini Experience*, the American psychiatrist Lee Sannella makes the useful distinction between the *kundalini* proper and what he calls the *physio-kundalini*, that is, the psychosomatic manifestations of awakening.[1]

The twentieth-century sage Ramana Maharshi, who, as far as anyone can tell, was genuinely enlightened, made the point that the *kundalini* rises from whatever *lakshya* (locus of concentration) an adept has chosen. In the same conversation with a visitor to his hermitage, the sage also equated the *kundalini* with the life energy (*prāna-shakti*).[2] Elsewhere Ramana Maharshi identifies the *kundalini* with the ultimate Reality itself. From the few comments he made about the Goddess power and associated concepts, it appears that he granted them the same reality as anything else in the orbit of finite existence. From the vantage-point of his own realization, however, they were all equally illusory. Since we are dealing here only with the empirical or finite dimension, we can take his statements as confirming the existence of the *kundalini*, the subtle channels (*nādī*), subtle centers (*cakra*), and so on. Those adepts who, in the process of their enlightenment, do not experience the characteristic phenomena of *kundalini* awakening could be said to have somehow bypassed them.

It makes sense to assume, with Lee Sannella, that those phenomena are the result of blockages in the subtle or etheric body, which is composed of a network of energy (*prāna*) filaments. These blockages prevent the free flow of the *kundalini-shakti* in the central channel, the *sushumnā-nādī*, which originates in the "root-prop center" (*mūlādhāra-cakra*) and terminates at the "thousand-spoked center" (*sahasrāra-cakra*). The former is located in the subtle body at a place corresponding to the perineum; the latter at a place corresponding to the crown of the head (i.e., the fontanel). The *kundalini* is thought to exist in the dormant state at the basal center where she must be awakened and invited to rise along the central channel to the top of the head where she reunites with pure Consciousness. This reunion is described as the communion of Shiva and Shakti, God and Goddess, or Consciousness and Energy.

On the complete ascent of the *kundalinī*, the individuated consciousness of the adept at least temporarily melts away in the state of *nirvikalpa-samādhi* or transconceptual ecstasy. While this state reveals our true nature—as the transcendental Being-Consciousness-Bliss (*sat-cid-ānanda*)—it excludes body awareness. It could therefore be considered an incomplete enlightenment. So long as the unconscious contains karmic seeds awaiting fruition, this elevated state of consciousness sooner or later is replaced again by the ordinary state of awareness. Through repeated awakening of the *kundalinī* and *nirvikalpa-samādhi*, the karmic seeds can be gradually thinned out.

Ultimately, the Tantric *yogin* seeks to "irrigate" the body with the nectar of immortality that oozes from the awakened thousand-petaled center. This esoteric process transfigures and transforms the ordinary physical body into a supraphysical energy body endowed with extraordinary capacities (*siddhi*) and immortality. For this to occur, the adept must transcend even *nirvikalpa-samādhi* and attain complete enlightenment in the waking state as well. This final ecstatic condition is not, strictly speaking, a state of consciousness. It *is* that which is Real. In the Tantric tradition, it is sometimes known as *sahaja-samādhi* or spontaneous ecstasy, which is constant and continuous. This realization has been summed up in the Buddhist Tantric formula "*samsāra* = *nirvāna*," or immanence equals transcendence.

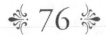

76

Who or What Is the Self in Self-Realization?

THE SOUTH INDIAN SAGE Ramana Maharshi (1879–1950) regularly reminded his visitors to ask themselves: Who am I? Well, who are we? Are we the body? Which part of the body are we? Or are we the entire body? If so, where does our body end? The skin? What about the electro-magnetic field that is part of the body and extends beyond it?

Above all, which body are we? The body that is now twenty, thirty, or sixty years old? Or the body of our childhood? Within the span of seven years, we are told, all the cells of the human body are completely replaced. This means that in one lifetime each of us comes to literally inhabit several bodies serially.

If we are not the body, are we the mind? If we are inclined to say yes, then we should ask ourselves this: Which mind are we? The barely existing mind of the infant that we once were? Or the confused, rebellious mind of adolescence? Or the mind that keeps changing even as our body is growing older? And, moreover, where does our own mind end and the "mind" of our particular culture begin? Who are we really? What or where is our identity?

Some 2,500 years ago, Gautama the Buddha asked himself these same penetrating questions. He found the following answer: Since the body-mind is constantly changing, it cannot possibly have a permanent identity. As he would put it: There is no self. Everything is *anātman* or devoid of a stable identity. Nature is a process of continuous transmutation. The ego-identity of the ordinary human being is a mechanism created through spiritual ignorance (*avidyā*). Out of this root ignorance all other distorted views about Reality arise.

The Hindu sages who composed the *Upanishads* and the *Bhagavad-Gītā* came up with a similar analysis of the situation. They, too, felt that the body-mind could not possibly be the identity of the human being. But, unlike the Buddha, they did not remain silent about what is beyond or prior to the body-mind and the universe. Instead they boldly affirmed that the identity of the human being—and indeed of every being—is unqualified

Being-Consciousness-Bliss (*sat-cid-ānanda*). Their teachings were based on their own spiritual realization (*adhyātma-sākshatkāra*), their own transcendence of the body-mind in the state of transconceptual ecstasy (*nirvikalpa-samādhi*).

Their philosophical ideas are collectively known as Vedānta ("*Vedas'* end") or Jnāna-Yoga, the path of liberating wisdom. They called that single transindividual Identity the *ātman* (meaning literally "self/oneself") or the *purusha* (meaning literally "man"). They also spoke of that One as *brahman* (from the root *brih*, meaning "to grow" or "to expand"), because that Identity is not only the Core of human consciousness but the eternal Foundation of the world at large.

The *ātman* of Vedānta is clearly quite distinct from the self or "I" that we ordinarily presume ourselves to be. The self or ego (*ahamkāra*), as Alan Watts noted, is a convenient fiction by which we bring unity or order to our experiences.[1] It is a fiction that can be very destructive, as when we build our life around "Number One." Then we are dealing with selfishness, self-centeredness, ego-centrism, or self-conceit.

By contrast, spiritual life is about radical self-transcendence, that is, going beyond the ego-fiction. This is not the same as altruism, which even at its purest is still a manifestation of the finite, unenlightened self or ego. The practice of radical self-transcendence can be described as conscious growth toward the transcendental or transpersonal Self-Identity, the *ātman*. Some call this "God-Consciousness."

The Self of Vedānta/Jnāna-Yoga is also completely different from the Self talked about by Jungian psychotherapists. The Jungian Self is the ego-transcending spiritual center of the mature human personality; it is not a superconscious transcendental Being.

The Self, or *ātman*, of Vedānta is by definition beyond space-time and the whole body-mind complex. It is not a property of the individual person. Therefore, the Self is never "my" self, nor is Self-realization "my" Self-realization. When Self-realization happens, "I" am not there! So long as we believe that we are a particular man or woman, with a particular character and distinct tendencies, habits, or likes and dislikes, we live out of the ego-fiction. Then we necessarily fear the loss of what we consider to be our "own"—our various material and intellectual possessions as well as our social relationships. Above all, we fear the death of the individual we believe ourselves to be.

But when there is genuine understanding or wisdom (*prajñā*), we begin to see a larger truth. We may even catch a glimpse of the Being-Consciousness-

Bliss (*sat-cid-ānanda*) that is the underlying Identity not only of "me" but of all beings who, from the unenlightened point of view, appear to be separate entities. Even describing that Ultimate as Being (*sat*), Consciousness (*cit*), and Bliss (*ānanda*) is saying too much. Hence some sages, especially in Buddhism, have preferred to call it "Emptiness" (*shūnyatā*). The wisest among them have remained silent.

This is obviously a very deep subject on which scores of volumes could and indeed have been written. All I intend to do in this short essay is remind us of its existence and of the mystery of our being in the world—a great matter that can profitably form the substance of many meditations.

❧ 77 ❧

Emptiness

THE ULTIMATE REALITY, by definition, transcends the mind that seeks to comprehend it. Therefore India's sages have since ancient times spoken of it as "formless" (*arūpa*), "unqualified" (*nirguna*), and "transconceptual" (*nirvikalpa*). At the same time, many of them have sympathized with their disciples' emotional and intellectual need for a less abstract description. Thus the Yoga literature is replete with metaphysical statements that paint pictures of the ultimate Reality, ascribing to it qualities that the ordinary mind deems positive, good, and desirable: light, infinity, eternity, omnipotence, grace, love, wisdom, forgiveness, protection, and so forth.

Also, instead of using a neuter noun to refer to that ultimate Singularity, the adepts name it after male and female deities. Dropping the neuter noun *brahman* widely used in the *Upanishads*, they speak of the ultimate Reality as Brahma, Vishnu, Shiva, Krishna, Pārvatī, Sarasvatī, Kālī, Rādhā, and so on. They invoke the One as "Creator," "Father," "Mother," "Friend," or "Beloved."

When asked what "it" is, Gautama the Buddha declined to speculate. Yet even he appears to have occasionally softened his nonmetaphysical stance, for we have a few passages in which he describes *nirvāna* in positive terms. This paved the way for the subsequent metaphysical developments of Mahāyāna Buddhism with its transcendental Buddhas and Bodhisattvas and their respective paradises. But the Mahāyāna teachers balanced this elaboration with a strong emphasis on emptiness (*shūnyatā*)—a concept also found in some schools of Hindu Yoga, notably that of the tenth-century *Yoga-Vāsishtha*.

Ever since the *Prajnā-Pāramitā-Sūtras*, or the scriptures on the perfection of wisdom, practitioners of Mahāyāna and Tantrayāna have sought to cultivate the recognition that all phenomena are empty (*shūnya*): Everything that we could possibly point to, talk about, or even merely think of is a conceptual construct. Hence, according to the masters of Mahāyāna and Tantrayāna, nothing that is composite has any essence (*sva-bhāva*); everything is "without self" (*nairātmya*). In its most developed form—that of the Madhyamaka school founded by Nāgārjuna—this teaching came to mean that nothing is independently real.

In his *Madhyamaka-Kārikā* (24.18), Nāgārjuna notes that it is the Buddha's teaching of "dependent origination (*pratītya-samutpāda*) that we call 'emptiness' (*shūnyatā*)." Everything arises in dependence on causes and conditions or what in modern ecology is known as the "web of life" or "interconnectedness." When we think of a star, for instance, we must admit that it is not so much a stable thing but a very complex *process* of limited duration. The same is true of our body, the mind, and every other conceivable thing. But in order to navigate in the world of appearances, we artificially construct a cosmos populated by stable things, as if these had inherent existence. The problem with this is that we begin to take them very seriously—including our body-mind—and start reacting either by attracting or rejecting them. In the case of our body, we even go so far as to identify with it, and as a result we suffer all kinds of negative consequences, notably the fear of death.

The cure, according to Mahāyāna and Tantrayāna, is to cultivate the vision of emptiness, realizing of course that "emptiness" itself is a mental construct and therefore empty of inherent existence. Practitioners who forget this truth are apt to take *shūnyatā* itself as a definitive view (*drishti*) rather than as an antidote to all abstractions, which is the intended purpose. This kind of thinking has led to accusations of nihilism: that nothing whatsoever is real at any level and that *nirvāna* therefore is a completely meaningless and undesirable goal. In fact, both nihilism and realism are erroneous. Already the Buddha declined to speculate about the nature of *nirvāna*; he simply wanted to point a way to its realization. The Madhyamaka school simply developed this fundamental teaching along rigorous logical lines, focusing on the art of refutation of all possible metaphysical standpoints.

But the language of emptiness is not meant to be merely a game of logic. Its real function is to shatter the conceptual mind and guide it to the truth about phenomena. For this emptiness must not only be understood intellectually but *experienced* through the cultivation of wisdom and compassion by means of the ten stages of the *bodhisattva* path. The inherent selflessness or emptiness of beings notwithstanding, a *bodhisattva* is altruistically dedicated to their liberation. This total dedication to the spiritual welfare of others is known as *bodhicitta*, or the enlightenment mind, which leads to the accumulation of merit (*punya*)—a type of energy that can then be used for practical service of others. The accumulation of merit is paralleled by the accumulation of wisdom (*prajnā*), which guarantees that a *bodhisattva's* help is effective.

Bodhicitta is activated through the study and practice of the six perfections (*pāramitā*) over numerous lifetimes:

1. Generosity (*dāna*), which consists in giving material assistance, teaching the Buddha's *dharma*, and granting protection from all kinds of fears
2. Morality (*shīla*), which is the strict observation of either the five lay or the 250 monastic vows
3. Patience (*kshānti*), which consists in the capacity to endure hardship and especially to remain indifferent to harm inflicted by others
4. Vigor (*vīrya*), which, apart from physical stamina comprises such yogic virtues as heedfulness (*apramāda*) and fortitude (*dhriti*)
5. Meditation (*dhyāna*), which is mental discipline leading to mastery of the whole range of higher states of mind
6. Wisdom (*prajnā*), which is the higher mental faculty of discerning the Real from the unreal

Sometimes four more perfections are named: skillful means (*upāya-kaushalya*), vow (*pranidhāna*), strength (*bala*), and knowledge (*jnāna*).

By means of the cultivation of the six or ten perfections, the path of the *bodhisattva* unfolds in ten stages (*bhūmi*):

1. Joyous stage (*pramuditā-bhūmi*), which is attained with the first perception of emptiness and in which the practitioner focuses on the perfection of generosity
2. Immaculate stage (*vimalā-bhūmi*), which coincides with overcoming all tendencies toward negative thoughts and actions, even in the dream state
3. Illuminating stage (*prabhākarī-bhūmi*), which is marked by the absence of duality in meditation and the perfection of patience
4. Blazing stage (*arcishmatī-bhūmi*), which gives the practitioner mastery of the thirty-seven "harmonies with enlightenment" amounting to extensive control of the mind, particularly in meditation
5. Very-difficult-to-conquer stage (*sudurjayā-bhūmi*), which leads to the perfection of equanimity and the capacity to remain in meditation for any length of time
6. Face-to-face stage (*abhimukhī-bhūmi*), which is so called because the practitioner understands directly the dependent arising of all phenomena and which would allow him or her to enter into *nirvāna*, were it not for the *bodhisattva* vow of liberating all sentient beings

7. Far-going stage (*dūrangamā-bhūmi*), which is a state of perfect spontaneity and leads to perfection in skillful means, enabling the practitioner to adapt his or her teachings to the varying needs and capacities of students

8. Immovable stage (*acalā-bhūmi*), which makes the practitioner's spiritual realization irrevocable and also gives him or her the ability to assume various forms to teach others

9. Good thoughts stage (*sādhumatī-bhūmi*), which is associated with the perfection of power (*bala*) and the capacity to understand all languages

10. Cloud-of-*dharma* stage (*dharma-megha-bhūmi*), which is so named because at this level, the practitioner spreads the Buddha's teaching like a cloud pouring rain and nourishing the Earth, and he or she acquires a perfect body and mind

Upon completion of the high-level contemplation at the cloud-of-*dharma* stage, the practitioner enters into full Buddhahood. This is sometimes referred to as the "eleventh stage." It is the level of total omniscience and omnipotence.

❧ 78 ❧
Liberation

ALL FORMS, BRANCHES, or schools of Yoga have the same final goal: liberation, enlightenment, freedom, the transcendence of the human condition, or the fulfillment of our highest potential. The Sanskrit language has many words to convey this "attainment" (in alphabetical order): *apavarga, ātma-jnāna, ātma-sātkarana, bodhi, kaivalya, moksha, mukti, nirvāna, siddhi, vimukti,* and so forth.

How liberation, or enlightenment, is to be understood differs from system to system. All schools of Yoga are in unanimous agreement that liberation, or freedom, is the most worthwhile pursuit to which we could dedicate ourselves. Every other objective is merely secondary, temporary, and not ultimately fulfilling. In other words, liberation is at the top of the value pyramid that, in Hindu Yoga, comprises the following four major human "goals" or "purposes" (*purusha-artha*): material welfare (*artha*), pleasure (*kāma*), morality (*dharma*), and spiritual freedom (*moksha*).

Almost all schools of Yoga, moreover, agree that enlightenment, or freedom, is our original or true nature. In other words, liberation is not something new that we must create or attain. Rather, it is what is the case when we cease to live in our respective conceptual prisms—be they factual frameworks, grand philosophies, belief systems, or mere opinions. In the liberated state, we are simply *real*. In the state we now regard as real, we are merely mistaken or inauthentic.

Liberation becomes self-evident when we have succeeded in lifting the spell of ignorance (*avidyā*), which is responsible for our misidentification with a particular body-mind. We are born in ignorance. This yogic notion corresponds to the Judeo-Christian belief that we are born in sin. Our sin is that we are oblivious of our spiritual nature and enamored of the body-mind and its physical and noetic environments. According to some interpretations within the Judeo-Christian tradition, sinning originated with Adam and Eve, which produced an inner corruption in human beings that is hereditarily passed from generation to generation. Rather, Yoga affirms that our spiritual ignorance is not "original" but an activity that we perpetuate in every moment. Also, in the yogic understanding, the "sin" of spiritual blindness is not an offense against God. Some branches and schools of Yoga do not even entertain the notion of a personal God. It is simply a serious shortcoming by which we conceal our true nature from ourselves. This is quite similar to the Greek interpretation of sin. The Greek word for "sin" is *hamartia*, meaning "missing the mark."

Out of spiritual ignorance, we constantly commit deeds that violate universal principles of morality and thus reap the karmic consequences of our misguided actions (and volitions), which in turn keep us ignorant of our real nature. In essence, however, we are free. This teaching corresponds to the fundamental Judeo-Christian belief that, beneath all our sins, we are intrinsically good, since God—who is by definition good—fashioned human beings in his image. For the Jew or Christian, God forgives the original sin and all subsequent sins when we feel genuine remorse for and turn away from our sinful conduct. In the Christian tradition, Jesus sacrificed himself for the sake of all sinners, which has led to the reductionistic doctrine in some Christian circles that in order to enjoy God's forgiveness we must simply believe in Jesus.

Yoga, too, calls for a turning-away from our usual (sinful) ways. Some forms of Yoga include in their theology the element of grace (*prasāda*), but all emphasize self-effort in the form of sustained practice of the yogic path. Gaudāpāda, in his *Māndūkya-Kārikā* (3.41), offers this striking simile:

> Controlling the mind is like the unrelenting effort that is necessary to empty the ocean, one drop at a time, with the help of the tip of a *kusha* grass.

Either through effort alone or through a combination of effort and grace, we can overcome our spiritual ignorance and actively shape our future destiny. If belief is involved in some schools of Yoga, it plays only a preliminary role. The accent is typically on wisdom (*jnāna*), even in the more sophisticated approaches of Bhakti-Yoga, the devotional path.

The impulse to attain freedom—or, in the *bhakti*-oriented schools, union with the Divine—underlies all yogic effort. Only in this way can the practitioner be assured of not getting stuck along the path. This impulse is known as *mumukshutva*, the desire for liberation, wholeness, perfection, or lasting happiness. With the sole exception of this desire, or impulse, all desires (*kāma*) relate to either the physical world or some subtle object or state, including heaven. Since all manifestation (*vyakta*)—whether coarse (*sthūla*) or subtle (*sūkshma*)—is finite, none of these desires can give us true fulfillment. They are, to put it differently, all part of the world of change (*samsāra*). The impulse to liberation, however, is directed toward the unmanifest (*avyakta*), infinite Reality.

Having kindled the impulse toward ultimate freedom and adopted an appropriate spiritual path, the practitioner gradually sheds ignorance (or sin) and simply awakens as the ever-present Real. Even this experience of awakening is merely a metaphor. From the perspective of the ultimate Reality (which has no perspective at all), nothing ever happened. We were never ignorant, self-divided, or unhappy, and therefore we also did not awaken. Whenever we talk about the fully liberated or enlightened being, we inevitably get trapped in paradoxes or doctrines. And yet, tens of thousands of adepts have risked opening their mouths in order to convey something of the Unthinkable or Unspeakable to (apparent) others.

When we examine the Hindu concept of liberation, or enlightenment, we find that it comes in two fundamental forms: bodiless liberation (*videha-mukti*) and living liberation (*jīvan-mukti*). The former type implies perfect transcendence not only of the human condition but of embodiment as such. It is a state of being that is utterly formless and wholly apart from the universe in all its many levels. This is the great spiritual ideal promulgated in the philosophical traditions of Mīmāmsā, Nyāya, Vaisheshika, Īshvara Krishna's school of Sāmkhya, some Vedānta teachers (like Bhāskara, Yādava, and Nimbārka), and apparently also Patanjali's school of Yoga.

The second type of liberation, *jīvan-mukti*, is the ideal favored by most teachers of Hindu, Buddhist, and Jaina Yoga. It can be said to be India's most important contribution to world spirituality. Living liberation, or liberation while still alive in a body, is the idea that it is possible to be inwardly absolutely free while yet simultaneously appearing as an embodied individual. Closely related to this notion is the so-called witnessing Consciousness (*sāk-shin*), which is the essential "quality" of the ultimate Reality, be it called "Self," "Spirit," "Truth," or "the Divine." For the sages of India, of course, both these notions are not merely abstract ideas but actual realities that are completely verifiable by anyone willing to undergo the rigors of the spiritual path.

Both forms of liberation have in common that they terminate our suffering (*duhkha*) along with our sense of individuation (*ahamkāra* or *as-mitā*). But whereas *videha-mukti* coincides with the death of the body-mind, in *jīvan-mukti* our flesh-and-blood existence continues without, however, in any way limiting our inner freedom. Bodiless liberation and embodied liberation are essentially the same. Those authorities who affirm the possibility of living liberation view it as a precursor to disembodied liberation. The liberated being, they assure us, remains quite unaffected by the presence or absence of a finite body-mind along with its personality and distinct life history.

Vidyāranya, a *yogin*-scholar of the fourteenth century, was the first to provide a detailed examination of the ideal of *jīvan-mukti* in his *Jīvanmukti-Viveka*. This great Sanskrit writer, who was a master of clarity, made the following pertinent observations (chapter 1):

> Well, what is this *jīvan-mukti*? What proof is there for it? How is it brought about? Of what use is its attainment? [In answer, one can] state: For a living person, bondage (*bandha*) consists in those qualities of the mind that are characterized by feelings of pleasure and pain, agency and enjoyment, etc. Bondage results from the [various] forms of the causes of affliction (*klesha*); living liberation (*jīvan-mukti*) [results] from their removal. Now is this bondage removed from the Witness (*sākshin*) or the mind? Certainly not the former, because removal [of bondage occurs] by means of knowledge of Truth (*tattva-jnāna*). But it also cannot be removed from the latter [i.e., the mind], because this is an impossibility. As the fluidity of water can be [by mixing earth with it], or as the heat of fire [can be controlled by other means], so can control be exercised over the mind's [sense of] agency, etc. Everywhere this is a common intrinsic condition. It is not [necessarily] thus. Although complete removal is not possible, neutralization (*abhibhava*) is possible. Just as watery liquidity can be neutralized by mixing [water] with earth, or fiery heat by means of *mani, mantra*, and so on, just so all the fluctuations (*vritti*) of the mind can be neutralized by means of the practice of Yoga.

In describing the condition of the *jīvan-mukta*, the embodied liberated being, Vidyāranya quotes profusely from the *Yoga-Vāsishtha*. This extensive Kashmiri work, which is presented as a dialogue between the Sage Vasishtha and Prince Rāma, states (5.90–98):

> He is a *jīvan-mukta* for whom, even though he is busy with ordinary life, all this ceases to exist and [only] the space [of ultimate Consciousness] remains.

> He is a true *jīvan-mukta* whose face neither flushes nor pales in pleasure or pain and who subsists on whatever comes his way.

He is a true *jīvan-mukta* who is awake when sleeping, who knows no waking, and whose knowledge is entirely free from any *vāsanā*.

He is a true *jīvan-mukta* who, though responsive to feelings such as attachment, hatred, fear, and other feelings, stands wholly pure within, like space.

He is a true *jīvan-mukta* whose real nature is not influenced by egotism and whose mind is not subjected to attachment, whether he remains active or is inactive.

He is a true *jīvan-mukta* whom the world does not fear and who does not fear the world, and who is free from joy, jealousy, and fear.

He is a true *jīvan-mukta* who is at peace with the ways of the world; who, though full of all learning and arts, is yet without any; and who, though endowed with mind, is without it.

He is a true *jīvan-mukta* who, though deeply immersed in all things, keeps his head cool, just as anyone would, when engaged in attending to other's affairs; and whose Self is whole.

After leaving the condition of living liberation, he enters into liberation after death, on the disintegration of the body by lapse of tenure, even as the wind comes to a standstill.

Depending on their operative *karma*—the so-called *prārabdha-karman*—the sages look and behave differently. Some, like the famous King Janaka, are very active; others prefer silence and the solitude of forests or mountains. Some let the body drop as it will; others undertake the gargantuan discipline of transmuting the body into light, as is the objective in some Tantric teachings. These external distinctions tell us nothing about the spiritual realization of those sages. All of them, however, can be expected to emanate a palpable peace that, in the words of Saint Paul, "passeth all understanding."

Notes

Chapter 1: What Is Yoga?

1. The word *yogī*, which is often found in the English literature, represents the nominative case of the Sanskrit stem *yogin*. For the sake of consistency and easy recognition, I have used the stem of Sanskrit words throughout this book. There are many different nominative case endings, which can be confusing to those not familiar with the Sanskrit language. For instance, the word *āsana* (seat or posture) becomes *āsanam* in the nominative; *yoga* (union) becomes *yogah*; *go* (cow) becomes *gauh*; etc.
2. See Georg Feuerstein, *The Yoga Tradition* (Prescott, Ariz.: Hohm Press, rev. ed., 2001).
3. For a review of the Indus-Sarasvati civilization, see Georg Feuerstein, S. Kak, and D. Frawley, *In Search of the Cradle of Civilization* (Wheaton, Ill.: Quest Books, 1995).
4. There are several complete translations of the *Rig-Veda* available in various Western languages. In English, the two-volume rendering by R. Griffith may be consulted with some reservations. See R. Griffith, *The Hymns of the Rig Veda* (Delhi: Motilal Banarsidass, repr. 1976). Most Western translators do not yet fully appreciate the spiritual depth of this archaic scripture. On this, see Sri Aurobindo, *On the Veda* (Pondicherry, India: Sri Aurobindo Ashram, 10th ed., 1977) and also Jeanine Miller, *The Vedas* (London: Rider, 1974).
5. For a good discussion and translation of the teachings of the *Upanishads*, see S. Radhakrishnan, ed. and trans., *The Principal Upanisads* (London: George Allen & Unwin, 1974).
6. Classical Yoga (or Pātanjala-yoga or *yoga-darshana*) is explained in chapters 61, 62, and 74 of the present volume. See also Georg Feuerstein, *The Philosophy of Classical Yoga* (Rochester, Vt.: Inner Traditions, 1996) and *The Yoga-Sūtra: A New Translation and Commentary* (Rochester, Vt.: Inner Traditions, 1989).
7. Many Indian scholars place Patanjali earlier, with the favored date being around 200 B.C.E., but the native tradition of the identity of the Yoga adept with his namesake the grammarian is highly doubtful.
8. Paul Brunton, *The Notebooks of Paul Brunton*. Vol. 1: *Perspectives: The Timeless Way of Wisdom* (Burdett, N.Y.: Larson Publications, 1984), p. 261.

Chapter 4: Yoga: For Whom?

1. For readers of my book *Structures of Consciousness* (Lower Lake, Calif.: Integral Publishing, 1987), which discusses the evolutionary stages mapped out by Jean Gebser, I would like to add the following observation: There is good evidence for a shift from a preeminently mythical (or mythological/analogical) to a more rational/logical (or what Gebser called "mental") style of thinking roughly around 500 B.C.E. We can see this in Greece as much as in India. This cognitive style, however, does not appear to have significantly altered our basic emotional make-up—our need for security and love and our capacity for anger, greed, envy, etc.
2. See Abraham H. Maslow, *The Farther Reaches of Human Nature* (Harmondsworth: Penguin Books, 1973).

3. Shri Yogendra, *Yoga Essays* (Santa Cruz, India: The Yoga Institute, 1978), p. 113.

CHAPTER 7: IS YOGA A RELIGION?

1. On "Christian Yoga," see J. M. Dechanet, *Christian Yoga* (London: Search Press, 1973); *Yoga and God: An Invitation to Christian Yoga* (St. Meinrad, Ind.: Abbey Press, 1975); Justin O'Brien, *Christianity and Yoga: A Meeting of Mystic Paths* (London: Arkana, 1989).

2. See, for instance, the Tamil adept Civavākkiyar cited in Kamil V. Zvelebil, *The Poets of the Powers* (Lower Lake, Calif.: Integral, 1993), p. 85.

CHAPTER 8: YOGA AS ART AND SCIENCE

1. B. K. S. Iyengar, *Light on the Yoga Sūtras of Patanjali* (London: Thorsons, 1993), p. xix.

2. Lucien Price, ed., *Dialogues of Alfred North Whitehead* (New York: Mentor Books, 1956), p. 143.

3. See, e.g., James Funderburk, *Science Studies Yoga* (Honesdale, Pa.: Himalayan International Institute, 1977).

4. B. K. S. Iyengar, *The Art of Yoga* (New Delhi: HarperCollins), p. xiii.

5. Ibid., p. 5.

6. Ibid., p.15.

CHAPTER 9: THE YOGA OF SCIENCE

1. Carl Friedrich von Weizsäcker, *Unity of Nature* (New York: Farrar, Strauss, Giroux, 1980), p. 13.

CHAPTER 11: YOGA IN HINDUISM, BUDDHISM, AND JAINISM

1. See, e.g., Jean-François Jarrige and R. H. Meadow, "The Antecedents of Civilization in the Indus Valley," *Scientific American*, 243: 122–133 (1980) and James G. Shaffer, "The Indus Valley, Baluchistan, and Helmand Traditions: Neolithic Through Bronze Age," in Robert Ehrich, ed., *Chronologies in Old World Archaeology* (Chicago: University of Chicago Press, 3d ed., 1992). See also Colin Renfrew, *Archaeology & Language: The Puzzle of Indo-European Origins* (Cambridge: Cambridge University Press, 1987); Navaratna S. Rajaram and David Frawley, *Vedic Aryans and the Origins of Civilization: A Literary and Scientific Perspective* (New Delhi: Voice of India, 2d ed., 1995); A. Kalyanaraman, *Aryatarangini: The Sage of the Indo-Aryans* (Bombay: Asia Publishing House, 1969), vol. 1.

CHAPTER 13: THE TREE OF HINDU YOGA

1. Sri Aurobindo, *The Synthesis of Yoga* (Pondicherry, India: Sri Aurobindo Ashram, 1976), p. 29.

2. Ibid., p. 29.

3. Ibid., p. 30.

4. Swami Satprakashananda, *Methods of Knowledge* (London: Kegan Paul, Trench, Trubner, 1932), p. 137.

5. Shyam Sundar Goswami, *Laya Yoga* (Rochester, Vt.: Inner Traditions International, 1996), p. 68.

CHAPTER 15: CROSSING THE BOUNDARY BETWEEN HINDUISM
AND BUDDHISM VIA TANTRA-YOGA

1. As part of my early interest in Buddhism, I translated Wolfgang Schumann's *Buddhism* into English and Sangharakshita's *Three Jewels* into German.
2. Mircea Eliade, *Yoga: Immortality and Freedom* (Princeton: Princeton University Press, 1973), p. 200.

CHAPTER 16: VAJRAYĀNA BUDDHIST YOGA

1. The Sanskrit word *vajra* can mean "thunderbolt," "diamond," and "adamantine." In the Vedic era, it referred to God Indra's weapon, the thunderbolt. In Tantra, it symbolizes both the ultimate Reality and compassion. As a scepter, it is one of two ritual implements of Buddhist *tāntrikas*, the other being the bell (*ghantā*), which stands for wisdom.
2. See Chögyal Namkhai Norbu, *The Crystal and the Way of Light: Sutra, Tantra and Dzogchen*. Ed. by John Shane (Ithaca, N.Y.: Snow Lion, 2000), p. 40.
3. Cited in Chögyal Namkhai Norbu, *The Crystal and the Way of Light*, p. 45.

CHAPTER 17: INTRODUCING THE GREAT LITERARY HERITAGE
OF HINDU YOGA

1. A more extensive bibliography can be found in my book *The Yoga Tradition* (Prescott, Ariz.: Hohm Press, 2d ed., 1991).

CHAPTER 18: YOGA SYMBOLISM

1. Sri Aurobindo, *On the Veda* (Pondicherry, India: Sri Aurobindo Ashram, 1956), p. 377.
2. See David Frawley, *Wisdom of the Ancient Seers: Mantras of the Rig Veda* (Salt Lake City, Utah: Passage Press, 1992); Jeanine Miller, *The Vedas: Harmony, Meditation, Fulfilment* (London: Rider, 1974); *The Vision of Cosmic Order in the Vedas* (London: Routledge & Kegan Paul, 1985).
3. See Willard Johnson, *Poetry and Speculation in the Ṛg Veda* (Berkeley: University of California Press, 1980).
4. Heinrich Zimmer, *Myths and Symbols in Indian Art and Civilization*. Edited by J. Campbell (Princeton, N.J.: Princeton University Press, 1972), p. 41.
5. See Sripad Amrit Dange, *Sexual Symbolism from the Vedic Ritual* (Delhi: Ajanta Publications, 1979).
6. See Georg Feuerstein, *Introduction to the Bhagavad-Gītā* (Wheaton, Ill.: Quest Books, 1983), pp. 64–67.

CHAPTER 20: THE TWELVE STEPS OF SPIRITUAL RECOVERY

1. See Georg Feuerstein, *Sacred Sexuality: Living the Vision of the Erotic Spirit* (Los Angeles: J. P. Tarcher, 1992).
2. See Jean Gebser, *The Ever-Present Origin* (Athens, Ohio: Ohio University Press, 1985).
3. See Karl Jaspers, *Vom Ursprung und Ziel der Geschichte* (Frankfurt: Fischer Bücherei, 1956).
4. See Adolf Jánaĉek, "The Message of Patanjali's Yoga-Sūtras," in Shri Yogendra, *Yoga in Modern Life* (Santa Cruz, India: The Yoga Institute, 1966), pp. 118ff.
5. See S. Freud, *The Psychopathology of Everyday Life* (The Hague: A. A. Brill, 1914).
6. See *Collected Works of C. G. Jung*. Volume 9. (Part 1): *Archetypes and the Collective*

Unconscious. Edited and translated by Gerhard Adler and R. F. C. Hull (Princeton: Princeton University Press, 1968).

7. Aldous Huxley, *The Doors of Perception/Heaven and Hell* (Harmondsworth, England: Penguin Books, 1959).
8. Ibid., p. 86.
9. See Jean Gebser, *Der Unsichtbare Ursprung* (The Invisible Origin) (Olten and Freiburg: Walter Verlag, 1970).

CHAPTER 21: HAPPINESS, WELL-BEING, AND REALITY

1. A masochist takes perverse pleasure in physical or emotional pain in specific situations but otherwise, like everyone else, seeks to reduce or avoid pain and suffering.
2. *Little Essays Drawn from the Writings of George Santayana*, by Logan Pearsall Smith with the collaboration of the author (Freeport, N.Y.: Books for Libraries Press, 1967), p. 251.

CHAPTER 24: LIFE IS AN EARTHQUAKE

1. *Mahāvagga* 1.6.19. The five "aggregates" (*skandha*) are form (*rūpa*), i.e., the body; sensation (*vedanā*); perception (*samjnā*); mental composite (*samskāra*), i.e., volition; and consciousness (*vijnāna*).
2. Omraam Mikhaël Aïvanhov, *"Know Thyself,"* Part 1 (Fréjus, France: Prosveta, 1992), p. 221.
3. Omraam Mikhaël Aïvanhov, *Cosmic Moral Laws* (Fréjus, France: Prosveta, 1984), p. 19.

CHAPTER 26: SPIRITUAL FRIENDSHIP

1. Quoted from Jamgon Kongtrul Lodro Taye, *Buddhist Ethics.* Trans. and ed. by The International Translation Committee (Ithaca, N.Y.: Snow Lion, 1998), p. 61.
2. Ibid., p. 61.
3. Quoted from Tsong-kha-pa, *The Great Treatise on the Stages of the Path to Enlightenment.* Trans. by the Lamrim Chenmo Translation Committee (Ithaca, N.Y.: Snow Lion, 2000), vol. 1, p. 72.

CHAPTER 28: THE GURU FUNCTION: BROADCASTING REALITY

1. Guy Claxton, *Wholly Human: Western and Eastern Visions of the Self and Its Perfection* (London: Routledge & Kegan Paul, 1981), p. 98.
2. Letter to Adi Da from anonymous student, 1986.
3. The Sanskrit word *darshana* means literally "vision" or "seeing" and here refers to the act of meditatively beholding the teacher to receive his or her blessings.
4. Ibid.
5. Guy Claxton, *op cit*, p. 98.
6. See Irina Tweedie, *The Chasm of Fire: A Woman's Experience of Liberation Through the Teaching of a Sufi Master* (Tisbury, England: Element Books, 1979). See also the unabridged version of the diary she kept during her discipleship with a Sufi teacher, entitled *Daughter of Fire: A Diary of a Spiritual Training with a Sufi Master* (Nevada City, Calif.: Blue Dolphin, 1986).
7. *Kula-Arnava-Tantra* (13.104, 108, 110). Trans. by Georg Feuerstein.
8. John Welwood, "On Spiritual Authority: Genuine and Counterfeit," in Dick Anthony, Bruce Ecker, and Ken Wilber, *Spiritual Choices: The Problem of Recognizing*

Authentic Paths to Inner Transformation (New York: Paragon House, 1987), pp. 299–300.

9. Ibid., p. 292.
10. Dick Anthony, Bruce Ecker, and Ken Wilber, *op cit*, p. 6.
11. Ram Dass, *Journey of Awakening: A Meditator's Guidebook* (New York: Bantam Books, 1978), p. 126.
12. Omraam Mikhaël Aïvanhov, *What Is a Spiritual Master?* (Fréjus, France: Prosveta, 1984), p. 70.

CHAPTER 31: GRACE HAS A PLACE IN YOGA
1. Swami Niranjanananda, *Yoga Sadhana Panorama* (Munger, Bihar: Bihar School of Yoga, 1997), vol. 2, p. 222.
2. B. K. S. Iyengar, *Light on the Yoga Sūtras of Patañjali* (London: Thorsons, 1996), p. 73.
3. Swami Niranjanananda, *op cit.*, p. 222.

CHAPTER 32: *TAPAS*, OR VOLUNTARY SELF-CHANGE
1. Commonly the Vedic Sanskrit word *bibharti* is rendered as "carries," but Jeanine Miller rightly chose "endures" to convey the patient spiritual work of *tapas*. See Georg Feuerstein and Jeanine Miller, *The Essence of Yoga* (Rochester, Vt.: Inner Traditions International, 1998), p. 97.

CHAPTER 33: THE ART OF PURIFICATION
1. Mikhaël Aïvanhov, *Light Is a Living Spirit* (Fréjus, France: Prosveta, 1987), pp. 91–92.
2. M. K. Gandhi, *An Autobiography: The Story of My Experiments with Truth* (Boston: Beacon Press, 1957), p. 332.
3. Swami Sivananda, *Practice of Yoga* (Sivanandanagar, India: Divine Life Society, 1970), p. 214.

CHAPTER 34: OBSTACLES ON THE PATH ACCORDING TO PATANJALI
1. In Sanskrit the word *ātman* can refer to either the ego-self (*ahamkāra*) or the transcendental Self, or Spirit. Thus this *Gītā* statement could also be interpreted in a more conventional sense: We can be our own worst enemy or our best friend.

CHAPTER 36: SILENCE IS GOLDEN: THE PRACTICE OF MAUNA
1. See Jean Gebser, *The Ever-Present Origin* (Athens: Ohio University Press, 1986).
2. Jean Klein, *Neither This Nor That I Am* (London: Watkins, 1981), p. 90.

CHAPTER 38: LIVING IN THE DARK AGE (KALI-YUGA)
1. See Karl Jaspers, *Vom Ursprung und Ziel der Geschichte* (Munich: Fischer Bucherei, 1956).
2. The Sanskrit term *rajas* stands for the dynamic quality in Nature, which is traditionally used to apply to both external and psychological manifestations.
3. The Sanskrit word *tamas* denotes "inertia," one of the three principal forces of Nature, the other two being *rajas* (the principle of dynamism) and *sattva* (the principle of lucidity). In the golden age, the *sattva* principle was overwhelmingly prevalent. It was increasingly undermined by the other two principles in subsequent world ages.
4. See Oswald Spengler, *Der Untergang des Abendlandes* (Munich: Beck, 1963).
5. See Jean Gebser, *The Ever-Present Origin* (Athens: Ohio University Press, 1985).

6. See, e.g., Sri Aurobindo, *The Life Divine* (Pondicherry, India: Sri Aurobindo Ashram, 1977), 2 vols. See also, e.g., P. Teilhard de Chardin, *The Future of Man* (London: Collins, 1964).
7. See Georg Feuerstein, *Structures of Consciousness: The Genius of Jean Gebser—An Introduction and Critique* (Lower Lake, Calif.: Integral Publishing, 1987).

CHAPTER 39: YOGA AND TERRORISM
1. Georg Feuerstein, Subhash Kak, and David Frawley, *In Search of the Cradle of Civilization* (Wheaton, Ill.: Quest Books, 1995), pp. 271–272.
2. See Matthew White, "Deaths by Mass Unpleasantness: Estimated Totals for the Entire 20th Century," http://users.erols.com/mwhite28/warstat8.htm.
3. C. G. Jung, "Approaching the Unconscious," in *Man and His Symbols*, ed. by Carl G. Jung (New York: Dell, 1968), p. 84.
4. *Harijan*, October 21, 1939, p. 325.
5. See www.tibet.ca/wtnarchive/2000/3/30_2.html.

CHAPTER 40: YOGA BEGINS AND ENDS WITH VIRTUOUS ACTION
1. Tsong-kha-pa, *The Great Treatise on the Stages of the Path to Enlightenment.* Transl. by The Lamrim Chenmo Translation Committee (Ithaca, N.Y.: Snow Lion, 2000), p. 210.
2. Tsongkhapa, *The Principal Teachings of Buddhism*, With a Commentary by Pabongka Rinpoche (Howell, N.Y.: Mahayana Sutra and Tantra Press, 1998), pp. 34–35.
3. On unconventional behavior prior or subsequent to enlightenment, see chapter 30 (Holy Madness).

CHAPTER 43: YOGA AND VEGETARIANISM
1. Quoted from the website of the International Vegetarian Union (IVU).
2. Ibid. (Letter received by the IVU on April 20, 2001.) Quoted from the website of the Department of Information and International Relations, Tibetan Administration, Dharamsala.
3. Dalai Lama. Interview. World Tibet Network, 26 December 2000.

CHAPTER 44: THE PRACTICE OF ECO-YOGA
1. See James G. Lovelock, *Gaia: A New Look at Life on Earth* (New York: Oxford University Press, 1979).
2. The term "Eco-Yoga" was coined by Henryk Skolimowski, *Dancing Shiva in the Ecological Age* (New Delhi: Clarion Books, 1991).

CHAPTER 48: COMPASSION
1. See Nathan Katz, *Buddhist Images of Human Perfection* (Delhi: Motilal Banarsidass, 1989).
2. Tenzin Gyatso [the Dalai Lama], *The World of Tibetan Buddhism* (Boston: Wisdom, 1995), pp. 64–65.

CHAPTER 50: ĀSANAS FOR THE BODY AND THE MIND
1. See Trisha Lamb Feuerstein, "The Health Benefits of Yoga," *Yoga World*, no. 16 (2001), pp. 6–7.
2. In writing the philosophical considerations in this section, I have benefited from Karl

Baier. In his article "On the Philosophical Dimensions of Asana" (which can be found at www.yrec.org/asana.html), Baier argues convincingly that the postures themselves contain a philosophical quality.

3. Ibid.
4. B. K. S. Iyengar, *The Tree of Yoga* (Boston: Shambhala, 1989), p. 48.
5. See B. K. S. Iyengar, "Yoga and Peace," in: *Aṣṭadala Yogamālā (Collected Works)*, vol. 1: *Articles, Lectures, Messages* (New Delhi: Allied Publishers Ltd., 2000), p. 147.

CHAPTER 51: SHAVA-ÂSANA, OR CORPSE POSTURE

1. *Ekāgratā*, or "one-pointedness," is composed of *eka* (one), *agra* (point), and the suffix *tā* ("-ness") or ("-ity"). It is the essential process in the technique of *dhāranā*, or "concentration."
2. See K. N. Udupa, *Stress and Its Management by Yoga* (Delhi: Motilal Banarsidass), 1985.
3. See K. K. Datey, et al., "Shavasana: A Yogic Exercise in the Management of Hypertension," *Angiology*, vol. 20 (1969), pp. 325–333.
4. See Chandra Patel, "Yoga and Biofeedback in the Management of Hypertension," *Lancet* (Nov. 1973), pp. 1053-1055; "Yoga and Biofeedback in the Management of Hypertension" [letter], *Lancet* (Nov. 1973), p. 1212; "Yoga and Biofeedback in Hypertension" [letter], *Lancet* (Dec. 1973), p. 1327; "Yoga and Biofeedback in Hypertension" [letter], *Lancet* (Dec. 1973), pp. 1440–1441; "12-Month Follow-up of Yoga and Biofeedback in the Management of Hypertension," *Lancet* (Jan. 1975), p. 7898; "Yoga and Bio-feedback in the Management of Hypertension," *Journal of Psychosomatic Research*, vol. 19, nos. 5–6 (1975), pp. 355–360; "Yoga and Biofeedback in the Management of Stress in Hypertensive Patients," *Clinical Science and Molecular Medicine* (June 1975), vol. 48, Suppl. 2, pp. 171S–174S; "Transcendental Meditation and Hypertension," *Lancet* (March 1976), p. 539; "Biofeedback-aided Relaxation and Meditation in the Management of Hypertension," *Biofeedback Self Regulation*, vol. 2, no. 1 (1977, pp. 1–41.
5. Swami Muktabodhananda Saraswati, *Hatha Yoga Pradipika: The Light on Hatha Yoga* (Munger, India: Bihar School of Yoga, 1985), p. 112.

CHAPTER 54: BUDDHI-YOGA

1. Here the word *ātman* does not refer to the transcendental Self but to the body as the ordinary person's form of identity.

CHAPTER 55: JNĀNA-YOGA: THE PATH OF WISDOM

1. René Descartes, *Discourse on Method*, trans. John Veitch (La Salle, Ill.: Open Court, 1946), p. 17.
2. *A Practical Guide to Integral Yoga: Extracts Compiled from the Writings of Sri Aurobindo and The Mother* (Pondicherry, India: Sri Aurobindo Ashram, 1955), pp. 241–242.
3. Paul Brunton, *The Notebooks of Paul Brunton*, vol. 1: *Perspectives: The Timeless Way of Wisdom* (Burdett, N.Y.: Larson, 1984), p. 263.
4. The Sanskrit word *buddhi* stems from the verbal root *budh*, meaning "to be awake."
5. The word *manas* is derived from the verbal root *man*, meaning "to think." This Sanskrit term is related to the Latin word *mens*.
6. *Brihad-Āranyaka-Upanishad* (3.9.26).

7. *Brihad-Āranyaka-Upanishad* (2.4.14).

Chapter 56: "That Art Thou"—The Essence of Nondualist Yoga

1. See Paul Brunton, *The Notebooks of Paul Brunton.* Vol. 10: *The Orient: Its Legacy to the West* (Burdett, N.Y.: Larson, 1987).
2. See Anthony J. Alston, trans., *The Thousand Teachings of Śamkara* [*Upadesha-Sahasrī*] (London: Shanti Sadan, 1990); Swami Chinmayananda, *Talks on Śankara's Vivekachoodamani* [*Viveka-Cūdāmani*] (Bombay: Central Chinmaya Mission Trust, 1976).
3. See Paul Brunton, *A Search in Secret India* (York Beach, Maine: Samuel Weiser, 1985). See also Arthur Osborne, *The Teachings of Ramana Maharshi* (York Beach, Maine: Samuel Weiser, 1995).
4. See Robert Powell, *The Wisdom of Sri Nisargadatta Maharaj* (New York: Globe Press Books, 1992).

Chapter 57: Discernment and Self-Transcendence

1. See Ken Wilber, *The Atman Project* (Wheaton, Ill.: Theosophical Publishing House, 1980).
2. These two sayings are respectively written in transliterated Sanskrit *idam nāham* and *tan nāham.*
3. *Neti* is composed the two words *na iti* (not thus). This is a classic Upanishadic maxim, which affirms our identity with the all-comprising Self.
4. This is a classic Upanishadic maxim, which affirms our identity with all-comprising Self.

Chapter 58: Karma-Yoga: The Way of Self-Transcending Action

1. M. K. Gandhi, *An Autobiography: The Story of My Experiments with Truth* (Boston: Beacon Press, 1957), p. 265.
2. Ibid., p. 504.
3. Ibid., p. 504.
4. See Robert A. McDermot, ed., *The Essential Aurobindo* (New York: Schocken Books, 1973), p. 116.

Chapter 59: Bhakti-Yoga: "Worship Me with Love"

1. The *anāhata-cakra*, which is also known as the *hrit-padma* (heart lotus), is one of seven principal psychoenergetic centers of the body.
2. See the translation by Swami Tyagisananda, *Narada Bhakti Sutras* (Mylapore, India: Ramakrishna Math, 5th ed. 1972). For further study, see the following works: Bhaktivedanta Swami, *The Nectar of Devotion* (New York: Bhaktivedanta Book Trust, 1979); Swami Sivananda, *Essence of Bhakti Yoga* (Sivanandanagar, India: Sivananda Literature Research institute, 1960); Swami Vivekananda, *Bhakti-Yoga* (Calcutta: Advaita Ashram, 1970), and Prem Prakash, *The Yoga of Spiritual Devotion: A Modern Translation of the Narada Bhakti Sutras* (Rochester, Vt.: Inner Traditions International, 1998).
3. For the playful relationship between Krishna and the cowherd girls, see David R. Kinsley, *The Divine Player: A Study of Kṛṣṇa Līlā* (Delhi: Banarsidass, 1979).
4. John Welwood, *Journey of the Heart: Intimate Relationship and the Path of Love* (New York: HarperCollins, 1990), p. 39.

CHAPTER 62: FAITH AND SURRENDER: A NEW LOOK
AT THE EIGHTFOLD PATH

1. See Paul Tillich's *The Courage to Be* (New Haven, Conn.: Yale University Press, 1952).
2. I owe this particular insight to Professor Paul Tillich.
3. See chapter 69 for a discussion of the employment of sexual energies in certain schools of Tantra.
4. This distinction was made by Adam Curie in his book *Mystics and Militants: A Study of Awareness, Identity, and Social Action* (London: Tavistock Publications, 1972).
5. *Ashtāvakra-Samhitā* 2.21 and 25.
6. *Ashtāvakra-Samhitā* 18.78 and 18.80.

CHAPTER 65: THE SACRED SYLLABLE *Om*

1. Max Müller, *Three Lectures on the Vedānta Philosophy* (London: Longmans, Green, and Co., 1894), p. 116.
2. Ibid.
3. See Swami Sankarananda, *The Rigvedic Culture of the Pre-Historic Indus* (Calcutta: Ramakrishna Vedanta Math, 1942), p. 75.
4. See Vihari-Lala Mitra, *The Yoga-Vasishtha-Maharamayana* (Calcutta: Bonnerjee and Co., 1891), vol. 1., p. 39. Apparently, Mitra got this idea from Ram Mohan Roy, the founder of Brahma Samaj.
5. Ibid., p. 46. In linking *om* with *Amen*, Mitra took his cue from the great Sanskrit scholar Rajendra-Lala Mitra.
6. See, e.g., Georg Feuerstein, Subhash Kak, and David Frawley, *In Search of the Cradle of Civilization: New Light on Ancient India* (Wheaton, Ill.: Quest Books, 1996).
7. Max Müller, *op cit*, p. 116.

CHAPTER 66: MUDRĀS: GESTURES OF WHOLENESS

1. For a more detailed discussion of *mudrās*, see Georg Feuerstein, *Tantra: The Path of Ecstasy* (Boston: Shambhala Publications, 1998), pp. 207–217.
2. See Yogamaharishi Dr. Swami Gitananda Giri, *Frankly Speaking* (Chinnamudaliarchavady, India: Satya Press, 1997), p. 136.
3. Ibid., p. 137.

CHAPTER 70: SEX, ASCETICISM, AND MYTHOLOGY

1. See, e.g., Bertrand Russell, *Unpopular Essays* (New York: Simon and Schuster, 1967), p. 150.

CHAPTER 71: PATHWAYS TO RELAXATION AND MEDITATION

1. See Judith Lasater, *Relax and Renew* (Berkeley, Calif.: Rodmell Press, 1995).
2. Herbert Benson, *The Relaxation Response* (New York: Avon Books, 1996), pp. 72-73.
3. Yoga Maharishi Dr. Swami Gitananda Giri, "Shava Asana—The Corpse Posture," *Yoga Life*, vol. 27, no. 5 (May 1996), pp. 3–12. *Yoga Life* is a monthly magazine published by the late Swami Gitananda's ashram. It always contains valuable information about Yoga practice, which is not easily found elsewhere.
4. Although Swami Gitananda did not explain *prashrita* (misspelled *prashritha*), it is derived from the prefix *pra* and the verbal root *shrī*, forming the stem *shraya*. However, since *prashaya* is usually used to convey bending forward deferentially, one might want to consider *uttāna-shaya* instead, which means "resting (with the face) upward."

CHAPTER 72: WHAT IS MEDITATION?

1. John H. Clark, *A Map of Mental States* (London: Routledge & Kegan Paul, 1983), p. 29.
2. Robert E. Ornstein, *The Psychology of Consciousness* (San Francisco: W.H. Freeman, 1972), p. 107.
3. John Welwood, ed., *The Meeting of the Ways: Explorations in East-West Psychology* (New York: Schocken Books, 1979), p. 117.
4. C. Maxwell Cade and Nona Coxhead, *The Awakened Mind: Biofeedback and the Development of Higher States of Awareness* (Longmead, England: Element Books, 1987), p. 95.
5. Daniel Goleman, "Meditation: Doorway to the Transpersonal," in Robert N. Walsh and Frances Vaughan, eds., *Beyond Ego: Transpersonal Dimensions in Psychology* (Los Angeles: J. P. Tarcher, 1980), p. 136.
6. See Jeanine Miller, *The Vedas: Harmony, Meditation and Fulfillment* (London: Rider, 1974).
7. Paul Brunton, *The Notebooks of Paul Brunton*, vol. 4, part 1: *Meditation* (Burdett, N.Y.: Larson, 1986), pp. 172–173.
8. See David W. Orme-Johnson and John T. Farrow, eds. *Scientific Research on the Transcendental Meditation and TM-Sidhi program: Collected Papers*, vol. 1 (Rheinweiler, Germany: Maharishi European Research University Press, 1977).

CHAPTER 73: PRAYER IN YOGA

1. Larry Dossey, *Healing Words* (New York: HarperCollins, 1993), pp. xvii–xviii.

CHAPTER 75: THE SERPENT POWER AND SPIRITUAL LIFE

1. See Lee Sannella, *The Kundalini Experience: Psychosis or Transcendence?* (Lower Lake, Calif.: Integral Publishing, 1992).
2. See *Talks with Sri Ramana Maharshi*, ed. by Sadhu Arunachala (Major A. W. Chadwick) (Tiruvannamalai, India: Sri Ramanasramam, 9th ed., 1994), p. 240.

CHAPTER 76: WHO OR WHAT IS THE SELF IN SELF-REALIZATION?

1. See Alan Watts, *Psychotherapy East and West* (New York: Mentor Books, 1961).

Glossary
Key Sanskrit Terms of Hindu Yoga

ABHYĀSA   Practice. See also *vairāgya*.

ĀCĀRYA (sometimes spelled *āchārya* in English)   A preceptor, instructor. See also *guru*.

ADVAITA (nonduality)   The truth and teaching that there is only one Reality (*ātman, brahman*), especially as found in the *Upanishads*. See also *Vedānta*.

AHAMKĀRA (I-maker)   The individuation principle, or ego, which must be transcended. See also *asmitā*. See also *buddhi, manas*.

AHIMSĀ (nonharming)   The single most important moral discipline (*yama*).

ĀKĀSHA (ether/space)   The first of the five material elements of which the physical universe is composed; also used to designate "inner" space, that is, the space of consciousness (called *cid-ākāsha*).

AMRITA (immortal/immortality)   A designation of the deathless Spirit (*ātman, purusha*); also the nectar of immortality that oozes from the psychoenergetic center at the crown of the head (*sahasrāra-cakra*, see *cakra*) when it is activated and transforms the body into a "divine body" (*divya-deha*).

ĀNANDA (bliss)   The condition of utter joy, which is an essential quality of the ultimate Reality (*tattva*).

ANGA (limb)   A fundamental category of the yogic path, such as *āsana, dhāranā, dhyāna, niyama, prānāyāma, pratyāhāra, samādhi, yama*; also the body (*deha, sharīra*).

ĀRANYAKA (that which pertains to the forest)   An early type of ritual text used by forest-dwelling renouncers. See also *Brahmana, Upanishad, Veda*.

ARJUNA (White)   One of the five Pāndava princes who fought in the great war depicted in the *Mahābhārata*, disciple of the God-man Krishna whose teachings can be found in the *Bhagavad-Gītā*.

ĀSANA (seat)   A physical posture (see also *anga, mudrā*); the third limb (*anga*) of Patanjali's eightfold path (*ashta-anga-yoga*); originally this meant only meditation posture, but subsequently, in Hatha-Yoga, this aspect of the yogic path was greatly developed.

ĀSHRAMA (that where effort is made)   A hermitage; also a stage of life, such as *brahmacarya*, householder, forest dweller, and complete renouncer (*samnyāsin*).

ASHTA-ANGA-YOGA, ASHTĀNGA-YOGA (eight-limbed union)   The eightfold Yoga of Patanjali, consisting of moral discipline (*yama*), self-restraint (*niyama*), posture (*āsana*), breath control (*prānāyāma*), sensory inhibition (*pratyāhāra*), concentration (*dhāranā*), meditation (*dhyāna*), and ecstasy (*samādhi*), leading to liberation (*kaivalya*).

ASMITĀ (I-am-ness)   A concept of Patanjali's eight-limbed Yoga, roughly synonymous with *ahamkāra*.

ĀTMAN (self)   The transcendental Self, or Spirit, which is eternal and superconscious; our true nature or identity; sometimes a distinction is made between the *ātman* as the individual self and the *parama-ātman* as the transcendental Self. See also *purusha*. See also *brahman*.

AVADHŪTA (he who has shed [everything])   A radical type of renouncer (*samnyāsin*) who often engages in unconventional behavior.

AVIDYĀ (ignorance)   The root cause of suffering (*duhkha*); also called *ajnāna*. See also *vidyā*.

ĀYURVEDA, ĀYUR-VEDA (life science)   One of India's traditional systems of medicine, the other being South India's Siddha medicine.

BANDHA (bond/bondage)   The fact that human beings are typically bound by ignorance (*avidyā*), which causes them to lead a life governed by karmic habit rather than inner freedom generated through wisdom (*vidyā, jnāna*).

BHAGAVAD-GĪTĀ (Lord's Song)   The oldest full-fledged Yoga book found embedded in the *Mahābhārata* and containing the teachings on Karma-Yoga (the path of self-transcending action), Sāmkhya-Yoga (the path of discerning the principles of existence correctly), and Bhakti-Yoga (the path of devotion), as given by the God-man Krishna to Prince Arjuna on the battlefield 3,500 years or more ago.

BHĀGAVATA-PURĀNA (Ancient [Tradition] of the Bhāgavatas)   A voluminous tenth-century scripture held sacred by the devotees of the Divine in the form of Vishnu, especially in his incarnate form as Krishna; also called *Shrīmad-Bhāgavata*.

BHAKTA (devotee)   A disciple practicing Bhakti-Yoga.

BHAKTI (devotion/love)   The love of the *bhakta* toward the Divine or the *guru* as a manifestation of the Divine; also the love of the Divine toward the devotee.

BHAKTI-SŪTRA (Aphorisms on Devotion)   An aphoristic work on devotional Yoga authored by Sage Nārada; another text by the same title is ascribed to Sage Shāndilya.

BHAKTI-YOGA (Yoga of devotion)   A major branch of the Yoga tradition, utilizing the feeling capacity to connect with the ultimate Reality conceived as a supreme Person (*uttama-purusha*).

BINDU (seed/point)   The creative potency of anything where all energies are focused; the dot (also called *tilaka*) worn on the forehead as indicative of the third eye.

BODHI (enlightenment)   The state of the awakened master, or *buddha*.

BODHISATTVA (enlightenment being)   In Mahāyāna Buddhist Yoga, the individual who, motivated by compassion (*karunā*), is committed to achieving enlightenment for the sake of all other beings.

BRAHMA (he who has grown expansive)   The Creator of the universe, the first principle (*tattva*) to emerge out of the ultimate Reality (*brahman*).

BRAHMACARYA (from *brahma* and *acarya* "brahmic conduct")   The discipline of chastity, which produces *ojas*.

BRAHMAN (that which has grown expansive)   The ultimate Reality (see also *ātman, purusha*).

BRĀHMANA   A brahmin, a member of the highest social class of traditional Indian society; also an early type of ritual text explicating the rituals and mythology of the four *Vedas*. See also *Āranyaka, Upanishad, Veda*.

BUDDHA (awakened)   A designation of the person who has attained enlightenment (*bodhi*) and therefore inner freedom; honorific title of Gautama, the founder of Buddhism, who lived in the sixth century B.C.E.

BUDDHI (she who is conscious, awake)   The higher mind, which is the seat of wisdom (*vidyā, jnāna*). See also *manas*.

CAKRA (wheel)   Literally, the wheel of a wagon; metaphorically, one of the psychoenergetic centers of the subtle body (*sūkshma-sharīra*); in Buddhist Yoga, five such centers are known, while in Hindu Yoga often seven or more such centers are mentioned: *mūla-ādhāra-cakra* (*mūlādhāra-cakra*) at the base of the spine, *svadhishthāna-cakra* at the genitals, *manipura-cakra* at the navel, *anāhata-cakra* at the heart, *vishuddha-* or *vishuddhi-cakra* at the throat, *ājnā-cakra* in the middle of the head, and *sahasrāra-cakra* at the top of the head.

CIN-MUDRĀ (consciousness seal)   A common hand gesture (*mudrā*) in meditation (*dhyāna*), which is formed by bringing the tips of the index finger and the thumb together, while the remaining fingers are kept straight.

CIT (consciousness)   The superconscious ultimate Reality (see *ātman, brahman*).

CITTA (that which is conscious)   Ordinary consciousness, the mind, as opposed to *cit*.

DARSHANA (seeing)   Vision in the literal and metaphorical sense; a system of philosophy, such as the *yoga-darshana* of Patanjali. See also *drishti*.

DEVA (he who is shining)   A male deity, such as Shiva, Vishnu, or Krishna, either in the sense of the ultimate Reality or a high angelic being.

DEVĪ (she who is shining)   A female deity such as Pārvatī, Lakshmī, or Rādhā, either in the sense of the ultimate Reality (in its feminine pole) or a high angelic being.

DHĀRANĀ (holding)   Concentration, the sixth limb (*anga*) of Patanjali's eight-limbed Yoga.

DHARMA (bearer)   A term of numerous meanings; often used in the sense of "law," "lawfulness," "virtue," "righteousness," "norm."

DHYĀNA (ideating)   Meditation, the seventh limb (*anga*) of Patanjali's eight-limbed Yoga.

DĪKSHĀ (initiation)   The act and condition of induction into the hidden aspects of Yoga or a particular lineage of teachers; all traditional Yoga is initiatory.

DRISHTI (view/sight)   Yogic gazing, such as at the tip of the nose or the spot between the eyebrows; see also *darshana*.

DUHKHA (bad axle space)   Suffering, a fundamental fact of life, caused by ignorance (*avidyā*) of our true nature (i.e., the Self or *ātman*).

GĀYATRĪ-MANTRA   A famous Vedic *mantra* recited particularly at sunrise: *tat savitur varenyam bhargo devasya dhīmahi dhiyo yo nah pracodayāt*, "Let us contemplate the most excellent splendor of God Savitri, so that he may inspire our visions."

GHERANDA-SAMHITĀ ([Sage] Gheranda's Compendium)   One of three major manuals of classical Hatha-Yoga, composed in the seventeenth century; see also *Hatha-Yoga-Pradīpikā, Shiva-Samhitā*.

GORAKSHA (Cow Protector)   Traditionally said to be the founding adept of Hatha-Yoga, a disciple of Matsyendra.

GRANTHI (knot)   Any one of three common blockages in the central pathway (*sushumnā-nādī*) preventing the full ascent of the serpent power (*kundalinī-shakti*); the three knots are known as *brahma-granthi* (at the lowest psychoenergetic center of the subtle body), the *vishnu-granthi* (at the heart), and the *rudra-granthi* (at the eyebrow center).

GUNA (quality)   A term that has numerous meanings, including "virtue"; often refers to any of the three primary "qualities" or constituents of Nature (*prakriti*): *tamas* (the principle of inertia), *rajas* (the dynamic principle), and *sattva* (the principle of lucidity).

GURU (he who is heavy, weighty)   A spiritual teacher. See also *ācārya*.

GURU-BHAKTI (teacher devotion)   A disciple's self-transcending devotion to the *guru*. See also *bhakti*.

GURU-GĪTĀ (Guru's Song)   A text in praise of the *guru*, often chanted in *āshramas*.

GURU-YOGA (Yoga [relating to] the teacher)   A yogic approach that makes the *guru* the fulcrum of a disciple's practice; all traditional forms of Yoga contain a strong element of *guru-yoga*.

HAMSA (swan/gander)   Apart from the literal meaning, this term also refers to the breath (*prāna*) as it moves within the body; the individuated consciousness (*jīva*) propelled by the breath. See *jīva-ātman*. See also *parama-hamsa*.

HATHA-YOGA (Forceful Yoga)   A major branch of Yoga, developed by Goraksha and other adepts c. 1000 C.E., and emphasizing the physical aspects of the transformative path, notably postures (*āsana*) and cleansing techniques (*shodhana*), but also breath control (*prānāyāma*).

HATHA-YOGA-PRADĪPIKĀ (Light on Hatha-Yoga)   One of three classical manuals on Hatha-Yoga, authored by Svātmārāma Yogendra in the fourteenth century.

HIRANYAGARBHA (Golden Germ)   The mythical founder of Yoga; the first cosmological principle (*tattva*) to emerge out of the infinite Reality; also called Brahma.

IDĀ-NĀDĪ (pale conduit)   The *prāna* current or arc ascending on the left side of the central channel (*sushumnā-nādī*) associated with the parasympathetic nervous system and having a cooling or calming effect on the mind when activated. See also *pingalā-nādī*.

ĪSHVARA (ruler)   The Lord; referring either to the Creator (see *Brahma*) or, in Patanjali's *yoga-darshana*, to a special transcendental Self (*purusha*).

ĪSHVARA-PRANIDHĀNA (dedication to the Lord)   In Patanjali's eight-limbed Yoga one of the practices of self-restraint (*niyama*). See also *Bhakti-Yoga*.

JAINA (sometimes Jain)   Pertaining to the *jīnas* (conquerors), the liberated adepts of Jainism; a member of Jainism, the spiritual tradition founded by Vardhamana Mahāvīra, a contemporary of Gautama the Buddha.

JAPA (muttering)   The recitation of *mantras*.

JĪVA-ĀTMAN, JĪVĀTMAN (individual self)   The individuated consciousness, as opposed to the ultimate Self (*parama-ātman*).

JĪVAN-MUKTA (he who is liberated while alive)   An adept who, while still embodied, has attained liberation (*moksha*).

JĪVAN-MUKTI (living liberation)   The state of liberation while being embodied; see also *videha-mukti*.

JNĀNA (knowledge/wisdom)   Both worldly knowledge or world-transcending wisdom, depending on the context. See also *prajñā*. See also *avidyā*.

JNĀNA-YOGA (Yoga of wisdom)   The path to liberation based on wisdom, or the direct intuition of the transcendental Self (*ātman*) through the steady application of discernment between the Real and the unreal and renunciation of what has been identified as unreal (or inconsequential to the achievement of liberation).

KAIVALYA (isolation)   The state of absolute freedom from conditioned existence, as explained in *ashta-anga-yoga*; in the nondualistic (*advaita*) traditions of India, this is usually called *moksha* or *mukti* (meaning "release" from the fetters of ignorance, or *avidyā*).

KĀLĪ   A Goddess embodying the fierce (dissolving) aspect of the Divine.

KALI-YUGA   The dark age of spiritual and moral decline, said to be current now; *kali* does not refer to the Goddess Kālī but to the losing throw of a die.

KĀMA (desire)   The appetite for sensual pleasure blocking the path to true bliss (*ānanda*); the only desire conducive to freedom is the impulse toward liberation, called *mumukshutva*.

KAPILA (He who is red)   A great sage, the quasi-mythical founder of the Sāmkhya tradition, who is said to have composed the *Sāmkhya-Sūtra* (which, however, appears to be of a much later date).

KARMAN, KARMA (action)   Activity of any kind, including ritual acts; said to be binding only so long as engaged in a self-centered way; the "karmic" consequence of one's actions; destiny.

KARMA-YOGA (Yoga of action)   The liberating path of self-transcending action.

KARUNĀ (compassion)   Universal sympathy; in Buddhist Yoga the complement of wisdom (*prajnā*).

KHECARĪ-MUDRĀ (space-walking seal)   The Tantric practice of curling the tongue back against the upper palate in order to seal the life energy (*prāna*). See also *mudrā*.

KOSHA (casing)   Any one of five "envelopes" surrounding the transcendental Self (*ātman*) and thus blocking its light: *anna-maya-kosha* (envelope made of food, the physical body), *prāna-maya-kosha* (envelope made of life force), *mano-maya-kosha* (envelope made of mind), *vijnāna-maya-kosha* (envelope made of consciousness), and *ānanda-maya-kosha* (envelope made of bliss); some older traditions regard the last *kosha* as identical with the Self (*ātman*).

KRISHNA (Puller)   An incarnation of God Vishnu, the God-man whose teachings can be found in the *Bhagavad-Gītā* and the *Bhāgavata-Purāna*.

KUMBHAKA (potlike)   Breath retention. See also *pūraka, recaka*.

KUNDALINĪ-SHAKTI (coiled power)   According to Tantra and Hatha-Yoga, the serpent power or spiritual energy, which exists in potential form at the lowest psychoenergetic center of the body (i.e., the *mūla-ādhāra-cakra*) and which must be awakened and guided to the center at the crown (i.e., the *sahasrāra-cakra*) for full enlightenment to occur.

KUNDALINĪ-YOGA   The yogic path focusing on the *kundalinī* process as a means of liberation.

LAYA-YOGA (Yoga of dissolution)   An advanced form or process of Tantric Yoga by which the energies associated with the various psychoenergetic centers (*cakra*) of the subtle body are gradually dissolved through the ascent of the serpent power (*kundalinī-shakti*).

LINGA (mark)   The phallus as a principle of creativity; a symbol of God Shiva. See also *yoni*.

MAHĀBHĀRATA (Great Bharata)   One of India's two great ancient epics telling of the great war between the Pāndavas and the Kauravas and serving as a repository for many spiritual and moral teachings.

MAHĀTMA (from *mahā-ātman*, great self)   An honorific title (meaning something like a great soul) bestowed on particularly meritorious individuals, such as Gandhi.

MAITHUNĀ (twinning)   The Tantric sexual ritual in which the participants view each other as Shiva and Shakti respectively.

MANAS (mind)   The lower mind, which is bound to the senses and yields information (*vijnāna*) rather than wisdom (*jnāna, vidyā*). See also *buddhi*.

MANDALA (circle)   A circular design symbolizing the cosmos and specific to a deity.

MANTRA (from the verbal root *man* "to think")   A sacred sound or phrase, such as *om*, *hūm*, or *om namah shivāya*, that has a transformative effect on the mind of the individual reciting it; to be ultimately effective, a mantra needs to be given in an initiatory context (*dīkshā*).

MANTRA-YOGA   The yogic path utilizing mantras as the primary means of liberation.

MARMAN (lethal [spot])   In Āyur-Veda and Yoga, a vital spot on the physical body where energy is concentrated or blocked. See also *granthi*.

MATSYENDRA (Lord of Fish)   An early Tantric master who founded the Yoginī-Kaula school and is remembered as a teacher of Goraksha.

MĀYĀ (she who measures)   The deluding or illusive power of the world; illusion by which the world is seen as separate from the ultimate singular Reality (*ātman*).

MOKSHA (release)   The condition of freedom from ignorance (*avidyā*) and the binding effect of karma; also called *mukti, kaivalya*.

MUDRĀ (seal)   A hand gesture (such as *cin-mudrā*) or whole-body gesture (such as *viparīta-karanī-mudrā*); also a designation of the feminine partner in the Tantric sexual ritual.

MUNI (he who is silent)   A sage.

NĀDA (sound)   The inner sound, as it can be heard through the practice of Nāda-Yoga or Kundalinī-Yoga.

NĀDA-YOGA (Yoga of the [inner] sound)   The Yoga or process of producing and intently listening to the inner sound as a means of concentration and ecstatic self-transcendence.

NĀDĪ (conduit)   One of 72,000 or more subtle channels along or through which the life force (*prāna*) circulates of which the three most important ones are the *idā-nādī*, *pingalā-nādī*, and *sushumnā-nādī*.

NĀDĪ-SHODHANA (channel cleansing)   The practice of purifying the conduits, especially by means of breath control (*prānāyāma*).

NĀRADA   A great sage associated with music, who taught Bhakti-Yoga and is attributed with the authorship of one of two *Bhakti-Sūtras*.

NĀTHA (lord)   Appellation of many North Indian masters of Yoga, in particular adepts of the Kānphāta (Split-ear) school allegedly founded by Goraksha.

NETI-NETI (not thus, not thus)   An Upanishadic expression meant to convey that the ultimate Reality is neither this nor that, that is, is beyond all description.

NIRODHA (restriction/control)   In Patanjali's eight-limbed Yoga, the very basis of the process of concentration, meditation, and ecstasy; in the first instance, the restriction of the "whirls of the mind" (*citta-vritti*).

NIYAMA ([self-]restraint)   The second limb of Patanjali's eightfold path, which consists of purity (*shauca*), contentment (*samtosha*), austerity (*tapas*), study (*svādhyāya*), and dedication to the Lord (*īshvara-pranidhāna*).

NYĀSA (placing)   The Tantric practice of infusing various body parts with life force (*prāna*) by touching or thinking of the respective physical area.

OJAS (vitality)   The subtle energy produced through practice, especially the discipline of chastity (*brahmacarya*).

OM   The original mantra symbolizing the ultimate Reality, which is prefixed to many mantric utterances.

PARAMA-ĀTMAN or PARAMĀTMAN (supreme self)   The transcendental Self, which is singular, as opposed to the individuated self (*jīva-ātman*) that exists in countless numbers in the form of living beings.

PARAMA-HAMSA, PARAMAHANSA (supreme swan)   An honorific title given to great adepts, such as Ramakrishna and Yogananda.

PATANJALI   Compiler of the *Yoga-Sūtra*, who lived around 150/200 C.E.

PINGALĀ-NĀDĪ (reddish conduit)   The *prāna* current or arc ascending on the right side of the central channel (*sushumnā-nādī*) and associated with the sympathetic nervous system and having an energizing effect on the mind when activated. See also *idā-nādī*.

PRAJÑĀ (wisdom)   The opposite of spiritual ignorance (*ajnāna, avidyā*); one of two means of liberation in Buddhist Yoga, the other being skillful means (*upāya*), i.e., compassion (*karunā*).

PRAKRITI (creatrix)   Nature, which is multilevel and, according to Patanjali's *yoga-darshana*, consists of an eternal dimension (called *pradhāna* or "foundation"), levels of subtle existence (called *sūkshma-parvan*), and the physical or coarse realm (called *sthūla-parvan*); all of Nature is deemed unconscious (*acit*), and therefore it is viewed as being in opposition to the transcendental Self or Spirit (*purusha*).

PRAKRITI-LAYA (merging into Nature)   A high-level state of existence that falls short of actual liberation (*kaivalya*); the being who has attained that state.

PRĀNA (life/breath)   Life in general; the life force sustaining the body; the breath as an external manifestation of the subtle life force.

PRĀNĀYĀMA (from *prāna* and *āyāma*, "life/breath extension")   Breath control, the fourth limb (*anga*) of Patanjali's eightfold path, consisting of conscious inhalation (*pūraka*), retention (*kumbhaka*), and exhalation (*recaka*); at an advanced state, breath retention occurs spontaneously for longer periods of time.

PRASĀDA (grace/clarity)   Divine grace; mental clarity.

PRATYĀHĀRA (withdrawal)   Sensory inhibition, the fifth limb (*anga*) of Patanjali's eightfold path.

PŪJĀ (worship)   Ritual worship, which is an important aspect of many forms of Yoga, notably Bhakti-Yoga and Tantra.

PŪRAKA (filling in)   Inhalation, an aspect of breath control (*prānāyāma*).

PURĀNA (Ancient [History])   A type of popular encyclopedia dealing with royal genealogy, cosmology, philosophy, and ritual; there are eighteen major and many more minor works of this nature.

PURUSHA (male)   The transcendental Self (*ātman*) or Spirit, a designation that is mostly used in Sāmkhya and Patanjali's *yoga-darshana*.

RĀDHĀ   The God-man Krishna's spouse; a name of the divine Mother.

RĀJA-YOGA (Royal Yoga)   A late medieval designation of Patanjali's eightfold *yoga-darshana*, also known as Classical Yoga.

RĀMA   An incarnation of God Vishnu preceding Krishna; the principal hero of the *Rāmāyana*.

RĀMĀYĀNA (Rāma's life)   One of India's two great national epics telling the story of Rāma; see also *Mahābhārata*.

RECAKA (expulsion)   Exhalation, an aspect of breath control (*prānāyāma*).

RIG-VEDA   See *Veda*.

RISHI (seer)   A category of Vedic sage; an honorific title of certain venerated masters, such as the South Indian sage Ramana, who is known as *maharshi* (from *maha* meaning "great" and *rishi*). See also *muni*.

SADHANA (accomplishing)   Spiritual discipline leading to *siddhi* (perfection or accomplishment); the term is specifically used in Tantra.

SAHAJA (together born)   A medieval term denoting the fact that the transcendental Reality and the empirical reality are not truly separate but coexist, or with the latter being an aspect or misperception of the former; often rendered as "spontaneous" or "spontaneity"; the *sahaja* state is the natural condition, that is, enlightenment or realization.

SAMADHI (putting together)   The ecstatic or unitive state in which the meditator becomes one with the object of meditation, the eighth and final limb (*anga*) of Patanjali's eightfold path; there are many types of *samadhi*, the most significant distinction being between *samprajnata* (conscious) and *asamprajnata* (supraconscious) ecstasy; only the latter leads to the dissolution of the karmic factors deep within the mind; beyond both types of ecstasy is enlightenment, which is also sometimes called *sahaja-samadhi* or the condition of "natural" or "spontaneous" ecstasy, where there is perfect continuity of superconscious throughout waking, dreaming, and sleeping.

SAMATVA or SAMATA (evenness)   The mental condition of harmony, balance.

SAMKHYA (Number/Enumeration)   One of the main traditions of Hinduism, which is concerned with the classification of the principles (*tattva*) of existence and their proper discernment in order to distinguish between Spirit (*purusha*) and the various aspects of Nature (*prakriti*); this influential system grew out of the ancient (pre-Buddhist) Samkhya-Yoga tradition and was codified in the *Samkhya-Karika* of Ishvara Krishna (c. 350 C.E.).

SAMNYASA (casting off)   The state of renunciation, which is the fourth and final stage of life (see *ashrama*) and consisting primarily in an inner turning away from what is understood to be finite and secondarily in an external letting go of finite things; see also *vairagya*.

SAMNYASIN (he who has cast off)   A renouncer.

SAMPRAJNATA-SAMADHI   See *samadhi*.

SAMSARA (confluence)   The finite world of change, as opposed to the ultimate Reality (*brahman* or *nirvana*).

SAMSKARA (activator)   The subconscious impression left behind by each act of volition, which, in turn, leads to renewed psychomental activity; the countless *samskaras* hidden in the depth of the mind are ultimately eliminated only in *asamprajnata-samadhi* (see *samadhi*).

SAMYAMA (constraint)   The combined practice of concentration (*dharana*), meditation (*dhyana*), and ecstasy (*samadhi*) in regard to the same object.

SAT (being/reality/truth)   The ultimate Reality (*atman* or *brahman*).

SAT-SANGA (true company/company of Truth)   The practice of frequenting the good company of saints, sages, Self-realized adepts, and their disciples, in whose company the ultimate Reality can be felt more palpably.

SATYA (truth/truthfulness)   Truth, a designation of the ultimate Reality; also the practice of truthfulness, which is an aspect of moral discipline (*yama*).

SHAKTI (power)   The ultimate Reality in its feminine aspect, or the power pole of the Divine. See also *kundalini-shakti*.

SHAKTI-PĀTA (descent of power)   The process of initiation, or spiritual baptism, by means of the benign transmission of an advanced or even enlightened adept (*siddha*), which awakens the *shakti* within a disciple, thereby initiating or enhancing the process of liberation.

SHANKARA (He who is benevolent)   The eighth-century adept who was the greatest proponent of nondualism (Advaita Vedānta) and whose philosophical school was probably responsible for the decline of Buddhism in India.

SHISHYA (student/disciple)   The initiated disciple of a guru.

SHIVA (He who is benign)   The Divine; a deity that has served *yogins* as an archetypal model throughout the ages.

SHIVA-SAMHITĀ (Shiva's Compendium)   One of three major manuals of classical Hatha-Yoga, probably composed in the eighteenth century.

SHIVA-SŪTRA (Shiva's Aphorisms)   Like the *Yoga-Sūtra* of Patanjali, a classical work on Yoga, as taught in the Shaivism of Kashmir; authored by Vasugupta (ninth century C.E.).

SHODHANA (cleansing/purification)   A fundamental aspect of all yogic paths; a category of purification practices in Hatha-Yoga.

SHRADDHĀ (faith)   An essential disposition on the yogic path, which must be distinguished from mere belief.

SHUDDHI (purification/purity)   The state of purity; a synonym of *shodhana*.

SIDDHA (accomplished)   An adept, often of Tantra; if fully Self-realized, the designation *mahā-siddha* or "great adept" is often used.

SIDDHA-YOGA (Yoga of the adepts)   A designation applied especially to the Yoga of Kashmiri Shaivism, as taught by Swami Muktananda (twentieth century).

SIDDHI (accomplishment/perfection)   Spiritual perfection, the attainment of flawless identity with the ultimate Reality (*ātman* or *brahman*); paranormal ability, of which the Yoga tradition knows many kinds.

SPANDA (vibration)   A key concept of Kashmir's Shaivism according to which the ultimate Reality itself "quivers," that is, is inherently creative rather than static (as conceived in Advaita Vedānta).

SUSHUMNĀ-NĀDI (very gracious channel)   The central *prāna* current or arc in or along which the serpent power (*kundalinī-shakti*) must ascend toward the psychoenergetic center (*cakra*) at the crown of the head in order to attain liberation (*moksha*).

SŪTRA (thread)   An aphoristic statement; a work consisting of aphoristic statements, such as Patanjali's *Yoga-Sūtra* or Vasugupta's *Shiva-Sūtra*.

SVĀDHYĀYA (one's own going into)   Study, an important aspect of the yogic path, listed among the practices of self-restraint (*niyama*) in Patanjali's eightfold Yoga; the recitation of *mantras* (see also *japa*).

TANTRA (continuity)   A type of Sanskrit work containing Tantric teachings; the tradition of Tantrism, which focuses on the *shakti* side of spiritual life and which originated in the early common era and achieved its classical features around 1000 C.E.; Tantrism has a right-hand (*dakshina*) or conservative and a left-hand (*vāma*) or unconventional/antinomian branch, with the latter utilizing, among other things, sexual rituals.

TAPAS (glow/heat)   Austerity, penance, which is an ingredient of all yogic approaches, since they all involve self-transcendence.

TATTVA (thatness)   A fact or reality; a particular category of existence such as the *ahamkāra*, *buddhi*, *manas*; the ultimate Reality (see also *ātman*, *brahman*).

TURĪYA (fourth), also called *cathurtha*   The transcendental Reality, which exceeds the three conventional states of consciousness, namely waking, sleeping, and dreaming.

UPANISHAD (sitting near)   A type of scripture representing the concluding portion of the revealed literature of Hinduism, hence the designation *Vedānta* for the teachings of these sacred works; see also *Āranyaka, Brāhmana, Veda*.

UPĀYA (means)   In Buddhist Yoga, the practice of compassion (*karunā*). See also *prajnā*.

VAIRĀGYA (dispassion)   The attitude of inner renunciation, the counterpole to *abhyāsa*. See also *samnyāsa*.

VĀSANĀ (trait)   The concatenation of subliminal activators (*samskāra*) deposited in the depth of the mind where they exert a binding effect.

VEDA (Knowledge)   The body of sacred wisdom found in the four Vedic hymnodies that form the source of Hinduism: *Rig-Veda, Yajur-Veda, Sāma-Veda*, and *Atharva-Veda*; also the collective name for these hymnodies. See also *Vedānta*.

VEDĀNTA (Veda's end)   The teachings forming the doctrinal conclusion of the revealed literature (*shruti*) of Hinduism. See also *Upanishad*. See also *Āranyaka, Brāhmana, Veda*.

VIDEHA-MUKTI (disembodied liberation)   The state of liberation without a physical or subtle body. See also *jīvan-mukti*.

VIDYĀ (knowledge/wisdom)   A synonym of *prajnā*.

VIJNĀNA BHIKSHU   A sixteenth-century Yoga master who authored several works on Yoga, including the *Yoga-Vārttika* (a comprehensive commentary on the *Yoga-Sūtra*) and *Yoga-Sāra-Samgraha* (a summary of Rāja-Yoga as taught by Patanjali).

VISHNU (Worker)   The deity who is worshiped by the Vaishnavas and who has had nine incarnations, including Rāma and Krishna, with the tenth incarnation (*avatāra*)— Kalki—coming at the close of the *kali-yuga*.

VIVEKA (discernment)   A most important aspect of the yogic path.

VRĀTYA (from *vrata* "vow")   A member of the sacred brotherhood in Vedic times in whose circles early yogic practices were developed.

VRITTI (whirl)   In Patanjali's *yoga-darshana*, specifically the five types of mental activity: valid cognition (*pramāna*), misconception (*viparyaya*), imagination (*vikalpa*), sleep (*nidrā*), and memory (*smriti*).

VYĀSA (Arranger)   Name of several great sages, but specifically referring to Veda Vyasa, who arranged the Vedic hymnodies in their current form and who also is attributed with the compilation of the *Purānas*, the *Mahābhārata*, and other works, including the *Yoga-Bhāshya* commentary on the *Yoga-Sutra*.

YAJNA (sacrifice)   Ritual sacrifice is fundamental to Hinduism; Yoga also knows of an inner sacrifice (as accomplished through meditation and self-surrender).

YĀJNAVALKYA   The most renowned sage of the early Upanishadic era.

YAMA (discipline)   The first limb (*anga*) of Patanjali's eightfold path, comprising moral precepts that have universal validity (such as nonharming and truthfulness); also the name of the Hindu deity of death.

YANTRA (device)   A geometric design representing the body of one's meditation deity, used for external and internal worship.

YOGA (union/discipline)   The unitive discipline by which inner freedom is sought;

spiritual practice, as practiced in Hinduism, Buddhism, and Jainism; the spiritual tradition specific to India; the specific school of Patanjali (see *ashta-anga-yoga*).

YOGA-DARSHANA (Yoga view/system)   Patanjali's Rāja-Yoga.

YOGA-SŪTRA (Aphorisms of Yoga)   Patanjali's aphoristic compilation forming the source of Rāja-Yoga, also called "Classical Yoga."

YOGIN   A male practitioner of Yoga.

YOGINĪ   A female practitioner of Yoga.

YONI (womb)   The perineum or female genitals, but also the source of the universe. See also *linga*.

YUGA (age/era)   A division of time. See *kali-yuga*.

Index

About the Author

GEORG FEUERSTEIN, Ph.D., M.Litt., became interested in Yoga at the age of fourteen and wrote his first book on the Yoga tradition at the age of nineteen. He has won an international reputation as an independent scholar in the area of Hindu esotericism and consciousness research. His original contribution to the study of spirituality, and especially to the dialogue between East and West, has been acknowledged by leading scholars, including Mircea Eliade, Jacob Needleman, Seshagiri Rao, Ninian Smart, and Huston Smith. He has received awards from the Leverhulme Trust Fund, A New American Place, and the British Academy, and for several years his work was sponsored by Laurance S. Rockefeller.

In addition to being the founder and president of the Yoga Research and Education Center in California, Dr. Feuerstein is editor-in-chief of the annual *International Journal of Yoga Therapy*, is in charge of YREC's 800-hour distance learning course on the philosophy, history, and literature of Yoga, and maintains a comprehensive website on Yoga (www.yrec.org).

Dr. Feuerstein has published more than thirty books and more than twenty edited volumes, as well as about two hundred articles and five hundred book reviews. Among his more important writings are *Holy Madness* (Paragon House, 1991), *Wholeness or Transcendence? Ancient Lessons for the Emerging Global Civilization* (Larson Publications, 1992), *In Search of the Cradle of Civilization* (Quest Books, 1995), *The Philosophy of Classical Yoga* (Inner Traditions, 1996), *Lucid Waking: Mindfulness and the Spiritual Potential of Humanity* (Inner Traditions, 1997), *The Shambhala Encyclopedia of Yoga* (Shambhala Publications, 1997), *Tantra: The Path of Ecstasy* (Shambhala Publications, 1998), and *The Yoga Tradition* (Hohm Press, 1998).

Georg Feuerstein lectures widely and leads teacher trainings on various aspects of the Yoga tradition. His passion is to make traditional yogic wisdom accessible to modern spiritual seekers and to foster the dialogue between traditions. He can be contacted by e-mail at mail@yrec.org.